Recent Results in Cancer Research 174

H.-J. Senn · U. Kapp (Eds.)

Cancer Prevention

With 48 Figures and 27 Tables

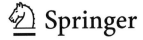 Springer

Prof. Dr. med. Hans-Jörg Senn
Prof. Dr. med. Ursula Kapp
Tumor-Zentrum ZeTuP St. Gallen/Chur
(Tumordiagnostik, Behandlung + Prävention)
Rorschacherstr. 150
CH-9006 St. Gallen
Schweiz

Library of Congress Control Number: 2006931793
ISSN 0080-0015
ISBN 10 3-540-37695-X   Springer Berlin Heidelberg New York
ISBN 13 978-3-540-37695-8   Springer Berlin Heidelberg New York

Springer is a part of Springer Science + Business Media
springer.com

Editor: Dr. Ute Heilmann, Heidelberg
Desk editor: Dörthe Mennecke-Bühler, Heidelberg
Production editor: Nadja Kroke, Leipzig
Cover design: Frido Steinen Broo, eStudio Calamar, Spain
Typesetting: LE-TeX Jelonek, Schmidt & Vöckler GbR, Leipzig
Printed on acid-free paper   SPIN 11683414   21/3100/YL – 5 4 3 2 1 0

Contents

List of Contributors

Adriana Albini, Director
Responsabile Ricerca Oncologica
Polo Scientifico e Tecnologico,
IRCCS Multimedica
Viale Fantoli 16/15
20138 Milano
Italy

Craig Allred
Department of Pathology
Baylor School of Medicine
One Baylor Plaza
Houston, TX 77030
USA

Hoda Anton-Culver, PhD
Professor
Department of Epidemiology
Chao Family Comprehensive Cancer Center
University of California, Irvine
Irvine, CA 92601
USA

Donna Badgwell, PhD
Department of Experimental Therapeutics
University of Texas
M.D. Anderson Cancer Center
Houston, TX 77030
USA

Gabriela Balogh, PhD
Breast Cancer Research Laboratory
Fox Chase Cancer Center
333 Cottman Avenue
Philadelphia, PA 19111
USA

Helmuth Bartsch, Prof.
Deutsches Krebsforschungszentrum (DKFZ)
Toxicology and Cancer Risk Factors
Im Neuenheimer Feld 280
69120 Heidelberg
Germany

Robert C. Bast, Jr., MD
M.D. Anderson Cancer Center
Unit 355
1515 Holcombe Boulevard
Houston, TX 77030-4009
USA

Roberto Benelli
SC Oncologia Sperimentale A
Instituto Nazionale per la Ricerca sul Cancro
Largo Rosanna Benzi 10
16132 Genova
Italy

Monica Bertagnolli, MD
Brigham and Women's Hospital
Dana Farber Cancer Institute
c/o Daria Christiansen
Room CA 104
75 Francis Street
Boston, MA 02115
USA

Candice Black, DO
Department of Pathology
Dartmouth Medical School
Hanover, NH 03755
USA

Molly Brewer
Division of Gynecologic Oncology
University of Arizona
Tucson, AZ 85724
USA

Nigel Bundred
University Department of Surgery
University Hospital of South Manchester
Whythenshaw Hospital
Manchester M23 9LT
UK

Dan Chan, PhD
Johns Hopkins Medical Center
Baltimore, MD 21205
USA

Robert B. Clarke
Cancer Research UK
Department of Medical Oncology
Christie Hospital
University of Manchester
Wilmslow Road
Manchester M20 4BX
UK

Jack Cuzick, Prof.
Cancer Research UK
Department of Epidemiology,
Mathematics and Statistics
Wolfson Institute of Preventive Medicine
Charterhouse Square
London EC1M 6BQ
UK

Mary Daley, MD
Fox Chase Cancer Center
333 Cottman Avenue
Philadelphia, PA 19111
USA

Heike Dally
Deutsches Krebsforschungszentrum (DKFZ)
Toxicology and Cancer Risk Factors
Im Neuenheimer Feld 280
69120 Heidelberg
Germany

Ethan Dmitrovsky, MD
Department of Pharmacology and Toxicology
Dartmouth Medical School
7650 Remsen
Hanover, NH 03755
USA

Konstantin H. Dragnev, MD
Department of Medicine
Dartmouth Medical School
Hanover, NH 03755
USA

Daniel S. Engeler, Dr. med
Department of Urology
Kantonsspital
9007 St. Gallen
Switzerland

Gareth Evans
Department of Medical Genetics
St. Mary's Hospital
Hathersage Road
Manchester M13 0JH
UK

Patrick J. Farmer, PhD
Department of Chemistry
Chao Family Comprehensive Cancer Center
University of California, Irvine
Irvine, CA 92601
USA

Qing Feng, PhD
Department of Pharmacology and Toxicology
Dartmouth Medical School
Hanover, NH 03755
USA

Sarah Freemantle, PhD
Research Assistant Professor
Department of Pharmacology and Toxicology
Dartmouth Medical School
Hanover, NH 03755
USA

Gerhard Fürstenberger, PhD
Deutsches Krebsforschungszentrum (DKFZ)
Research Program Cell and Tumor Biology
Im Neuenheimer Feld 280
69120 Heidelberg
Germany

Cedric F. Garland, PhD
Department of Family and Preventive Medicine
0631C
University of California, San Diego
9500 Gilman Drive
La Jolla, CA 92093-0631
USA

Edward D. Gorham, PhD
Department of Family and Preventive Medicine
0631C
University of California, San Diego
9500 Gilman Drive
La Jolla, CA 92093-0631
USA

William B. Grant, PhD
Sunlight, Nutrition and Health Research Center
(SUNARC)
2115 Van Ness Avenue, MB 101
San Francisco, CA 94109-2510
USA

Peter Greenwald, MD, PhD
Division of Cancer Prevention
National Cancer Institute
National Institutes of Health
6130 Executive Boulevard
Suite 2040
Bethesda, MD 20892-7309
USA

Mary A. Hernandez, RN
Department of Experimental Therapeutics
University of Texas
M.D. Anderson Cancer Center
Houston, TX 77030
USA

Rebecca Heulings, BS
Breast Cancer Research Laboratory
Fox Chase Cancer Center
333 Cottman Avenue
Philadelphia, PA 19111
USA

Anthony Howell, Prof.
CRUK Department of Medical Oncology
Christie Hospital
University of Manchester
Wilmslow Road
Manchester M20 4BX
UK

Ursula Kapp, Prof. Dr. med
Tumor-Zentrum ZeTuP St. Gallen/Chur
Rorschacherstrasse 15
9006 St. Gallen
Switzerland

Sutisak Kitareewan, PhD
Instructor
Department of Pharmacology and Toxicology
Dartmouth Medical School
Hanover, NH 03755
USA

Victor A. Levin, MD
Neuro-Oncology Unit 431
University of Texas
M.D. Anderson Cancer Center
P.O. Box 301402
Houston, TX 77230-1402
USA

Anna Lokshin, PhD
University of Pittsburgh,
Cancer Institute
Pittsburgh, PA 15232
USA

Karen Lu
Department of Gynecologic Oncology
University of Texas
M.D. Anderson Cancer Center
Houston, TX 77030
USA

Zhen Lu, MD
Department of Experimental Therapeutics
University of Texas
M.D. Anderson Cancer Center
Houston, TX 77030
USA

Yan Ma, PhD
Department of Pharmacology and Toxicology
Dartmouth Medical School
Hanover, NH 03755
USA

Ali Mahdavi, MD
Division of Gynecologic Oncology
Chao Family Comprehensive Cancer Center
University of California, Irvine
101 The City Drive
Building 56, Room 262
Orange, CA 92868-3298
USA

Daniel Mailo, PhD
Breast Cancer Research Laboratory
Fox Chase Cancer Center
333 Cottman Avenue
Philadelphia, PA 19111
USA

Friedrich Marks, Prof., PhD
Deutsches Krebsforschungszentrum (DKFZ)
Research Program Cell and Tumor Biology
Im Neuenheimer Feld 280
69120 Heidelberg
Germany

Vincent Memoli, MD
Department of Pathology
Dartmouth Medical School
Hanover, NH 03755
USA

Frank L. Meyskens, Prof.
University of California, Irvine
101 The City Drive South
Building 25, Suite 191, Route 81
Orange, CA 92868
USA

Gordon B. Mills, MD, PhD
Department of Molecular Therapeutics
University of Texas
M.D. Anderson Cancer Center
Houston, TX 77030
USA

Bradley J. Monk, MD
Division of Gynecologic Oncology
Chao Family Comprehensive Cancer Center
University of California, Irvine
101 The City Drive
Building 56, Room 262
Orange, CA 92868-3298
USA

Karin Müller-Decker, PhD
Deutsches Krebsforschungszentrum (DKFZ)
Research Program Cell and Tumor Biology
Im Neuenheimer Feld 280
69120 Heidelberg
Germany

Hoyoku Nishino, Prof.
Department of Biochemistry and Molecular
Biology
Graduate School of Medical Science
Kyoto Prefectural University of Medicine
Kyoto 602-8566
Japan

Douglas M. Noonan
Dipartimento di Scienze Biologiche e Cliniche,
Università dell'Insubria
Via Ravasi 2
21100 Varese
Italy

William Nugent, MD
Department of Surgery
Dartmouth Medical School
Hanover, NH 03755
USA

Robert Ozols, MD
Fox Chase Cancer Center
333 Cottman Avenue
Philadelphia, PA 19111
USA

Michael Pollak, Prof., MD
General Jewish Hospital
Medicine and Oncology
3755 Chemin de la Côte-Ste. Catherine
Montreal, Quebec H3T IE2
Canada

Odilia Popanda, PhD
Deutsches Krebsforschungszentrum (DKFZ)
Toxicology and Cancer Risk Factors
Im Neuenheimer Feld 280
69120 Heidelberg
Germany

Karl Pummer, Prof. Dr. med.
Department of Urology
Medical University of Graz
8036 Graz
Austria

Gad Rennert, MD, PhD
CHS National Cancer Control Center
Carmel Medical Center
7 Michal Street
Haifa 34362
Israel

James R. Rigas, MD
Department of Medicine
Dartmouth Medical School
Hanover, NH 03755
USA

Angela Risch, PhD
Deutsches Krebsforschungszentrum (DKFZ)
Toxicology and Cancer Risk Factors
Im Neuenheimer Feld 280
69120 Heidelberg
Germany

Cheryl L. Rock, PhD, RD
Department of Family and Preventive Medicine
and Cancer Prevention and Control Program
University of California, San Diego
9500 Gilman Drive
Department 0901
La Jolla, CA 92093-0901
USA

Stefan Rose-John, Prof. Dr.
Biochemisches Institut
Christian-Albrechts-Universität zu Kiel
Olshausenstrasse 40
24098 Kiel
Germany

Irma H. Russo, MD
Breast Cancer Research Laboratory
Fox Chase Cancer Center
333 Cottman Avenue
Philadelphia, PA 19111
USA

Jose Russo, MD
Breast Cancer Research Laboratory
Fox Chase Cancer Center
333 Cottman Avenue
Philadelphia, PA 19111
USA

Patricia A. Russo, BA
Breast Cancer Research Laboratory
Fox Chase Cancer Center
333 Cottman Avenue
Philadelphia, PA 19111
USA

Richard Santen
Division of Endocrinology and Metabolism
University of Virginia
P.O. Box 801416
Aurbach Medical Research Building
450 Ray Hunt Drive
Charlottesville, VA 22908
USA

Peter Schmezer, PhD
Deutsches Krebsforschungszentrum (DKFZ)
Toxicology and Cancer Risk Factors
Im Neuenheimer Feld 280
69120 Heidelberg
Germany

Hans-Peter Schmid, Prof. Dr. med.
Department of Urology
Kantonsspital
9007 St. Gallen
Switzerland

Bernd J. Schmitz-Dräger, Prof. Dr. med.
Euromed Clinic
Europa-Allee 1
90763 Fürth
Germany

Heidi Schooltink, Dr. rer. nat.
Biochemisches Institut
Christian-Albrechts-Universität zu Kiel
Olshausenstrasse 40
24098 Kiel
Germany

Hans-Jörg Senn, Prof. Dr. med.
Tumor-Zentrum ZeTuP St. Gallen/Chur
Rorschacherstrasse 15
9006 St. Gallen
Switzerland

Sumit J. Shah, PhD
Department of Pharmacology and Toxicology
Dartmouth Medical School
Hanover, NH 03755
USA

Craig Sinclair
The Cancer Council Victoria
1 Rathdowne Street
Carlton, Victoria 3053
Australia

Steven Skates, PhD
Massachusetts General Hospital
and Harvard Medical School
Boston, MA 02115
USA

Sun Yang, PhD, PharmD
Assistant Project Scientist
Department of Medicine, (Hematology/
Oncology)
Chao Family Comprehensive Cancer Center
University of California, Irvine
Irvine, CA 92601
USA

Yinhua Yu, MD
Department of Experimental Therapeutics
University of Texas
M.D. Anderson Cancer Center
Houston, TX 77030
USA

Zhen Zhang, PhD
Johns Hopkins Medical Center
Baltimore, MD 21205
USA

Changping Zou, PhD
Division of Gynecologic Oncology
University of Arizona
Tucson, AZ 85724
USA

Part I

Genetic Risk Profiles and Biomarkers in Cancer Prevention

1 A Favorable View: Progress in Cancer Prevention and Screening

Peter Greenwald

Recent Results in Cancer Research, Vol. 174
© Springer-Verlag Berlin Heidelberg 2007

Abstract

Clifton Leaf, in his article "Why We're Losing the War on Cancer," presents criticisms of past research approaches and the small impact of this research thus far on producing cures or substantially extending the life of many cancer patients. It is true that gains in long-term survival for people with advanced cancers have been modest, hindered in part by the heterogeneity of tumors, which allows the cancers to persist using alternate molecular pathways and so evade many cancer therapeutics. In contrast, clinical trials have demonstrated that it is possible to reduce the incidence or improve cancer survival through prevention and early detection. Strides have been made in preventing or detecting early the four deadliest cancers in the United States (i.e., lung, breast, prostate, and colorectal). For example, 7-year follow-up data from the Breast Cancer Prevention Trial (BCPT) provides evidence that tamoxifen reduces the occurrence of invasive breast tumors by more than 40%; recent studies using aromatase inhibitors and raloxifene are also promising. The Prostate Cancer Prevention Trial (PCPT) showed that finasteride reduced prostate cancer incidence by 25%, and the ongoing Selenium and Vitamin E Cancer Prevention Trial (SELECT) is investigating selenium and vitamin E for prostate cancer prevention based on encouraging results from earlier studies. Living a healthy lifestyle, including regular physical activity, avoiding obesity, and eating primarily a plant-based diet has been associated with a lower risk of colorectal cancer. In addition, noninvasive stool DNA tests for early detection are being studied, which may lessen the reluctance of people to be screened for colorectal polyps and cancer. Behavioral and medical approaches for smoking prevention are ways to reduce the incidence of lung cancer, with antinicotine vaccines on the horizon that may help former smokers to avoid relapse. The US National Lung Screening Trial is testing whether early detection via spiral CT screening will reduce lung cancer mortality. Prevention and earlier detection offer efficient and practical strategies to reduce the cancer burden. Several of the suggestions Mr. Leaf makes, such as developing interdisciplinary collaborations and allocating resources to research earlier in the process of carcinogenesis, have become an integral strategy in the National Cancer Institute's (NCI) approach in the past decade, specifically in the realm of cancer prevention and early detection. For example, an aggressive program to identify biomarkers for earlier detection of cancer – the NCI's Early Detection Research Detection (EDRN) – has identified three promising biomarkers since its establishment in 2000. It collaborates with the National Institute of Standards and Technology and extramural scientists to develop validation standards and to identify the best technologies to use for systematic investigations. If these biomarkers can be validated, they might help to reduce cancer mortality.

Introduction

Since the initiation of the commonly known War on Cancer in 1972, there has been an unprecedented focus on the cancer burden in the United States, and how to reduce its impact on public health. The National Cancer Act of 1971 resulted in strategic planning to mobilize the research and academic communities, with the backing of the resources of the federal government, to address the significant mortality and morbidity caused by cancer. The Act set in motion a systematic federal response that became the War on Cancer. Now, 30 years later, it is correct and appropriate for a realistic assessment of the progress made and areas of research likely to continue progress in the future. For the most part, Clifton Leaf, in his article on the War on Cancer, has provided a fair assessment of the overall success of the war on cancer, at least regarding progress for attaining a cure for every cancer (Leaf 2004). There are, however, significant parts of the cancer story that have been overlooked: prevention, screening, and detection. In these important strategic research initiatives, there are hopeful signs that suggest progress will be more tangible in the next 5–10 years. For example, cancer incidence rates for all cancer sites combined increased during the first years of the war on cancer from the mid-1970s through 1992, decreased from 1992 through 1995, and have remained stable between 1996 and 2002 (Weir et al. 2003; Edwards et al. 2005). Mortality rates for all cancer sites decreased by 1.1% annually from 1993 through 2002, and for the majority of the 15 most common cancers (Edwards et al. 2005). There are, however, specific cancer sites – breast and lung cancers in women – where incidence or mortality rates have increased in the past decade. In addition, cancer incidence and mortality rates remain disparate among various geographic, racial, economic, and age-related groups. Understanding what strategies have provided the benefit of reduced incidence and mortality rates is critical to understanding how future success will be achieved in the war on cancer. These include, foremost, the role of cancer prevention strategies – both society-wide adoption of healthy lifestyle choices and chemoprevention – and an increased use of population-wide screening programs to identify those at high risk of developing cancer and those with cancer at the earliest, and most treatable, stages. In addition, the recent development of better diagnostic tools using emerging technologies, such as biomarker identification and validation and "-omics" methodologies, have had a role in equipping cancer researchers with the tools needed to prevent, diagnose, and treat existing disease. By reviewing progress at the cancer sites that represent the majority of cases of cancer in the United States – lung, colorectal, breast, and prostate – it is clear that progress has been, and continues to be, made in the war against cancer.

Lung Cancer

Lung cancer is the leading cause of cancer mortality and the second most common cancer among men and women in the United States, but recent trends indicating reductions in mortality and incidence are encouraging (Page et al. 2000). From 1992 to 2002, incidence rates for lung cancer have declined approximately 20% in men but only 1% in women; mortality rates have declined in the same period approximately 2% overall (i.e., for both men and women) (Edwards et al. 2005). Progress against lung cancer, which is predominantly caused by smoking tobacco, is an example of using a multipronged strategy integrating lifestyle and medical approaches, and governmental regulation, to address a significant public health problem. These are strategies developed in the war on cancer. Beginning with clinical intervention studies in the 1980s, it became apparent that educating the public and intervening to help people quit smoking was a significant step for reducing the incidence and mortality from lung cancer. The Community Intervention Trial for Smoking Cessation (COMMIT) and the American Stop Smoking Intervention Study (ASSIST) showed that individual interventions have modest success in helping smokers quit, but that strong tobacco-control policies at the state level with enhanced tobacco control programs could dramatically reduce smoking (COMMIT Research Group 1991; Stillman et al. 2003). Subsequently, increasing the federal and state tax on tobacco products; enacting legislation aimed at reducing youth smoking; reducing exposure to environmental smoke in workplaces, restaurants, or other public spaces; and employing a greater number of media campaigns that focus on anti-smoking campaigns, particularly among youth, have been implemented.

Progress against lung cancer is also being made in medical approaches to smoking prevention. Anti-nicotine vaccines are being developed that have the effect of blocking nicotine before it reaches the brain, thus relieving the addictive power of the compound. Early clinical studies (i.e., phase I trials) have shown that these vaccines have low toxicity (Cerny 2005), and phase II trials are underway. The promise of a safe, effective vaccine that can provide smokers with another avenue for cessation is compelling. Other encouraging research findings have been reported in chemoprevention of lung cancer in current or former smokers who exhibit evidence of bronchial dysplasia, a precursor lesion associated with future lung cancer. A phase IIb trial in Vancouver investigated the ability of an-ethole dithiolethione (ADT) to inhibit or reverse bronchial dysplasia (Lam et al. 2002). ADT triggers the production of glutathione-s-transferase (GST), one of the body's natural defense mechanisms against carcinogens. In the trial, ADT, compared to placebo in 112 current and former smokers, reduced the number and rate of progression of dysplastic lesions, a significant finding that is currently being investigated in larger chemoprevention trials (Lam et al. 2002). The ability to reverse damage initiated by exposure to tobacco smoke in the lung could improve the benefit of smoking cessation beyond the modest benefits (approximately one-half of all lung cancer cases in the United States occur in former smokers) seen to date (Burns 2000).

Screening for lung cancer, such as in all cancers, represents an opportunity to identify precursors of cancer, overt cancer, and cellular characteristics (i.e., genetic and epigenetic) that confer increased or decreased risk factor(s) for cancer. At present, there is no lung-cancer screening test that has been shown to reduce mortality from lung cancer. To investigate the utility of a new lung screening tool, spiral computed tomography (CT), against the standard chest x-ray, NCI is conducting the National Lung Screening Trial (NLST), a randomized controlled trial (RCT), to determine which screening method has the greatest impact on mortality from lung cancer (Gohagan et al. 2004). The NLST has enrolled more than 50,000 current or former smokers in the RCT, which is designed to provide three an-nual screenings by each method. Results should be available by 2009.

As a strategic model in the war on cancer, the focus on reducing the incidence and mortality from lung cancer has produced some significant, though modest, successes. It is encouraging to health professionals that the strategies put in place during the past decades are beginning to show real reductions in the rates of lung cancer incidence and mortality, as well as in the numbers of adults and young people smoking. This long-term strategy should show more impressive results in the next decade if the strategies continue to be implemented. One of the areas of some concern, however, is the recent increase in lung cancer among women. This must be considered in view of the societal changes that occurred during the past decades as more women began to smoke cigarettes in the 1960s and 1970s. The lack of progress in the incidence of lung cancer among women might be explained by the fact that what is being seen in data from the early 2000s is the result of women catching up to incidence rates seen in men because of increased use of tobacco products in the past three decades. To illustrate, between 1965 and 1998, the ratio of men smoking and women smoking increased from approximately 2 to 1 in 1965 to 3 to 2 in 1998 (U.S. Department of Health and Human Services 2001). The same report notes the increased smoking rates among American teenagers, especially teenage girls. Continued focus on prevention and intervention initiatives in place might be seen in reducing incidence in women and teenagers during the next decade. Lung cancer develops over a long period of time – possibly as much as 20–30 years – and there is a lag between the success of interventions and actual progress.

Breast Cancer

Female breast cancer incidence rates increased by 0.4% per year from 1987 to 2002, a slower rate of increase than in the previous time period, which saw an increase of 3.7% per year from 1980 through 1987 (Edwards et al. 2005). Mortality rates, however, decreased 2.3% annually from 1990 to 2002. These modest gains resulting from basic and clinical research have improved the understanding of breast cancer etiology and risk factors. The encouraging lessons in research that led to these modest gains also portend the reasonable expectation of further gains in the future. The tamoxifen story is an appropriate case study on the need for increasing knowledge at the clinical level through years of research to develop a proof-of-principle that directed further investigations in animal models and humans before translation to large clinical trials. This time-consuming process is yielding tangible benefits in the search for prevention strategies and treatments against a cancer that is highly visible in the lay press and was increasing dramatically in the 1980s. Early clinical studies of tamoxifen, a selective estrogen receptor modulator (SERM), indicated it occupies the estrogen receptor site in breast tissue, thereby blocking the effects of endogenous estrogen and decreasing epithelial cell proliferation (Overmoyer 1999). Estrogen was known to increase cell proliferation, a critical physiological event in the initiation and growth of cancer in the breast. Tamoxifen had been shown in clinical and animal studies to inhibit the growth of human cancer cells in vitro, to inhibit the development of mammary tumors in mice inoculated with mouse mammary tumor virus, and to prevent tumor development and growth in rats (Nayfield et al. 1991; Furr and Jordan 1984; Greenwald et al. 1993). Based on these findings, the NCI supported a series of clinical studies through the National Surgical Adjuvant Bowel and Breast Project (NSABP) that showed that tamoxifen reduced recurrences of breast cancer and that women with previous breast cancer were also less likely to develop breast cancer in the opposite breast (Fisher et al. 1989). A larger RCT of tamoxifen was initiated by the NSABP – the Breast Cancer Prevention Trial (BCPT) – to compare tamoxifen against placebo for 5 years in more than 13,000 high-risk, pre- and postmenopausal women (Fisher et al. 1998). The BCPT was stopped after 3.6 years when data showed a statistically significant benefit of tamoxifen, including a 49% reduction in breast cancer incidence compared with the control group and a 69% reduction in the occurrence of estrogen receptor-positive (ER+) tumors compared to no difference in the occurrence of es-

trogen receptor-negative (ER−) tumors (Fisher et al. 1998). At the same time as results from the BCPT were being released, the publication of results from the Multiple Outcomes of Raloxifene Evaluation (MORE) osteoporosis trial indicated that the SERM raloxifene reduced the incidence of breast cancer by 74% without an associated increased risk for endometrial cancer seen in the tamoxifen trials (Cummings et al. 1999). The Study of Tamoxifen and Raloxifene (STAR) trial, which is designed to determine whether raloxifene is more or less effective than tamoxifen in reducing invasive breast cancer in women and to assess the occurrence of noninvasive breast cancer, endometrial cancer, cardiovascular events, and bone fractures, will enroll 22,000 high-risk, postmenopausal women, age 35 and older, in a double-blind trial that will be completed in 2006 (Vogel et al. 2002).

The success of the SERM trials has led to a progression of investigations to find agents that build on tamoxifen's success. Aromatase Inhibitors (AIs) influence the action of estrogen on breast tissue by blocking the conversion of androgens to estrone or estradiol. This allows the interruption of the negative consequences associated with estrogen exposure in breast tissue at an earlier physiologic moment than that of SERMs. A third-generation AI, anastrozole (Arimidex), was compared to tamoxifen in the Arimidex, Tamoxifen, Alone or in Combination (ATAC) trial and was significantly better than tamoxifen alone with regard to disease-free survival, time to recurrence, and reduction of the incidence of contralateral breast cancer (Baum et al. 2002).

Although the trials of SERMs and AIs have shown impressive reductions in recurrence and invasive cancer in the contralateral breast, cancer researchers continue to develop strategies to address those cancers that do not respond to anti-estrogen therapy. Preclinical studies have shown that tumors with increased expression and signaling through erbB Type 1 growth factor receptors, such as the epidermal growth factor receptor (EGFR) and HER2, do not respond to anti-estrogen therapy (Agrawal et al. 2005). Approximately 45% of breast cancer cells express EGFR. Newer compounds such as Gefitinib (Iressa) and erlotinib (Tarceva) proved promising in preclinical trials and are currently being investigated in clinical trials; early results suggest that EGRF-specific tyrosine kinase inhibitors, such as Gefitinib and erlotinib, might be beneficial against ER+ tumors that resist anti-estrogen therapy (Agrawal et al. 2005).

Past research and clinical studies have shown progress against ER+ breast cancer; to date, progress against ER− breast cancer has been slight. ER− breast tumors generally are more aggressive and few therapies exist for preventing progression of tumors that are not hormone-dependent. Recent attempts to develop a better understanding of ER− hormone-resistant tumors have included a strategy of changing the ER− phenotype to the ER+ phenotype, which will better respond to therapy, or targeting unique molecular signatures of ER− tumors, such as the cathepsin D pathway that is overexpressed in these tumors (Rochefort et al. 2003). Treatment results from three NSABP RCTs of postoperative chemotherapy in women with ER− tumors and negative axillary lymph nodes have demonstrated that a combination of methotrexate and 5-fluorouracil (MF) is more effective than surgery alone, that cyclophosphamide with MF (CMF) is more effective than MF, and that CMF and doxorubicin (Adriamycin) with cyclophosphamide (AC) are equally beneficial (Fisher et al. 2004). In addition, a recent small clinical study has shown that some progress is being made against ER− tumors with the use of paclitaxel, a taxane-containing drug used in women with early-stage breast cancer (Poole 2004). Further studies are planned using paclitaxel in combination with Gemcitabine. These findings are encouraging news for those women with the more aggressive ER− tumors and represent significant progress in the understanding of differences among breast cancer tumors.

The use of nonhormonal chemopreventive agents for breast cancer prevention or treatment is progressing as more is learned about the mechanisms involved in breast carcinogenesis. Farnesyl transferase inhibitors (FTIs) are being investigated in phase I trials to study their ability to control cell division downstream of the erbBs such as Ras and MEK, or in erbB-associated signaling networks such as Src kinase that affect tumor cell motility and invasiveness (Wakeling 2005). Statins and FTIs are also being investigated for their ability to induce G1 arrest; studies

in breast cancer cell lines are ongoing, and results indicate that these compounds are responsible for inhibition of the proteasome and upregulation of p21 (Efuet and Keyomarski 2006).

This basic research, coupled with findings from clinical trials, has shown that breast cancer can be detected and treated to reduce morbidity and mortality. As for each of the cancers, prevention is the best strategy for reducing incidence. To reduce the risk of breast cancer, results from population and basic research studies indicate that maintaining a healthy weight and avoiding lifetime weight gain, increasing vigorous physical activity, and limiting alcohol use are beneficial strategies.

Colorectal Cancer

Colorectal cancer incidence rates decreased by 10.4% in men and 2.9% in women between 1992 and 2002; mortality rates decreased by 5.5% among men and 6.6% among women during the same time period (Edwards et al. 2005). Lifestyle prevention strategies that have been identified in epidemiological and clinical studies to reduce the risk of colorectal cancer include increasing physical activity, increasing the intake of vegetables and fruits, limiting the intake of red meat and alcohol, and maintaining a healthy weight and avoiding obesity (American Cancer Society 2006). Much of the basic science and treatment of colorectal cancer has been discovered by the study of patients with familial adenomatous polyposis (FAP), a genetic disorder associated with mutations in the APC gene that results, if left untreated, in colorectal cancer in almost 100% of cases. Application of what was learned in FAP patients has been translated to strategies for the general population, including screening studies for polyps. One of the earliest clinical trials of the treatment of polyps to reduce the incidence of colorectal cancer was the National Polyp Study (NPS), a longitudinal surveillance study of adenoma patients. The NPS included approximately 1,400 patients who had a colonoscopy and removal of one or more polyps. After an average followup of 5.9 years, an assessment of the incidence of colorectal cancer among participants was conducted. Compared to reference groups, the NPS investigators reported a reduction in the incidence of colorectal cancer at 3, 6, and 9 years of 90%, 88%, and 76%, respectively, as shown in Fig. 1 (Winawer et al. 1993).

Results from trials such as the NPS focused attention on preventing colorectal cancer by preventing polyp formation or recurrence. They also established colonoscopy as the gold standard to identify and collect polyps for diagnostic purposes. At the time, other screening tools were being used to test for colorectal cancer, including fecal occult blood tests and sigmoidoscopy. Colorectal screening has been a story of some success in reducing mortality rates partly through detection of colorectal cancer at earlier stages than in the past. Consequently, there has been increased focus on assessing screening tools and developing improved methods for screening. The American Gastroenterological Association recently produced a review of emerging screening and diagnostic technologies, with recommendations for future research (Regueiro 2005). Colorectal screening provides one example of the types of progress that have occurred in the war on cancer, and the focused research that can impact mortality rates if the right screening method can be developed and applied to the general population. Traditional screening methods include both invasive (e.g., colonoscopy and sigmoidoscopy) and noninvasive methods (e.g., fecal occult blood tests). Assessments of screening behavior indicate that mass-screening tools gain wide acceptance if they are noninvasive and sensitive enough to offer assurance that the results are dependable. These criteria might be met by emerging screening technologies and methods, such as stool (fecal) DNA (fDNA), and messenger RNA (mRNA) tests. Testing by fDNA would be ideal because it is noninvasive, the sample can be collected at home and mailed to a laboratory for analysis, and the number of markers tested can be unlimited (Regueiro 2005). Although sensitivity is poor with fDNA at this time, if it can be substantially improved, those patients with suspect tests would be referred for colonoscopy or other confirming tests; thus, colorectal screening might become more acceptable to more of the public. Improvements in technology, such as computed tomographic (CT) colonography, also have the promise of noninvasive screening, but require bowel preparation and current costs make it prohibitive for population screening at this time. The goal of population screening can be met by continuing to develop and refine noninvasive screening tests. At the present time, there are an estimated 42 million Americans 50 years and older who have not had a colorectal cancer screening test. By bringing these individuals into the screening system, it is likely that significant numbers of colorectal cancer cases can have earlier diagnosis and better prognosis.

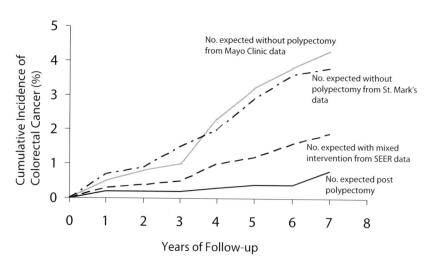

Fig. 1 National Polyp Study: Polypectomy Reduces Colorectal Cancer Incidence (Source: Winawer et al. 1993)

Prostate Cancer

Prostate cancer is the leading cancer diagnosed among US men and the second leading cause of cancer mortality. Prostate cancer mortality has declined only by approximately 11% from 1997 to 2002 (Edwards et al. 2005). Our understanding of prostate cancer etiology and risk factors has increased dramatically since the advent of the war on cancer. For example, in the 1980s, experimental and animal studies suggested that high levels of circulating androgens – steroid hormones that control the development and maintenance of masculine characteristics – promote prostate cell proliferation and inhibit prostate cell death (Brawley et al. 1994). Because proliferation and growth of prostate cells is stimulated by dihydrotestosterone (DHT), a product of testosterone conversion by the enzyme 5-α-reductase, inhibition of this enzyme was considered a viable strategy for mediating prostate cell growth and possible carcinogenesis. Finasteride, a 5-α-reductase inhibitor, was the subject of clinical studies and was found to inhibit the growth of prostate cancer cells in vitro (Brawley et al. 1994) and to reduce prostatic DHT by as much as 90% and serum DHT by 60%–80%, without binding to the prostate androgen receptor (Rittmaster 1994). As evidence accumulated that finasteride mediated prostate carcinogenesis, it was approved for the treatment of benign prostatic hyperplasia (Feigl et al. 1995).

Based on these encouraging clinical studies and small human trials of finasteride, in 1993 the NCI began the Prostate Cancer Prevention Trial (PCPT), the first phase III population-based, double-blind, RCT to assess whether the risk of prostate cancer could be reduced (Thompson et al. 2003). The PCPT was designed to compare finasteride against placebo and utilized the network of research centers known as the Community Clinical Oncology Program (CCOP), which was established in 1983 by the NCI as a creative mechanism to improve the accrual of patients to NCI phase III clinical trials, encourage community-based oncologists to participate in clinical research, and provide an avenue for disseminating new information on state-of-the-art cancer treatment outside the traditional cancer centers and research-oriented medical centers.

The PCPT enrolled 18,882 healthy men, age 55 and older, with normal digital rectal examination (DRE) and serum prostatic specific antigen (PSA), and was designed as a 10-year study in which one-half of the men received finasteride (5 mg/day) and one-half received a placebo (Feigl et al. 1995). The primary goal of the PCPT was to determine whether finasteride reduced the incidence of biopsy-proven prostate cancer compared to placebo. Secondary goals were to assess side effects of finasteride in healthy participants, to determine whether long-term finasteride use is acceptable for healthy participants, and to assess the effect of finasteride on DRE and PSA. To reduce the chance of bias in disease assessment, as finasteride can cause a reduction of prostate gland size and PSA level, study participants were required to undergo a prostate biopsy after completing the preventative drug regimen (Feigl et al. 1995). The PCPT was ended early, in June 2003, after a finding that finasteride reduced the prevalence of prostate cancer by 24.8% compared to placebo (Thompson et al. 2003). Participants in the finasteride group who did develop prostate cancer, however, had a slightly higher incidence of reported high-grade tumors (i.e., tumors of Gleason grade 7–10), which is under discussion as to whether this is a study artifact or something attributable to treatment.

As the PCPT was being conducted and reporting results with finasteride, two large-scale clinical intervention studies with prostate cancer as a secondary endpoint were reporting reduced prostate cancer risk with bioactive food components (BFCs). The most active form of vitamin E, α-tocopherol, was shown to reduce the risk of metastatic or fatal prostate cancer in the Health Professionals Follow-Up Study (Chan et al. 1999) and the Alpha-Tocopherol Beta-Carotene Cancer Prevention Study (ATBC) (Alpha-Tocopherol Beta-Carotene Cancer Prevention Study 1994). In addition, selenium was being studied in a skin cancer prevention trial, with secondary analysis of the data showing that participants who were given daily selenium-enriched brewer's yeast supplements (200-g/day) had a 63% reduced risk of prostate cancer (Clark et al. 1996). Selenium was also being studied in epidemiological studies of toenail and blood levels. For example, a study of selenium levels in toenails reported a

65% reduced risk of advanced prostate cancer in those with the highest levels of toenail selenium (Yoshizawa et al. 1998). In addition, a cohort study using analysis of quartiles of blood selenium levels indicated that prostate cancer was reduced by 50% in the highest quartile, and advanced prostate cancer was reduced by 70% (Nomura et al. 2000).

To follow up on the encouraging secondary-endpoint analyses from these large trials, the NCI, working with CCOP members and other institutions, funded the Selenium and Vitamin E Cancer Prevention Trial (SELECT). SELECT is coordinated by CCOP member Southwest Oncology Group and includes more than 400 sites throughout the United States, Puerto Rico, and Canada. It is the largest prostate prevention trial ever conducted and is a randomized, prospective, double-blind study designed to determine whether a 7- to 12-year regime of daily selenium and/or vitamin E supplements and/or placebo in a four-arm intervention design will decrease the risk of prostate cancer in healthy men (see Fig. 2) (Klein et al. 2001). Enrollment in SELECT began in 2001, and the accrual target goal of approximately 32,000 men was met during 2005. Final results are not anticipated until 2013.

Study supplements in SELECT include 200 μg of 1-selenomethionine, 400 mg of racemic α-tocopherol, and an optional multivitamin that does not contain selenium or vitamin E. Unlike the PCPT, SELECT will not require a biopsy at the end of the trial period; biopsies will be performed at the discretion of the physician. Routine clinical evaluations, however, which include a yearly DRE and a PSA test, will be performed (Klein et al. 2001). Secondary goals of SELECT are to assess the effect of selenium and vitamin E on the incidence of lung and colon cancer and on survival rates of participants diagnosed with lung and colon cancer. In addition, SELECT will examine the molecular genetics of cancer risk, explore possible associations between diet and cancer, assess age-related memory loss, and assess participants' quality of life. For more information, visit the NCI SELECT Web Site at http://www.nci.nih.gov/select.

Bioactive Food Components

In discussing progress in the war on cancer, nutrition is one area of cancer prevention that has emerged in the past 30 years that should play a

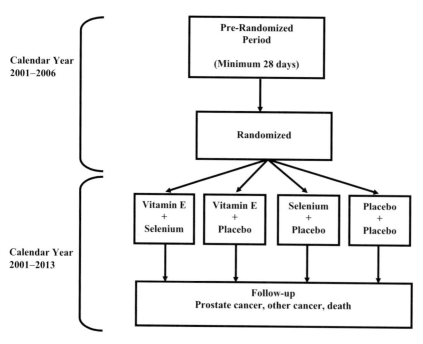

Fig. 2 Diagram of the schema for the Selenium and Vitamin E Cancer Prevention Trial (SELECT) (Klein et al. 2001)

significant future role in reducing the incidence and mortality from this disease. BFCs, natural or synthetic, have been studied in basic research that includes animal models. While it is true that much of the basic and animal research does not have immediate application for reducing human disease, the accumulated knowledge gained plays an important role in subsequent human prevention and treatment regimens. In nutrition research, it is important to have basic research to understand, among other important questions, the mechanisms responsible for actions of foods identified in population studies as potentially causative for cancer risk. Promising BFCs for chemoprevention include those that contain selenium (e.g., plants and animals depending on soil content), lycopene (e.g., tomatoes), indole-3-carbinol (I3C) (e.g., broccoli and cauliflower), and (-)-epigallocatechin-3-gallate (EGCG) (e.g., green tea). For prostate cancer chemoprevention at NCI using BFCs, there is a wide array of compounds being investigated that have promise for reducing prostate cancer risk (see Table 1). Investigating BFCs in clinical studies is based on knowledge gained through basic and animal research that have identified mechanisms-of-action that suggest how specific compounds may interrupt the process of carcinogenesis. This is a critical step in the scientific process for recommending that compounds proceed to possible further investigations in humans and to become part of recommendations for dietary interventions. For example, the biological activity of selenium is through selenoproteins, compounds that influence various molecular targets and pathways. Selenium also acts as an antioxidant in

the thioredoxin systems, acting as a constituent of the selenoenzyme thioredoxin reductase (TR). TR reduces thioredoxin, which causes reduced activity of nuclear transcription factor (NF$\kappa\beta$), an inducible oncogenic factor that causes induction of genes involved in a number of physiological processes, including those associated with cytokines, growth factors, cell adhesion molecules, and immunoreceptors (Milner et al. 2001). It also has a direct genetic effect in the inhibition of DNA synthesis and can induce DNA strand breakage by increasing cdc2/cdk2 kinase activities and arresting cell growth in S/G$_2$/M. Selenium also is involved in influencing apoptosis by fas ligand and p38 stress kinase induction (Fleming et al. 2001). In a Min mice study, mice fed selenium-enriched broccoli indicated that selenium-enriched broccoli enhanced the binding of transcription factor p53, NFκB, and AP-1 to their cis-acting elements, thus reducing tumorigenesis (Zeng et al. 2003). Each of these basic scientific studies provides information that might help to explain selenium's anticarcinogenic action regarding prostate cancer.

The carotenoid lycopene, found in tomatoes and tomato products, also has been suggested in animal and clinical studies to reduce the risk of prostate cancer by various mechanisms, including acting as an antioxidant, interfering with growth factor receptor signaling and cell cycle progression, and upregulating connexin 43, which allows direct intercellular gap junctional communication (Heber and Lu 2002). A review of population studies on tomato products, lycopene, and prostate cancer risk found that eating one serving of lycopene-containing foods per

Table 1 Food-derived chemopreventive agents for prostate cancer prevention (Source: National Cancer Institute data, 2006)

Agent	Preclinical		Clinical (phase)		
	Efficacy	Toxicology	I	II	III
Lycopene	X	X	X	X	
Selenomethionine	X	X	X	X	X
Soy isoflavones (genistein)	X	X	X	X	
Vitamin D analog	X	X	X	X	
Indole-3-carbinol analog	X	X	X	X	
Green tea catechins	X	X	X	X	X

day is associated with lower prostate cancer risk (Miller et al. 2002).

Vitamin D, an essential nutrient produced in the skin as a product of sun exposure and through consumption of foods such as dairy products and seafood, and vitamin D homologues have been investigated for their chemopreventive properties related to colorectal, prostate, and breast cancers. The active form of vitamin D – 1,25-hydroxy-cholecalciferol (1,25(OH)$_2$D) – binds intracellularly to cytoplasmic vitamin D receptor (VDR), which is found widely dispersed throughout the body; the resulting 1,25(OH)$_2$D–VDR complex is recognized to interact with nuclear vitamin D-responsive DNA elements (VDRE) and thereby either initiates or represses nuclear transcription of various target genes (Giovannucci 1998). Studies in breast cancer cell lines indicate that vitamin D depresses cell proliferation by upregulating endonuclease and downregulating genes (e.g., GRP-78, α-prothymosin, and calmodulin), directly regulates BRCA-1 expression via VDR-induced transcriptional activation of the BRCA-1 promoter, and induces apoptosis (Furuya et al. 2001; Campbell et al. 2000). Vitamin D also has been investigated in prostate and colorectal cancer cell lines and found to have numerous mechanisms of action that suggest it is important as a chemopreventive agent. These findings have been investigated in animal studies and clinical trials. For example, results of a RCT of vitamin D and calcium supplementation showed that high serum levels of 1,25(OH)$_2$D and calcium together are associated with a reduced risk of colorectal adenoma recurrence (Grau et al. 2003).

Genistein, an isoflavone found in soy food products, is being investigated in chemoprevention trials for breast and prostate cancers. It has been shown to induce cell cycle arrest and apoptosis in numerous cancer cell lines, including ER+ and ER– human breast carcinoma, prostate cancer, colon cancer, and lung cancer (Milner et al. 2001). Potential mechanisms of action of genistein include the upregulation of p21WAF[1], a growth-inhibiting protein that restrains the activity of cyclin-dependent kinases; inactivation of bcl-2, an anti-apoptotic gene, through phosphorylation; G$_2$/M cell cycle arrest and apoptosis; inhibition of a protein tyrosine kinase resulting in inhibition of cell growth; and inhibition of the anti-apoptotic transcription factor. These

actions make genistein a potentially useful BFC for reducing the risk of hormone-dependent cancers, especially for its potential to affect ER– breast cancer.

Other BFCs that are being investigated for their chemopreventive properties are (-), a constituent of green tea and in lesser amounts in black and white tea; and related indole compounds found in cruciferous vegetables such as broccoli and cauliflower; and phenylethyl isothiocyanate (PEITC) and related isothiocyanates, such as sulforaphane; and dithiolthione and other thiol-containing compounds, also found in cruciferous vegetables (Greenwald and Clifford 1995). EGCG has a selective growth inhibitory effect, operating on cancerous cells but not on normal cells; other green tea polyphenols (i.e., cathechins) act synergistically with EGCG to reduce cancer risk by the same mechanism. I3C has been shown in human trials to have anti-proliferative effects on prostate cells, as well as downregulation of DNA synthesis pathways. PEITC inhibits cellular damage caused by nitrosamines. This basic research is being investigated in small clinical trials to determine if they have utility as chemopreventive agents. Without identifying the specific compounds found in foods that have potential as anti-cancer agents, cancer researchers would have less of an understanding of the results of population studies on diet and nutrition. It is unlikely that there ever will be one diet-derived pill to prevent cancer, but the basic research investigations can lead to recommendations for a cancer-reducing diet and supplemental BFCs that will help to maintain a healthy immune and metabolic system to ward off potential cancer-inducing assaults, whether they come from the diet or the environment. An unprecedented opportunity exists for expanded use of foods and BFCs to achieve genetic potential, increase positive production of a healthy environment, and reduce the risk of disease.

Future Prospects

Future progress in the war on cancer will occur in areas that have proven successful during the past 30 years, as well as through continued development of new ways to identify people at risk and to intervene with prevention strategies that are based on sound scientific principles. Treatment modalities will continue to be developed for those people who are diagnosed with cancer. Promising new therapies should reduce the mortality rates from site-specific cancers during the next decade. There is, however, an imperative to reduce the number of people who get cancer and this can be achieved through lifestyle and medical strategies for prevention. One of the weakest links in the cancer prevention, diagnosis, and treatment continuum has been the predilection to wait until cancer is found before developing a strategy to defeat it. It is now understood that significant future progress in reducing the incidence of cancer will be achieved only through prevention efforts, and on this front, much has been learned throughout the past 3 decades. An important strategy for reducing morbidity and mortality from cancer in those who will get it is diagnosing cancer at the earliest stages of initiation (e.g., precancerous cells), which offers an opportunity to intervene with targeted drugs that keep the cancer cells from growing and spreading. Areas that can be identified as promising for continuing progress in the war on cancer, based on assessments of their success in the past are described below.

To ensure efforts continue in tobacco control, the medical community will need to advocate public policies that promote healthy lifestyles, including encouragement for tobacco cessation. Reducing smoking, especially among youth, can reduce the incidence and mortality from lung cancer, as well as moderate the impact of tobacco use on cardiovascular and other diseases. In concert with tobacco-control efforts, there is emerging evidence of the impact of obesity on cancer and cardiovascular disease incidence and mortality. For example, a prospective study of more than 900,000 Americans found that overweight or obesity contributes to 15%–20% of cancer deaths; given the increasing numbers of obese Americans, encouraging weight control could significantly impact cancer mortality and be a broadly effective lifestyle approach to cancer prevention (Calle et al. 2003). Efforts to encourage healthy diets, with increased attention to regular physical activity for people of all ages, can help people avoid obesity and overweight, and generally improve health. Efforts, such as the 5-A-Day For Better Health Initiative, established

and maintained since 1991 by a cooperative effort among the NCI, the US Centers for Disease Control and Prevention (CDC), and state health departments, is a cooperative, community-based effort that has shown steady progress in improving the diet of the American public. For example, intervention studies at 5-A-Day demonstration sites indicated that there was an average effective increase of 0.62 servings per day, a considerable increase among the US population in a decade. The authors of the evaluation recognized that the success of the program was related directly to the strength of the established partnerships and the number of initiatives conducted by members of the partnership (Potter et al. 2000). In addition, the number of consumers aware of the 5-A-Day messages increased from 8% to 20% during the evaluation period. Because clinical research and trials during the evaluation period continue to accumulate evidence that high consumption of vegetables and fruits is strongly associated with reductions in cancer risk, raising awareness to increase consumption is likely to be a valid strategy for cancer prevention and for improved public health. The 5-A-Day program is the type of intervention program that, in the future, will highlight the role of diet and nutrition in disease prevention and control, and can positively impact cancer awareness and prevention.

The future for cancer prevention clinical trials also looks encouraging as knowledge gained in the past is being investigated in medical and public health settings. Trials mentioned earlier (e.g., SELECT and STAR) will add immeasurably to the knowledge needed to make clinical recommendations to physicians, who will pass these decisions on to patients. Translating findings from the trials to the clinic has become an important focus of the NCI. Future prospects in this area are bright, because much of the challenge of the early days of the war on cancer was accumulating so much basic research knowledge that often there was difficulty in developing applications that could be recommended to patients. This problem has been alleviated somewhat as clinical trials for cancer prevention have involved community-based clinicians in recruiting patients and conducting trials at the community level. This model, as seen in the SELECT trial, shows a maturation of cancer prevention clinical studies that open a pathway to dissemination in the design of the trial.

The future of cancer prevention, and progress against cancer in general, is benefiting from emerging technologies for the screening of those at risk of cancer, earlier diagnosis, and treatment. Screening technologies, as discussed in the section on colorectal cancer, are being developed for other site-specific cancers. For example, breast cancer screening by mammography is still the accepted screening modality, although an imperfect tool. The use of magnetic resonance, positron emission tomography (PET), and magnetic resonance spectroscopy (MRS) are being used with some success (Smith and Andreopoulou 2004). Computerized imaging, known as computer-aided detection and diagnosis, in concert with mammography has been shown to increase the ability of radiologists to diagnose the early signs of breast cancer (Giger 2004). Although newer technologies at this point are not realistic for population-wide use, there are promising developments in the ability to identify those patients at higher risk that could benefit from these technologies.

Genetic and molecular biology have been integrated with cancer prevention research as knowledge of individual differences regarding cancer risk has been established. Genetic polymorphisms – variations in nucleotides within the same gene – have been found that are associated with cancer risk at various sites. The associations are complicated, but ongoing basic research is making progress toward identifying specific polymorphisms that might increase or decrease cancer risk. To illustrate, polymorphisms in the P450-CYP1A1 gene are associated with an increased risk of lung cancer with increased consumption of cruciferous vegetables, but decreased risk of breast cancer (Wargovich 2003). Understanding variability among individuals is a significant challenge that can be addressed with emerging technologies. The P450 gene also has a polymorphism that is associated with breast cancer and the intake of lignans, plant compounds metabolized to produce phytoestrogens. The CYP17 polymorphism appears to reduce the risk of breast cancer in premenopausal women with high levels of lignan consumption (McCann et al. 2002).

Significant progress is also being gained from the study of biomarkers for cancer risk prediction and early detection. The NCI's Early Detection Research Network (EDRN), established in 1998 with 18 biomarker development laboratories, is a collaborative effort of the NCI, academic, and private research institutions for the systematic identification, development, and validation of novel biomarkers that distinguish the characteristics of cancer cells. The EDRN is focusing on four cancer sites: (1) breast and gynecologic cancers, (2) gastrointestinal and other associated cancers, (3) lung and upper aerodigestive cancers, and (4) prostate and urologic cancers. Currently, the EDRN is proceeding on the validation of three promising biomarkers and many more are in the earliest phase of development. More information on the EDRN may be found at the NCI Web Site at http://www3.cancer.gov/prevention/cbrg/edrn/.

There is a wealth of new technologies that are being investigated in cancer research that can add significantly to progress in the next decade, including gene expression profiling, tissue microarrays, and proteomics. Of these, gene expression profiling allows rapid identification of literally thousands of differentially expressed genes, which may allow the detection and definition of changes in gene expression that can be correlated with precancerous conditions and perhaps indicate risk for progression to full-blown cancer. Serial analysis of gene expression (SAGE) is used to describe gene expression profiles of cell types with comparisons to cancer cells, identify the presence of malignant tissue, and follow progression of tumors as they grow or react to therapy. The increasing amounts of information available on the behavior and biology of normal and malignant cells will only accelerate development of more predictive assays that could be used in chemoprevention or intervention research.

Conclusion

There has been substantial progress in the war on cancer, and recent improvements in some cancer sites, regarding incidence and mortality, should be encouraging. There is still much to be known, but the types of systematic investigations conducted in the past have given us a wealth of knowledge that is being applied to cancer screening, diagnosis, and treatment. Cancer prevention has an important role in the fight against cancer. For progress to continue, cancer prevention must be built into the mainstream of major research institutions and become a part of clinical practice. Training cancer prevention researchers in new approaches and multidisciplinary collaborations with technologists, computer specialists, and investigators in fields outside oncology can make a substantial difference in developing approaches to better prevent cancer and improve patient outcomes.

References

American Cancer Society. http://www.cancer.org/docroot/home/index.asp. Accessed 30 January 2006

Agrawal A, Gutteridge E, Gee JM, Nicholson RI, Robertson JF (2005) Overview of tyrosine kinase inhibitors in clinical breast cancer. Endocr Relat Cancer 12 [Suppl 1]:S135–S144

Alpha-Tocopherol, Beta Carotene Cancer Prevention Study Group (1994) The effect of vitamin E and beta carotene on the incidence of lung cancer and other cancers in male smokers. N Engl J Med 330:1029–1035

Baum M, Budzar AU, Cuzick J, Forbes J, Houghton JH, Klijn JG, Sahmoud T (2002) Anastrozole alone or in combination with tamoxifen versus tamoxifen alone for adjuvant treatment of postmenopausal women with early breast cancer: first results of the ATAC randomised trial. Lancet 359:2131–2139

Brawley OW, Ford LG, Thompson I, Perlman JA, Kramer BS (1994) 5-Alpha-reductase inhibition and prostate cancer prevention. Cancer Epidemiol Biomarkers Prev 3:177–182

Burns DM (2000) Primary prevention, smoking, and smoking cessation: implications for future trends in lung cancer prevention. Cancer 89:2506–2509

Calle EE, Rodriguez C, Walker-Thurmond K, Thun MJ (2003) Overweight, obesity, and mortality from cancer in a prospectively studied cohort of U.S. adults. N Engl J Med 348:1625–1638

Campbell MJ, Gombart AF, Kwok SH, Park S, Koeffler HP (2000) The anti-proliferative effects of 1alpha,25(OH)2D3 on breast and prostate cancer cells are associated with induction of BRCA1 gene expression. Oncogene 19:5091–5097

Cerny T (2005) Anti-nicotine vaccination: where are we? Recent Results Cancer Res 166:167–175

Chan JM, Stampfer MJ, Ma J, Rimm EB, Willett WC, Giovannucci EL (1999) Supplemental vitamin E intake and prostate cancer risk in a large cohort of men in the United States. Cancer Epidemiol Biomarkers Prev 8:893–899

Clark LC, Combs GF Jr, Turnbull BW, Slate EH, Chalker DK, Chow J, Davis LS, Glover RA, Graham GF, Gross EG, Krongrad A, Lesher JL Jr, Park HK, Sanders BB Jr, Smith CL, Taylor JR (1996) Effects of selenium supplementation for cancer prevention in patients with carcinoma of the skin. A randomized controlled trial. Nutritional Prevention of Cancer Study Group. JAMA 276:1957–1963

COMMIT Research Group (1991) Community Intervention Trial for Smoking Cessation (COMMIT): summary of design and intervention. J Natl Cancer Inst 83:1620–1628

Cummings SR, Eckert S, Krueger KA, Grady D, Powles TJ, Cauley JA, Norton L, Nickelsen T, Bjarnason NH, Morrow M, Lippman ME, Black D, Glusman JE, Costa A, Jordan VC (1999) The effect of raloxifene on risk of breast cancer in postmenopausal women: results from the MORE randomized trial. Multiple Outcomes of Raloxifene Evaluation. JAMA 281:2189–2197

Edwards BK, Brown ML, Wingo PA, Howe HL, Ward E, Ries LA, Schrag D, Jamison PM, Jemal A, Wu XC, Friedman C, Harlan L, Warren J, Anderson RN, Pickle LW (2005) Annual report to the nation on the status of cancer, 1975–2002, featuring population-based trends in cancer treatment. J Nat Cancer Inst 97:1407–1427

Efuet ET, Keyomarsi K (2006) Farnesyl and geranylgeranyl transferase inhibitors induce G1 arrest by targeting the proteasome. Cancer Res 66:1040–1051

Feigl P, Blumenstein B, Thompson I, Crowley J, Wolf M, Kramer BS, Coltman CA Jr, Brawley OW, Ford LG (1995) Design of the Prostate Cancer Prevention Trial (PCPT). Control Clin Trials 16:150–163

Fisher B, Costantino J, Redmond C, Poisson R, Bowman D, Couture J, Dimitrov NV, Wolmark N, Wickerham DL, Fisher ER (1989) A randomized clinical trial evaluating tamoxifen in the treatment of patients with node-negative breast cancer who have estrogen-receptor-positive tumors. N Engl J Med 320:479–484

Fisher B, Costantino JP, Wickerham DL, Redmond CK, Kavanah M, Cronin WM, Vogel V, Robidoux A, Dimitrov N, Atkins J, Daly M, Wieand S, Tan-Chiu E, Ford L, Wolmark N (1998) Tamoxifen for prevention of breast cancer: report of the National Surgical Adjuvant Breast and Bowel Project P-1 Study. J Natl Cancer Inst 90:1371–1388

Fisher B, Jeong JH, Anderson S, Wolmark N (2004) Treatment of axillary lymph node-negative, estrogen receptor-negative breast cancer: updated findings from National Surgical Adjuvant Breast and Bowel Project clinical trials. J Natl Cancer Inst 96:1823–1831

Fleming J, Ghose A, Harrison PR (2001) Molecular mechanisms of cancer prevention by selenium compounds. Nutr Cancer 40:42–49

Furr BJ, Jordan VC (1984) The pharmacology and clinical uses of tamoxifen. Pharmacol Ther 25:127–205

Furuya Y, Ohta S, Shimazaki J (1996) Induction of apoptosis in androgen-independent mouse mammary cell line by 1, 25-dihydroxyvitamin D3. Int J Cancer 68:143–148

Giger ML (2004) Computerized analysis of images in the detection and diagnosis of breast cancer. Semin Ultrasound CT MR 25:411–418

Giovannucci E (1998) Dietary influences of 1,25(OH)2 vitamin D in relation to prostate cancer: a hypothesis. Cancer Causes Control 9:567–582

Gohagan J, Marcus P, Fagerstrom R, Pinsky P, Kramer B, Prorok P (2004) Baseline findings of a randomized feasibility trial of lung cancer screening with spiral CT scan vs chest radiograph: the Lung Screening Study of the National Cancer Institute. Chest 126:114–121

Grau MV, Baron JA, Sandler RS, Haile RW, Beach ML, Church TR, Heber D (2003) Vitamin D, calcium supplementation, and colorectal adenomas: results of a randomized trial. J Natl Cancer Inst 95:1765–1771

Greenwald P, Clifford CK (1995) Dietary prevention. In: Greenwald P, Kramer BS, Weed DK (eds) Cancer Prevention and Control. Marcel Dekker, New York, pp 302–327

Greenwald P, Kramer B, Weed D (1993) Expanding horizons in breast and prostate cancer prevention and early detection. The 1992 Samuel C. Harvey Lecture. J Cancer Educ 8:91–107

Heber D, Lu QY (2002) Overview of mechanisms of action of lycopene. Exp Biol Med 227:920–923

Klein EA, Thompson IM, Lippman SM, Goodman PJ, Albanes D, Taylor PR, Coltman C (2001) SELECT: the next prostate cancer prevention trial. Selenium and Vitamin E Cancer Prevention Trial. J Urol 166:1311–1315

Lam S, MacAulay C, Le Riche JC, Dyachkova Y, Coldman A, Guillaud M, Hawk E, Christen MO, Gazdar AF (2002) A randomized phase IIb trial of anethole dithiolthione in smokers with bronchial dysplasia. J Natl Cancer Inst 94:1001–1009

Leaf C (2004) Why we're losing the war on cancer (and how to win it). Fortune 149:76–82, 84–6, 88 passim

McCann SE, Moysich KB, Freudenheim JL, Ambrosone CB, Shields PG (2002) The risk of breast cancer associated with dietary lignans differs by CYP17 genotype in women. J Nutr 132:3036–3041

Miller EC, Giovannucci E, Erdman JW Jr, Bahnson R, Schwartz SJ, Clinton SK (2002) Tomato products, lycopene, and prostate cancer risk. Urol Clin North Am 29:83–93

Milner JA, McDonald SS, Anderson DE, Greenwald P (2001) Molecular targets for nutrients involved with cancer prevention. Nutr Cancer 41:1–16

Nayfield SG, Karp JE, Ford LG, Dorr FA, Kramer BS (1991) Potential role of tamoxifen in prevention of breast cancer. J Natl Cancer Inst 83:1450–1459

Nomura AM, Lee J, Stemmermann GN, Combs GF Jr (2000) Serum selenium and subsequent risk of prostate cancer. Cancer Epidemiol Biomarkers Prev 9:883–887

Overmoyer BA (1999) The breast cancer prevention trial (P-1 study). The role of tamoxifen in preventing breast cancer. Cleve Clin J Med 66:33–40

Page GP, Green JL, Lackland D (2000) Epidemiology of lung cancer with special reference to genetics, bioassays, women, and developing countries. Semin Respir Crit Care Med 21:365–373

Poole C (2004) Adjuvant chemotherapy for early-stage breast cancer: the tAnGo trial. Oncology (Williston Park) 18:23–26

Potter JD, Finnegan JR, Guinard JX (2000) 5-A-Day for Better Health Program evaluation report. NIH Publication No. 01–4904. Bethesda, MD, National Institutes of Health, National Cancer Institute

Regueiro CR (2005) AGA Future Trends Committee report: colorectal cancer: a qualitative review of emerging screening and diagnostic technologies. Gastroenterology 129:1083–1103

Rittmaster RS (1994) Finasteride. N Engl J Med 330:120–125

Rochefort H, Glondu M, Sahla ME, Platet N, Garcia M (2003) How to target estrogen receptor-negative breast cancer? Endocr Relat Cancer 10:261–266

Smith JA, Andreopoulou E (2004) An overview of the status of imaging screening technology for breast cancer. Ann Oncol 15 [Suppl 1]:I18–I26

Stillman FA, Hartman AM, Graubard BI, Gilpin EA, Murray DM, Gibson JT (2003) Evaluation of the American Stop Smoking Intervention Study (AS-SIST): a report of outcomes. J Natl Cancer Inst 95:1681–1691

Thompson IM, Tangen C, Goodman P (2003) The Prostate Cancer Prevention Trial: design, status, and promise. World J Urol 21:28–30

U.S. Department of Health and Human Services (2001) Women and Smoking: A Report of the Surgeon General. U.S. Department of Health and Human Services, Public Health Service, Office of the Assistant Secretary for Health, Office on Smoking and Health, Washington, DC

Vogel VG, Costantino JP, Wickerham DL, Cronin WM, Wolmark N (2002) The study of tamoxifen and raloxifene: preliminary enrollment data from a randomized breast cancer risk reduction trial. Clin Breast Cancer 3:153–159

Wakeling AE (2005) Inhibitors of growth factor signalling. Endocr Relat Cancer 12 [Suppl 1]:S183–S187

Wargovich MJ, Cunningham JE (2003) Diet, individual responsiveness and cancer prevention. J Nutr 133:2400S–2403S

Weir HK, Thun MJ, Hankey BF, Ries LA, Howe HL, Wingo PA, Jemal A, Ward E, Anderson RN, Edwards BK (2003) Annual report to the nation on the status of cancer, 1975–2000, featuring the uses of surveillance data for cancer prevention and control. J Nat Cancer Inst 95:1276–1299

Winawer SJ, Zauber AG, Ho MN, O'Brien MJ, Gottlieb LS, Sternberg SS, Waye JD, Schapiro M, Bond JH, Panish JF (1993) Prevention of colorectal cancer by colonoscopic polypectomy. The National Polyp Study Workgroup. N Engl J Med 329:1977–1981

Yoshizawa K, Willett WC, Morris SJ, Stampfer MJ, Spiegelman D, Rimm EB, Giovannucci E (1998) Study of prediagnostic selenium level in toenails and the risk of advanced prostate cancer. J Natl Cancer Inst 90:1219–1224

Zeng H, Davis CD, Finley JW (2003) Effect of selenium-enriched broccoli diet on differential gene expression in min mouse liver(1,2). J Nutr Biochem 14:227–231

2 Genetic Risk Profiles for Cancer Susceptibility and Therapy Response

Helmut Bartsch, Heike Dally, Odilia Popanda, Angela Risch, Peter Schmezer

Recent Results in Cancer Research, Vol. 174
© Springer-Verlag Berlin Heidelberg 2007

Abstract

Cells in the body are permanently attacked by DNA-reactive species, both from intracellular and environmental sources. Inherited and acquired deficiencies in host defense mechanisms against DNA damage (metabolic and DNA repair enzymes) can modify cancer susceptibility as well as therapy response. Genetic profiles should help to identify high-risk individuals who subsequently can be enrolled in preventive measures or treated by tailored therapy regimens. Some of our attempts to define such risk profiles are presented. Cancer susceptibility: Single nucleotide polymorphisms (SNPs) in metabolic and repair genes were investigated in a hospital-based lung cancer case–control study. When evaluating the risk associated with different genotypes for N-acetyltransferases (Wikman et al. 2001) and glutathione-S-transferases (Risch et al. 2001), it is mandatory to distinguish between the three major histological subtypes of lung tumors. A promoter polymorphism of the myeloperoxidase gene MPO was shown to decrease lung cancer susceptibility mainly in small cell lung cancer (SCLC) (Dally et al. 2002). The CYP3A4*1B allele was also linked to an increased SCLC risk and in smoking women increased the risk of lung cancer eightfold (Dally et al. 2003b). Polymorphisms in DNA repair genes were shown to modulate lung cancer risk in smokers, and reduced DNA repair capacity elevated the disease risk (Rajaee-Behbahani et al. 2001). Investigations of several DNA repair gene variants revealed that lung cancer risk was only moderately affected by a single variant but was enhanced up to approximately threefold by specific risk allele combinations (Popanda et al. 2004). Therapy response: Inter-individual differences in therapy response are consistently observed with cancer chemotherapeutic agents. Initial results from ongoing studies showed that certain polymorphisms in drug transporter genes (ABCB1) differentially affect response outcome in histological subgroups of lung cancer. Stronger beneficial effects were seen in non-small cell lung cancer (NSCLC) patients following gemcitabine and in SCLC patients following etoposide-based treatment. Several DNA repair parameters (polymorphisms, RNA expression, and DNA repair capacity) were measured in vitro in lymphocytes of patients before radiotherapy and correlated with the occurrence of acute side effects (radio-hypersensitivity). Our initial analysis of several repair gene variants in breast cancer patients (n=446) who received radiotherapy revealed no association of single polymorphisms and the development of side effects (moist desquamation of the irradiated normal skin). The risk for this side effect was, however, strongly reduced in normal weight women carrying a combination of XRCC1 399Gln and APE1 148Glu alleles, indicating that these variants afford some protection against radio-hypersensitivity (Chang-Claude et al. 2005). Based on these data we conclude that specific metabolic and DNA repair gene variants can affect cancer risk and therapy outcome. Predisposition to hereditary cancer syndromes is dominated by the strong effects of some high-penetrance tumor susceptibility genes, while predisposition to sporadic cancer is influenced by the combination of multiple low-penetrance genes, of which as a major challenge, many disease-relevant combinations remain to be identified. Before translating these findings into clinical use and application for public health measures, large population-based studies and validation of the results will be required.

Introduction

Cells in the body are permanently attacked by DNA-reactive species, both from intracellular and environmental sources. Inherited and acquired deficiencies in host defense mechanisms against such DNA damage, e.g., metabolic and DNA repair enzymes, are expected to modify cancer susceptibility (Bartsch and Hietanen 1996; Vineis 2004) as well as therapy response (Eichelbaum et al. 2006). Variations in an individual's metabolic and DNA repair phenotype have now been related to genetic polymorphisms, and many genes encoding carcinogen-metabolizing and DNA-repair enzymes have been identified and sequenced. Consequently, allelic variants (SNPs) that give rise to the observed variation opened new possibilities of studies on individual variability in cancer susceptibility that has been observed by epidemiologists. Scientists became aware that environmental and genetic factors interact in complex diseases.

The incorporation of studies of polymorphisms in metabolic and DNA repair genes into cancer epidemiology is particularly important for at least three reasons: (i) the identification of a subpopulation of subjects who are more susceptible to environmentally induced cancer would increase the power of epidemiological studies; (ii) the role of an etiological agent is strengthened when the enzyme(s) involved in its metabolism and damage removal are known; and (iii) metabolic polymorphisms may be particularly significant in relation to low-level exposures (Vineis et al. 1994), influencing the process of risk assessment and of setting acceptable limits of exposure, which should take individual susceptibility into account.

Genes and their products that are involved in cancer susceptibility may also modulate therapeutic outcome of anti-cancer drugs (Spitz et al. 2005). Interindividual differences in therapy response are consistently observed with most chemotherapeutic agents or regimens. Pharmacogenetic investigations are trying to link inherited genetic differences to the therapy response by specific drugs. The best recognized examples are genetic polymorphisms of drug-metabolizing enzymes, which affect 30% of all drugs (Eichelbaum et al. 2006), but inherited variations in DNA repair, in drug transporter genes and other drug target genes also likely contribute to the variability in the outcome of cancer treatment (Efferth and Volm 2005; Lee et al. 2005).

Given the number and variability in expression of carcinogen-metabolizing and DNA repair genes and the complexity of human carcinogen exposures, assessment of a single polymorphic enzyme (genotype) for risk prediction or therapy outcome is not sufficient. Therefore, so-called genetic risk profiles are being established taking into account genetic variation of a variety of genes and their products that affect the multistage carcinogenesis process. The utility of such profiles has been shown for instance for enzymes encoded by DNA repair genes that constantly monitor the genome to repair damaged nucleotide residues resulting from environmental and endogenous exposures. Inherited SNPs of DNA repair genes thus can also contribute to variations in DNA repair capacity and hence susceptibility to carcinogens. Recent studies suggested that the combined effect of multiple variant alleles may be more important than the investigation of a single SNP in modulating DNA repair capacity (Matullo et al. 2003; Mohrenweiser et al. 2003). A theoretical model was developed that underlies the rational for individualizing radiotherapy (Burnet et al. 1998). The gaussian distribution of the dose-response curve comprising sensitive and resistant subjects is likely to originate from the combined effects of several low-penetrance genes (Vineis 2004). Genetic profiles should help to identify high-risk individuals for environmentally induced cancer who subsequently can be enrolled in preventive measures. This type of approach may also help clinicians in the future to individualize and optimize anti-cancer drug therapy or radiotherapy and to predict side effects. Some of our current attempts to define such risk profiles are summarized below with special reference to polymorphic genes modulating tobacco smoke-induced lung cancer risk, chemotherapy response in lung cancer patients, and side effects in patients receiving radiotherapy.

Genetic Risk Profiles for Cancer Susceptibility

Genetic Variation in Metabolic Genes and Lung Cancer Risk

We have carried out analyses of a hospital-based case–control study, investigating lung cancer risk, for a number of genetic polymorphisms in metabolic genes, such as those coding for phase I activating and phase II conjugating enzymes. Genotype-specific modulation of lung cancer risk would not normally be expected unless there is environmental exposure to pro-carcinogens; therefore smoking and other environmental exposures must be taken into account. Clinically and etiologically there are important distinctions to be made between different histological tumor types. Given that some studies find an increased lung cancer risk for women compared to men, it is also interesting to stratify by gender where biologically plausible (Risch et al. 1993). Below we detail examples of our analyses where data were stratified by histology and gender.

Stratification by Lung Cancer Histology

Our studies on genetic polymorphisms and lung cancer risk show the importance of stratifying the analyses by lung cancer histology. Etiologically, small cell lung cancer (SCLC) and squamous cell carcinoma (SCC) have the strongest association with smoking because these tumors are found almost exclusively in smokers, whereas adenocarcinoma also develops in a significant number of non-smokers (Muscat and Wynder 1995). Recently, mutational and epigenetic evidence has even been found for independent pathways for lung adenocarcinomas arising in smokers and never smokers (Toyooka et al. 2006). In addition, the histogenesis of SCLC is completely different from that of NSCLC because it morphologically and immunohistochemically belongs to the neuroendocrine tumors (Kayser 1992; Brambilla et al. 2005).

The MPO-463 polymorphism is a good example, showing that separate analysis of different histological types of lung cancer is important in risk assessment. MPO-463 has functional significance for metabolism and DNA binding

of carcinogens present in tobacco smoke. We conducted a case–control study with 625 ever-smoking lung cancer patients that included 228 adenocarcinomas, 224 SCC and 135 SCLC, as well as 340 ever-smoking hospital-based controls. MPO genotyping was performed with capillary PCR followed by fluorescence-based melting curve analysis. Carriers of the MPO-463A variant genotypes showed a protective effect approaching significance (odds ratio [OR], 0.75; 95% CI, 0.55–1.01) when all lung cancer cases were compared with controls. Among histological types of lung cancer, a weak protective effect was found for both adenocarcinoma (OR, 0.81; CI, 0.55–1.19) and SCC (OR, 0.82; CI, 0.56–1.21) that was stronger and significant for SCLC (OR, 0.58; CI, 0.36–0.95; p=0.029) (Dally et al. 2002) (see Fig. 1).

Since 1997, controversial results have been published regarding the MPO-463A allele and its impact on lung cancer. This seems to be mainly due to differing proportions of histological types of lung cancer as well as differences in the number of never-smokers among cases and controls in several studies. The MPO genotype frequencies may also differ in nonmalignant lung diseases. As lung tumor development is frequently preceded by chronic inflammation of the lung (Mayne et al. 1999), with recruitment of large numbers of neutrophils to the lung and local release of MPO (Grattendick et al. 2002), future case–control studies investigating MPO genotype and lung cancer risk would ideally include information on previous lung diseases for both cases and controls. In conclusion, further (large) case–control studies should preferentially analyze smokers, include a separate analysis of histological types of lung cancer, and in such studies clinical assessment of and statistical adjustment for inflammatory nonmalignant lung diseases would be desirable (Dally et al. 2003a).

The highly polymorphic N-acetyltransferases (NAT1 and NAT2) are involved in both activation and inactivation reactions of numerous carcinogens, such as tobacco-derived aromatic amines. The potential effect of the NAT genotypes in individual susceptibility to lung cancer was examined in a hospital based case–control study consisting of 392 Caucasian lung cancer patients (152 adenocarcinomas, 173 SCC, and 67 other primary lung tumors) and 351 controls.

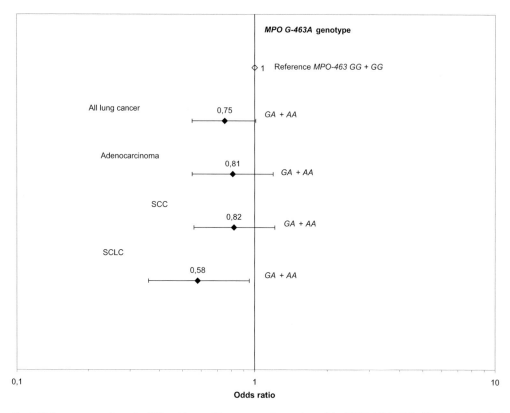

Fig. 1 Risk, among smokers, for different types of lung cancer for carriers of the MPO-463A allele. The study included 340 ever-smoking hospital controls, 625 ever-smoking lung cancer patients with 228 adenocarcinomas, 224 squamous cell carcinomas, and 135 small cell lung cancer cases (see also Dally et al. 2002)

In addition to the wild type allele NAT1*4, seven variant NAT1 alleles (NAT1*3, *10, *11, *14, *15, *17, and *22) were analyzed. Fluorescent-based melting curve analysis (LightCycler, Roche Diagnostics, Mannheim, Germany) was applied for the detection of the polymorphic NAT1 sites at nt 1088 and nt 1095. For NAT1, one or two NAT1*10 alleles identified fast NAT1 acetylators, whereas NAT*14, *15, *17, or *22 defined slow acetylators. Individuals with a NAT1*10 allele combined with a "slow allele" were considered intermediate acetylators. The NAT2 polymorphic sites at nt 481, 590, 803, and 857 were detected by either PCR-RFLP or LightCycler-based analyses. For NAT2, carriers of at least one wild type allele were considered fast acetylators. Multivariate logistic regression analyses were performed taking into account levels of smoking, age, gender, and occupational exposure (Wikman et al. 2001).

An increased risk for adenocarcinoma among the NAT1 putative fast acetylators (OR, 1.92; CI, 1.16–3.16) was found but could not be detected for SCC or the total case group (see Fig. 2). NAT2 genotypes alone appeared not to modify individual lung cancer risk; however, individuals with combined NAT1 fast and NAT2 slow genotype had significantly elevated adenocarcinoma risk (OR, 2.22; CI, 1.03–4.81), which was higher than that observed for NAT1 and AC alone (Wikman et al. 2001). This data clearly shows the importance of separating different histological lung tumor subtypes in studies on genetic susceptibility factors and implicates the NAT1*10 allele as a risk factor for adenocarcinoma.

Glutathione-S-transferase polymorphisms were also investigated as possible lung cancer risk factors. In our case–control study (389 Caucasian lung cancer patients, including 151 adeno-

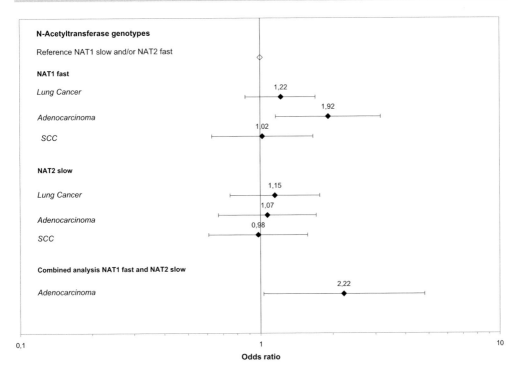

Fig. 2 Lung cancer risk for NAT1 fast and/or NAT2 slow acetylators for different types of non-small cell lung cancer. The study included 392 Caucasian lung cancer patients (152 adenocarcinomas, 173 squamous cell carcinomas and 67 other primary lung tumors) compared to 351 controls (see also Risch et al. 2001)

carcinomas and 172 SCCs, and 353 hospital controls without malignant disease), genotype frequencies for GSTM1, GSTM3, GSTP1, and GSTT1 were determined by PCR/RFLP-based methods. While adjusted odds ratios (OR) indicated no significantly increased risk for lung cancer overall due to any single GST genotype, the risk alleles for GSTM1, GSTM3, and GSTP1, conferring reduced enzyme activity, were present at higher frequency in SCC- than among adenocarcinoma patients (Risch et al. 2001). This is consistent with a reduced detoxification of carcinogenic polycyclic aromatic hydrocarbons from cigarette smoke that are more important for the development of SCC than of adenocarcinoma. An exploratory data analysis also identified statistically significantly increased ORs for the combinations GSTT1 non-null and GSTP1 GG or AG for lung cancer overall (OR, 2.23; CI, 1.11–4.45) and for SCC (OR, 2.69; CI, 1.03–6.99). For lung cancer overall, and especially among SCC patients, the GSTT1-null genotype was underrepresented (SCC 11.2% vs controls 19%, p=0.026; OR, 0.57; CI, 0.30–1.06). In conclusion, GST genotypes may act differently, either by detoxifying harmful tobacco carcinogens and/or by eliminating lung cancer chemopreventive agents. The latter role for GSTT1 would explain the observed lower risk of SCC associated with GSTT1-null.

The CYP3A isozymes play a pivotal role in the metabolism of numerous xenobiotics, including tobacco smoke constituents. The human CYP3A4 enzyme is involved in tobacco-specific nitrosamine- and BaP-metabolism, leading to genotoxic intermediates with subsequent DNA-adduct formation. Both CYP3A4 and CYP3A5 are present in human lung and show selective expression in specific lung cells (Raunio et al. 2005). An A to G point mutation in the nifedipine-specific response element in the promoter of CYP3A4 (CYP3A4*1B) has been associated with a twofold higher promoter activity and twofold higher CYP3A4 protein level. In a case–control study with 801 Caucasian lung cancer patients that included 330 adenocarcinomas, 260 SCCs, 171 SCLCs, and 432 Caucasian hospital-based controls, we investigated the influence of genetic polymorphisms in CYP3A isozymes on lung cancer risk. CYP3A genotyping was performed by capillary PCR followed by fluorescence-based melting curve analysis. After adjustment for gender, age, smoking, and occupational exposure, a significantly increased risk of contracting the smoking-related SCLC was observed for CYP3A4*1B carriers (OR, 2.25; CI, 1.11–4.55), while the risk was not significantly increased for lung cancer overall. No effect was observed for adenocarcinoma or SCC (see Fig. 3). No modification of lung cancer risk overall or histological types by the CYP3A5 genotype was found for the CYP3A5*1 allele carriers compared to CYP3A5 *3/*3 carriers (not shown). Individuals carrying the CYP3A5*1 homozygous genotype

had a greater than 3.9-fold increased risk either obtained for lung cancer overall and for all histological types, but ORs had large confidence intervals (not shown).

Stratification by Gender

In the past, gender differences in genetic susceptibility for lung cancer have been described for genetic factors including several genetic polymorphisms (Dresler et al. 2000; Pauk et al. 2005). A recent report by Larsen et al. showed a significant underrepresentation of the homozygous GSTP1 Ile105Val genotype in NSCLC compared with controls (OR, 0.73; CI, 0.53–1.00; p=0.050) and the effect was stronger in females (OR, 0.57; CI, 0.34–0.98; p=0.04) (Larsen et al. 2006).

Besides xenobiotic metabolism, CYP3A4 is also involved in steroid metabolism, thereby generating the putative carcinogen 16α-hydrox-

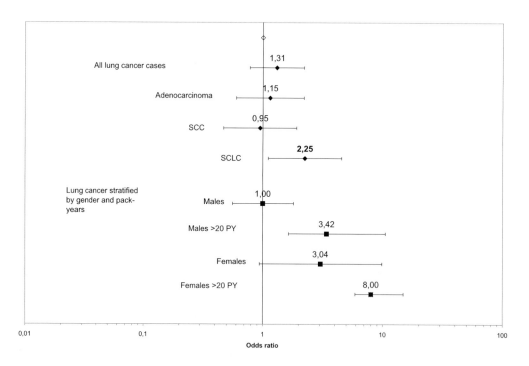

Fig. 3 CYP3A4 genotype-dependent risk for different histological types of lung cancer and for lung cancer stratified by gender and pack-years. The study included 432 hospital controls, 801 lung cancer patients with 330 adenocarcinomas, 260 squamous cell carcinomas, and 171 small cell lung cancer cases (see also Dally et al. 2003b). CYP3A4*1A/*1A reference genotype; CYP3A4*1B allele carriers including only one adenocarcinoma patient with a CYP3A4*1B/*1B genotype. *CYP3A4*1A/*1A reference genotype = pale diamond; CYP3A4*1B allele carriers including only one adenocarcinoma patient with a CYP3A4*1B/*1B genotype = dark diamond and dark square

yestrone in humans (Huang et al. 1998). A gender-stratified analysis was carried out to detect whether CYP3A genotypes affect lung cancer risk differently in males and females. We found an increased risk approaching significance for female CYP3A4*1B carriers (OR, 3.04; CI, 0.94–9.90; p=0.06), while male carriers were not affected (OR, 1.00; CI, 0.56–1.81) (see Fig. 3).

Our data suggest that smoking strengthens this gender-specific lung cancer risk. Heavier smoking men (≥20 PY) with the CYP3A4*1B allele had a significant OR for lung cancer of 3.42 (CI, 1.65–7.14; p=0.001) compared to *1A/*1A carriers with lower tobacco exposure (<20 PY). For women, the respective OR was 8.00 (CI, 2.12–30.30; p=0.005) (see Fig. 3).

Genetic Variation in DNA Repair Genes and Cancer Risk

The ability to repair DNA lesions is thought to be an important host factor contributing to individual cancer susceptibility. Different direct and indirect methods such as host-cell reactivation and comet assay or characterization of variants in DNA repair genes have been used in molecular epidemiological studies to identify subjects who are at high risk. Overall, the results in many studies showed positive and consistent associations between DNA repair capacity and cancer occurrence, mainly with odds ratios in the range of 2–10 (Berwick and Vineis 2000, 2005).

Modulation of Lung Cancer Risk by Genetic Variation in DNA Repair Genes

Many SNPs have been described in DNA repair genes, indicating that DNA repair pathways and activities are affected by a high degree of genetic variation (Mohrenweiser et al. 2003). Data on the functional impact of these polymorphisms is still limited, but there is sufficient evidence to show that many of the genetic variants can modify DNA repair activity, thus contributing to an increase in mutation rate, genetic instability, and cancer risk. We have investigated the effects of several polymorphisms in DNA repair genes on lung cancer risk including XPA (-4G/

A), XPD (Lys751Gln and Asp312Asn), XRCC1 (Arg399Gln), APE1 (Asp148Glu), and XRCC3 (Thr241Met) (Popanda et al. 2004).

Polymorphisms were analyzed in a case–control study including 463 lung cancer cases (among them 204 adenocarcinomas and 212 SCCs) and 460 tumor-free hospital controls. Genotypes were determined using PCR-based melting point analysis of sequence-specific probes (LightCycler technology). Odds ratios (OR) adjusted for age, gender, smoking, and occupational exposure were calculated.

In general, single polymorphisms were found to be weakly associated with lung cancer risk in our study population (see Fig. 4). For homozygous individuals carrying the Glu variant of APE1, a protective effect was found (OR, 0.77; CI, 0.51–1.16). Individuals homozygous for the variants XPA (-4A) (OR, 1.53; CI, 0.94–2.5), XPD 751Gln (OR, 1.39; CI, 0.90–2.14) or XRCC3 241Met (OR, 1.29; CI, 0.85–1.98) showed a slightly higher risk for lung cancer overall (see Fig. 4). In the subgroup of adenocarcinoma cases, adjusted ORs were found to be increased for individuals homozygous for XPA (-4A) (OR, 1.62; CI, 0.91–2.88) and XRCC3 241Met (OR, 1.65; CI, 0.99–2.75).

DNA is repaired via different repair pathways, each being specific for a defined type of DNA lesions (Hoeijmakers 2001). The genetic variants we have selected for our analysis are part of three DNA repair pathways, namely nucleotide excision repair (XPD, XPA), base excision repair (XRCC1, APE1), and DNA double-strand break repair (XRCC3). As an individual is characterized by many genetic variants (Mohrenweiser et al. 2003), we determined combined effects of variant alleles (Popanda et al. 2004) and identified 54 patients and controls who were homozygous for two or three of the potential risk alleles (i.e., the variants in nucleotide excision repair, XPA (-4A) and XPD 751Gln, and in homologous recombination, XRCC3-241Met). ORs were significantly increased when all patients (OR, 2.37; CI, 1.26–4.48) (see Fig. 4), patients with squamous cell carcinoma (OR, 2.83; CI, 1.17–6.85), and with adenocarcinoma (OR, 3.05; CI, 1.49–6.23) were analyzed. Combinations of polymorphisms in genes involved in the same repair pathway (XPA+XPD or XRCC1+APE1) affected

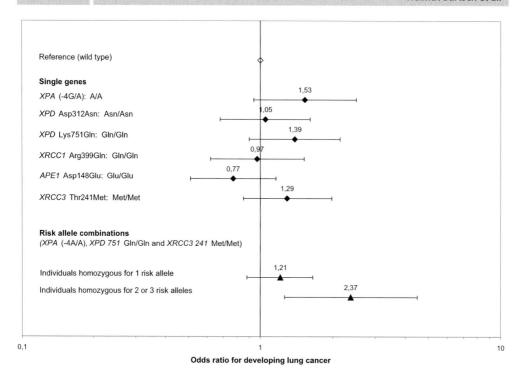

Fig. 4 Lung cancer risk for homozygous carriers of one or more risk alleles in DNA repair. Effects on cancer risk are shown for single variant alleles and for the combinations of two or three potential risk alleles (see also Popanda et al. 2004)

lung cancer risk only in patients with squamous cell carcinoma.

DNA repair, which is activated in the presence of DNA damage, is an important cellular defense mechanism against adverse effects caused by endogenous and environmental carcinogens. Thus, a functional defect in DNA repair capacity caused by a variant of a low penetrance gene will become apparent when measured in the presence of damaged DNA. In epidemiological studies, this requires detailed knowledge to which classes of environmental carcinogens individuals are exposed so as to assess a possible risk modification by genetic variants (Wild 2005). For example, the analysis of lung cancer patients with adenocarcinoma is presented here for the XPA (-4G/A) polymorphism (see Fig. 5) (Butkiewicz et al. 2004). A nearly threefold increased risk for adenocarcinoma was associated with the XPA AA genotype when individuals were occupationally exposed (OR, 2.95; CI, 1.42–6.14) or were heavy smokers with more than 20 pack-years (OR, 2.52;

CI, 1.17–5.42). In contrast, no genotype-dependent increase in OR was found for nonexposed individuals or light smokers. This significant effect of the XPA polymorphism in heavy smokers and occupationally exposed individuals suggests a strong gene–environment interaction for this gene.

The relatively low impact of single variant alleles on cancer risk that we and others have consistently found contrasts with the markedly increased risk associated with a reduced phenotypic DNA repair capacity (reviewed in Berwick and Vineis 2000; Mohrenweiser et al. 2003; Spitz et al. 2003). The DNA repair capacity determined in carcinogen (bleomycin) -treated human lymphocytes in vitro (see next chapter) is an integrative measure of the functional impact of all repair variants, contributing to the repair of DNA damage after a specific genotoxic exposure. In case of exposure to carcinogenic mixtures such as occurs in tobacco smokers, specific gene–gene interactions either within one repair pathway or

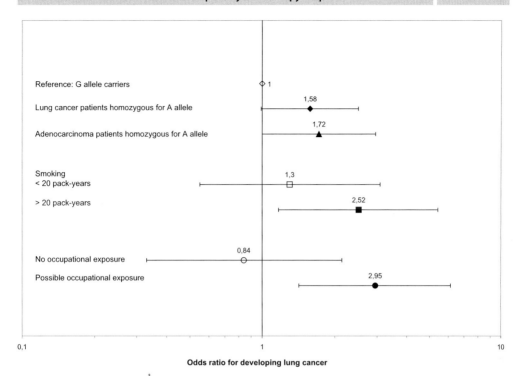

Fig. 5 Lung cancer risk for homozygous carriers of the (-4G/A) polymorphism in the XPA gene. An increased risk for adenocarcinoma associated with the XPA AA genotype was observed for heavy smokers and occupationally exposed individuals. No genotype-dependent increase in OR was found for those smoking less than 20 pack-years or for nonexposed individuals (see also Butkiewicz et al. 2004)

between different pathways are required. Our results on combined genotypes indicate that lung cancer risk is considerably enhanced by specific combinations of variant alleles. The interaction of several (or many) variant repair proteins, each with only slightly reduced functional activity, may be necessary to significantly decrease DNA repair activity and to increase cancer risk. However, given the huge number of possible genotype combinations in our cohort, only some individuals with a specific genotype combination could be studied. Validation of our results in larger population-based studies including a wider range of genetic variants is required. In our ongoing studies, we are also measuring phenotypic DNA repair capacity, which reflects complex DNA repair genotype combinations and which cannot be easily characterized by today's genotyping methods.

Phenotypic Variation in DNA Repair and Cancer Risk

We developed and validated a microgel electrophoresis (comet) assay to measure DNA repair capacity in cryopreserved peripheral blood lymphocytes from lung cancer patients and hospital-based controls without cancer (Schmezer et al. 2001). After thawing, phytohemagglutinin-stimulated cells were treated with bleomycin at 20 µg/ml for 30 min and the extent of DNA damage, expressed as mutagen sensitivity and DNA repair capacity, are determined by microgel electrophoresis. Repeated analysis of peripheral blood lymphocytes from the same individual demonstrated good reproducibility of the assay even for up to 12 months after cryopreservation.

Lymphocytes from 160 patients with non-small cell lung cancer and 180 tumor-free hospital controls were investigated. Mutagen sensitivity defined as the tail moment of bleomycin-treated cells, without allowing time for DNA repair, was significantly higher in lung cancer patients (p<0.0001) than in controls (Rajaee-Behbahani et al. 2001). DNA repair capacity was analyzed after allowing 15 min repair time. Lymphocytes of patients showed a reduced DNA repair capacity when compared to cells of controls (67% vs 79.3%; p<0.0004). Neither in the patients nor in the control group did we observe any correlation between mutagen sensitivity and DNA repair capacity with age or gender. The median values of DNA repair capacity and sensitivity in controls were used as the cut-off points to calculate odds ratios. After adjustment for age, gender, and smoking status, the cases versus controls had a more than twofold reduction in DNA repair capacity and a fourfold increase in mutagen sensitivity. Bleomycin sensitivity and DNA repair capacity were found to be independent susceptibility markers for non-small cell lung cancer.

Our results revealed the comet assay to be a sensitive and fast tool that can be applied both to native and cryopreserved peripheral blood lymphocytes. It is suitable to determine individual mutagen sensitivity and DNA repair capacity in whole cells, thus allowing the assessment of complex phenotypes of integrated response to DNA damage. Important parts of the assay such as scanning of the fluorescence images have been successfully automated (Iwakawa et al. 2005; Schunck et al. 2004), thus allowing high assay reproducibility and application in large-scale epidemiological studies. Validation of this assay in large prospective studies for the identification of high-risk subjects for non-small cell lung cancer is now warranted.

Further analyses of specific repair pathways or single repair enzymes can help to identify major factors that contribute to the observed differences in cellular DNA repair capacity among individuals within a population. We have therefore investigated the activity of poly(ADP-ribose) polymerase (PARP), a key enzyme in DNA strand-break repair. This nuclear enzyme is catalytically activated by strand breaks. Using $NAD^{(+)}$ as a precursor, it catalyzes the formation of ADP-ribose polymers, which are attached to various proteins (Bürkle 2001, 2005). We investigated whether differences in the activity of PARP

are associated with the risk for laryngeal cancer. In a case–control study on genetic, lifestyle, and occupational risk factors for laryngeal cancer, PARP activity was assessed as DNA damage-induced poly(ADP-ribose) formation in human peripheral blood lymphocytes by quantitative immunofluorescence analysis (Rajaee-Behbahani et al. 2002). Polymer formation was determined as the cellular response to bleomycin-induced DNA damage in lymphocytes from 69 laryngeal cancer patients and 125 healthy controls. The frequency of mutagen-induced polymer formation, measured as mean pixel intensity, was significantly lower in cases than in controls, and it was not influenced by either smoking, age, or sex. There was no significant difference between cases and controls in basal polymer formation, i.e., in cells that were not treated with bleomycin. When the highest tertile of polymer formation was used as the reference, the odds ratio for the lowest tertile of bleomycin-induced polymer formation was 3.8 (CI, 1.4–10.5; p=0.01). Peripheral blood lymphocytes from laryngeal cancer patients thus showed significantly less bleomycin-induced poly(ADP-ribose) formation. Our results suggest that a reduced capacity of somatic cells to synthesize poly(ADP-ribose) might be associated with an increased risk for laryngeal cancer, an observation that has also been made for other types of cancer such as breast cancer in women (Hu et al. 1997). A PARP variant (ADPRT V762A) that leads to altered enzyme function was significantly associated with increased prostate cancer risk (Lockett et al. 2004).

Genetic Risk Profiles for Therapy Response

Chemotherapy Response

Drug-metabolizing enzymes are responsible for the activation or detoxification of cytotoxic drugs including chemotherapeutics. Genetic variability between individuals in the pharmacokinetics of cancer chemotherapy plays an important role in therapeutic efficacy and safety (Scripture et al. 2005). Some prominent examples of the impact of genetic polymorphisms in anticancer drug metabolizing enzymes on response outcome have been described. Polymorphisms in thiopurine methyltransferase (TPMT) have been associated with mercaptopurine's efficacy and toxicity. Acute lymphoblastic leukemia patients with at least one mutant TPMT allele, which results in intermediate levels of TPMT activity, tend to have an improved response to mercaptopurine therapy and better chances of being cured, compared with patients who have two wild type TPMT alleles. On the other hand, patients with reduced TPMT activity are at higher risk of developing a thiopurine-related second tumor (Relling et al. 1999; Relling and Dervieux 2001). Thymidylate synthase (TS) activity is associated with better antitumor response to 5-fluorouracil (5-FU), which is widely used in the treatment of breast and colorectal cancer. TS activity is regulated by a variable number of tandem repeats in the enhancer/promoter region of the TS gene. Patients who have a homozygous genotype with three tandem repeats have higher TS activity and lower probability of responding to 5-FU therapy than patients with two tandem repeats (Villafrana et al. 2001; Relling and Dervieux 2001). Irinotecan is used to treat various solid tumors, such as colon cancer and lung cancer. A variant number of dinucleotide repeat sequences in the promotor for uridine 5'-diphosphate glucuronosyltransferase 1A1 (UGT1A1) influences the glucuronidation of SN-38, the active metabolite of irinotecan, which is associated with severe toxicity, including diarrhea and myelosuppression (Relling and Dervieux 2001; Candelaria et al. 2005).

There is an increasing number of publications that investigate the impact of genetic polymorphisms on response outcome in tumor therapy, especially on survival. There is a lack of clinical trials proving that pharmacogenetic testing before treatment helps to find the appropriate drug and dose for the individual patient, thereby improving therapeutic response outcome and/or reducing adverse drug reactions (Eichelbaum et al. 2006). However, pharmacogenetics in clinical cancer therapy has recently attracted increasing interest. At the Mayo Clinic, a microarray able to genotype more than 100,000 SNPs is used to investigate the genetic basis for differential responses to antihypertensive drugs to identify genes influencing drug response and ultimately tailor antihypertensive therapy for individual patients. The Roche AmpliChip CYP450 Test was cleared for diagnostic use in Europe and the United States in 2005 to identify SNPs in CYP2D6 and CYP2C19, which help to metabolize up to 25% of all prescription drugs, including those for cardiovascular disease and depression (Lipshutz 2005).

For the past decades, a widely used chemotherapy protocol for SCLC patients with extensive disease is the combination of carboplatin and etoposide. Other established drugs in SCLC polychemotherapy include combinations of cyclophosphamide, doxorubicin, and/or vincristine. Until recently, chemotherapeutic treatment of NSCLC has been neglected, as in contrast to SCLC, this histological type of lung cancer is relatively insensitive to standard cytotoxic agents. In the last few years, interest in the chemotherapy of NSCLC has rapidly increased, mostly because a number of new drugs – including paclitaxel, docetaxel, vinorelbine, gemcitabine, topotecan, and irinotecan – have emerged as active against this tumor. A number of clinical studies were conducted to identify an ideal chemotherapy regimen for advanced NSCLC, but to date, there is no accepted standard of care.

Currently, lung cancer therapy strategy is predominantly dependent on tumor stage and the performance status of the patient (Zochbauer-Muller et al. 1999; Jassem 1999; Thomas et al. 2002). Several molecular markers are considered to predict chemotherapy response in lung cancer patients (Rosell et al. 2004; Fischer and Lahm 2004), but only a very limited number of studies have been published showing any influence of genetic polymorphisms on response outcome in lung cancer treatment (Gautschi et al. 2006; Alberola et al. 2004).

In an ongoing pharmacogenetic study, the influence of certain SNPs and haplotypes on chemotherapy response outcome and survival in patients with primary lung cancer is being investigated. These concern enzymes that metabolize and transport anticancer agents used in lung cancer treatment. In addition, the influence of repair enzymes, especially those that play a critical role in platinum resistance is being analyzed. All patients receive a first-line chemotherapy. Chemotherapy response is assessed after the second cycle to detect mainly host factor-related mechanisms of resistance and to exclude, as far as possible, acquired mechanisms of resistance in the tumor developed during treatment.

A statistically significant association was found for SNPs in the ABCB1 transporter gene with chemotherapy response as well as with survival. The observations indicate that for a certain fraction of NSCLC patients with a gemcitabine-based therapy who are carriers of the variant alleles, treatment will be less effective compared to homozygous wild type carriers with the same treatment. These results imply that dose considerations in phase I and phase II trials should include relevant SNPs in drug transporters and that there is a need to identify such polymorphisms. An adapted dose, based on the patient's genetic make-up, may improve chemotherapy response and prolong life, and this should be evaluated in a multicenter clinical trial comparing genetically adaptive chemotherapy with conventional treatment (unpublished data).

Radiotherapy: Biomarkers of Sensitivity to Ionizing Radiation

Normal tissue reactions after therapeutic ionizing radiation (IR) differ considerably among patients and may require interruption of therapy. As this variability cannot be explained by radiation modalities, intrinsic genetic factors have been postulated to affect individual radiosensitivity (Andreassen et al. 2002). Given the high variability of treatment response in patients, predictive assays in the clinic are greatly needed, because hypersensitive patients could be identified prior to therapy and harmful side effects prevented. For patients with normal radiosensitivity, more efficient treatment schedules could be developed, improving tumor therapy (Peters and McKay 2001). During therapeutic treatment with IR, DNA single-strand breaks, oxidative DNA modifications, and DNA double-strand breaks are induced. In order to avoid death of damaged cells or fixation of mutations after cell replication, these DNA lesions are removed by specific cellular DNA repair mechanisms (Hoeijmakers 2001). Differences in DNA repair efficiency between individuals are therefore thought to be responsible for the variability in radiation response. This hypothesis is supported by associations found between cellular radiosensitivity measured as DNA repair capacity in vitro and clinical radiosensitivity in vivo, especially for patients with specific DNA repair gene defects (see Andreassen et al. 2002). In our study on biomarkers for radiosensitivity, we concentrated on DNA repair as an important part of the cellular radiation response. In two molecular epidemiological studies, we explored cellular DNA repair capacity, mRNA expression, and genetic variants of DNA repair and repair-related genes as possible biomarkers of radiosensitivity.

DNA Repair Capacity and mRNA Expression of Repair and Repair-Related Genes

The cellular capacity to repair IR-induced DNA damage plays a critical role for both the susceptibility of patients to side effects after radiotherapy and their subsequent cancer risk. Whether DNA repair capacity determined in vitro is correlated with the occurrence of acute side effects in radiotherapy patients was evaluated in a prospective study of 478 female breast cancer patients receiving adjuvant radiotherapy of the breast after breast-conserving surgery. Acute skin toxicity was documented systematically using a modified version of the common toxicity criteria (Twardella et al. 2003). Prognostic personal and treatment characteristics were identified for the entire cohort. Cryo-preserved lymphocytes from a subgroup of 113 study participants were γ-irradiated with 5 Gy in vitro and analyzed using the alkaline comet assay (Popanda et al. 2003). Reproducibility of this assay was determined by repeated analysis of cells from healthy donors and coefficients of variation were calculated to be between 0.16 and 0.3. The various parameters determined to characterize the individual DNA repair capacity showed large differences between patients. Eleven patients were identified with considerably enhanced DNA damage induction, and seven patients exhibited severely reduced DNA repair capacity after 15 and 30 min.

Using proportional hazards analysis to account for cumulative biologically effective IR dose, the hazard for the development of acute skin reactions (moist desquamation) associated with DNA repair capacity was modeled. Our results revealed that the examined comet assay parameters were not significantly associated with risk of acute skin toxicity. Of the 478 participants, 84 presented with acute reactions by the end of treatment. While higher body mass index was significantly associated with an increased risk for acute reactions when adjusted for treating hospital and photon beam quality, individual repair parameters as determined by the alkaline comet assay were, however, not informative enough. More comprehensive analyses including late effects of radiotherapy and repair kinetics optimized for different IR-induced DNA lesions are warranted.

In another prospective molecular epidemiology study, we analyzed constitutive mRNA expression of DNA repair or repair-related genes in radiotherapy patients to see whether gene expression patterns are predictive for therapy-related acute side effects. Therefore, prostate cancer patients (n=406) receiving intensity-modulated radiotherapy were recruited, and adverse effects were monitored during therapy using common toxicity criteria (US NIH 1999). For expression analyses, samples from 58 patients were selected according to their observed degree of clinical side effects to radiotherapy. Expression profiles were generated from PBL using customized cDNA-arrays that carried probes for 143 DNA repair or repair-related genes (Mayer et al. 2002). In addition, expression of selected genes was confirmed by quantitative RT-PCR. Constitutive mRNA expression profiles were analyzed for predicting acute clinical radiosensitivity (Hümmerich et al. 2006). Cluster analysis identified 19 differentially expressed genes. Many of these genes are involved in DNA double-strand break repair. Expression levels of these genes differed up to sevenfold from the mean of all patients, whereas expression levels of housekeeping genes varied only up to twofold. High expression of the identified genes was associated with a lack of clinical radiation sensitivity. Constitutive expression of DNA repair-related genes may affect the development of acute side effects in radiotherapy patients, and high expression levels of these genes seem to support protection from adverse reactions.

Associations of Acute Side Effects of Radiotherapy and Polymorphisms in Genes Involved in the Repair of Radiation-Induced DNA Damage

Here, we evaluated the association of the risk of acute skin reactions following radiotherapy with polymorphisms in the base excision repair genes XRCC1 (Arg194Trp, Arg280His, and Arg399Gln) and APE1 (Asp148Glu), the nucleotide excision repair gene XPD (Lys751Gln and Asp312Asn), the DNA double-strand break-repair genes XRCC2 (Arg188His) and XRCC3 (Thr241Met), and the DNA repair-related genes TP53 (Arg72Pro, p53PIN3) and p21 (Ser31Arg).

We conducted a prospective study of 446 female patients with breast cancer who received radiotherapy after breast-conserving surgery. All the patients were administered a typical breast-radiation treatment with an average biologically effective radiation dose (BED) of 54.0 Gy ± 4.8 Gy with a range from 35.5 Gy to 64.5 Gy (Twardella et al. 2003). BED was calculated to account for differences in fractionation and overall treatment time. The clinical radiation reaction developing in the skin within the radiation field of the breast was documented at regular time intervals during treatment and the severity of acute side effects was assessed using a classification system based on the common toxicity criteria (CTC) of the US NIH (1999). Seventy-seven of the 446 participants presented with increased acute toxicity (at least one moist desquamation or interruption of RT due to toxicity) by the end of treatment (Popanda et al. 2003; Twardella et al. 2003). For statistical evaluation, development of acute skin reactions associated with DNA repair gene polymorphisms was modeled using Cox proportional hazards, accounting for cumulative biologically effective radiation dose.

Overall results showed that the development of acute toxicity was not associated with the genetic variants studied, although the hazard ratios (HR) for the base excision repair genes were generally below 1 (Chang-Claude et al. 2005; Tan et al. 2005). However, risks were differential by body mass index, an independent risk factor for radiosensitivity. Among normal weight patients only, both carriers of the APE1 148Glu and the XRCC1 399Gln allele had decreased risk of acute skin reactions after radiotherapy (HR, 0.49 and

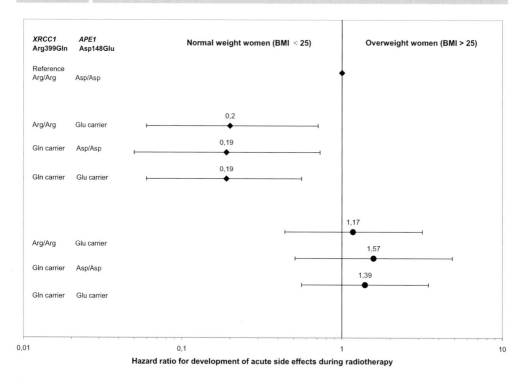

Fig. 6 Genetic variants in DNA repair, acute side effects of radiotherapy and body mass index. Risks to develop acute side effects of radiotherapy were differential by body mass index (see also Chang-Claude et al. 2005). Among normal-weight patients, carriers of both the XRCC1 399Gln and the APE1 148Glu alleles had decreased risk of acute skin reactions after radiotherapy. This protective effect was not observed in overweight patients (p interaction =0.009)

0.51, respectively) (see Fig. 6). The results for XRCC1 were confirmed by haplotype analysis. When considering combined effects, we observed that, compared to homozygote carriers of the wild type allele in both genes, the risk was most strongly reduced in carriers of both APE1 148Glu and XRCC1 399Gln alleles with normal weight (HR, 0.19; CI, 0.06–0.56) but not in those with overweight (HR, 1.39; CI, 0.56–3.45) (p for interaction 0.009) (see Fig. 6). A similar, but not significant difference in radiosensitivity in normal and overweight patients was observed for carriers of TP53 72Pro and p21 31Ser. No effect on radiosensitivity could be found for the polymorphisms in DNA double-strand break-repair genes.

Thus, in patients with normal weight the presence of the XRCC1 399Gln or APE1 148Glu alleles might afford some protection against acute radio-hypersensitivity. However, because of our limited analysis further DNA repair gene vari-ants including haplotype and combination analysis need to be investigated. In addition, late effects of radiotherapy should be included in order to evaluate whether a set of specific profile of genetic variants can serve as a predictive biomarker for radiosensitivity.

Conclusions and Future Perspectives

Genetic risk profiles should help to identify high-risk individuals for environmentally induced cancer who subsequently can be enrolled in preventive measures. Such an approach may also help clinicians in future to individualize and optimize anti-cancer drug therapy or radiotherapy and to predict side effects. At present, our results show that single allelic variants of low-penetrance genes affect cancer susceptibility mainly in specific subgroups, especially when the analyses are stratified by histological types of lung cancer, tobacco consumption, body weight, or gender. Nevertheless, it seems that, for complex biological endpoints such as cancer or therapy outcome, single allelic variants are not sufficient as predictive biomarkers because cancer susceptibility, efficacy of cancer chemotherapy, and resistance as well as drug-related toxicity in normal tissues, are multifactorial in nature and modulated by complex gene–gene and gene–environment interactions. Sophisticated approaches such as integrated drug metabolizing and repair pathway profiling or even genome-wide linkage analyses may improve the predictive power compared with genotyping of single genes (Matsuzaki et al. 2004; Evans and Relling 2004; Nebert and Vesell 2004). There is a great need for prospective clinical trials that evaluate therapies adapted to the patients' individual genetic background. Therefore, the implementation of pharmacogenetics into clinical routine diagnostics including genotype-based recommendations for treatment decisions and risk assessment is a challenge for the future.

Studies that used mouse models of human cancer confirmed the existence of numerous tumor-susceptibility genes and demonstrated that their individual effects are underestimated as they were highly dependent on genetic background and microenvironment (Fijneman 2005). A major challenge will therefore be to establish signatures that reflect phenotypic representation of genetic variation in networks of low-penetrance susceptibility genes. We developed and validated a microgel electrophoresis (comet) assay to measure DNA repair capacity with high assay reproducibility. It may serve as a sensitive and fast tool to assess complex phenotypes of integrated response to DNA damage and to identify informative signatures of genetic variation by phenotype–genotype comparison. Such developments will hopefully offer new possibilities to improve cancer screening programs, prevent tumor initiation, and intervene in tumor progression in a patient-tailored manner.

Acknowledgements

Studies in part supported by the Deutsche Krebshilfe, the Verein zur Förderung der Krebsforschung in Deutschland e.V. and the Bundesamt für Strahlenschutz. We thank Birgit Jäger, Reinhard Gliniorz, Otto Zelezny and Peter Waas for skilled technical assistance. We sincerely acknowledge the contributions by our collaborators: L. Edler, Biostatistik, DKFZ; P. Drings, H. Dienemann, K. W. Kayser, V Schulz, Thoraxklinik Heidelberg-Rohrbach; A. Bach, M.C. von Brevern, Axaron Bioscience AG, Heidelberg, A. Bürkle, Abtl. Molekulare Toxikologie, Universität Konstanz; H. Becher, Abteilung Tropenhygiene und öffentl. Gesundheitswesen, Universität Heidelberg; H. Ramroth, Abteilung Klinische Epidemiologie, DKFZ; A. Dietz, Abteilung Otolaryngologie, Kopf-Hals-Chirurgie, Universität Heidelberg; J. Chang-Claude, Klinische Epidemiologie und J. Debus, Strahlentherapeutische Onkologie, DKFZ. Susanna Fuladdjusch is thanked for excellent secretarial help.

References

Alberola V, Sarries C, Rosell R, Taron M, de las Peñas R, Camps C, Massuti B, Insa A, Garcia-Gomez R, Isla D, Artal A, Muñoz MA, Cobo M, Bover I, Gonzalez-Larriba JL, Terrasa J, Almenar D, Barcelo R, Diz P, Sanchez-Ronco M, Sanchez JJ (2004) Effect of the methylenetetrahydrofolate reductase C677T polymorphism on patients with cisplatin/gemcitabine-treated stage IV non-small-cell lung cancer. Clin Lung Cancer 5:360–365

Andreassen CN, Alsner J, Overgaard J (2002) Does variability in normal tissue reactions after radiotherapy have a genetic basis – where and how to look for it? Radiother Oncol 64:131–140

Bartsch H, Hietanen E (1996) The role of individual susceptibility in cancer burden related to environmental exposure. Environ Health Perspect 104:569–577

Berwick M, Vineis P (2000) Markers of DNA repair and susceptibility to cancer in humans: an epidemiologic review. J Natl Cancer Inst 92:874–897

Berwick M, Vineis P (2005) Measuring DNA repair capacity: small steps. J Natl Cancer Inst 97:84–85

Brambilla E, Brambilla C, Lanhiejoul S (2005) Impact of molecular pathology on the clinical management of lung cancer. Respiration 72:229–232

Bürkle A (2001) Poly(APD-ribosyl)ation, a DNA damage-driven protein modification and regulator of genomic instability. Cancer Lett 163:1–5

Bürkle A (2005) Poly(ADP-ribose). The most elaborate metabolite of NAD+. FEBS J 272:4576–4589

Burnet NG, Johansen J, Turesson I, Nyman J, Peacock JH (1998) Describing patients' normal tissue reactions: concerning the possibility of individualising radiotherapy dose prescriptions based on potential predictive assays of normal tissue radiosensitivity. Int J Cancer 79:606–613

Butkiewicz D, Popanda O, Risch A, Edler L, Dienemann H, Schulz V, Kayser K, Drings P, Bartsch H, Schmezer P (2004) Association between the risk for lung adenocarcinoma and a (-4) G-to-A polymorphism in the XPA gene. Cancer Epidemiol Biomarkers Prev 13:2242–2246

Candelaria M, Taja-Chayeb L, Arce-Salinas C, Vidal-Millan S, Serrano-Olvera A, Duenas-Gonzalez A (2005) Genetic determinants of cancer drug efficacy and toxicity: practical considerations and perspectives. Anticancer Drugs 16:923–933

Chang-Claude J, Popanda O, Tan X-L, Kropp S, Helmbold I, von Fournier D, Haase W, Sautter-Bihl ML, Wenz F, Schmezer P, Ambrosone CB (2005) Association between polymorphisms in the DNA repair genes, XRCC1, APE1, and XPD and acute side effects of radiotherapy in breast cancer patients. Clin Cancer Res 11:4802–4809

Dally H, Gassner K, Jäger B, Schmezer P, Spiegelhalder B, Edler L, Drings P, Dienemann H, Schulz V, Kayser K, Bartsch H, Risch A (2002) Myeloperoxidase (MPO) genotype and lung cancer histologic types: the MPO-463 A allele is associated with reduced risk for small cell lung cancer in smokers. Int J Cancer 102:530–535

Dally H, Bartsch H, Risch A (2003a). Correspondence re: Feyler et al., Point: myeloperoxidase (-463)G → A polymorphism and lung cancer risk. Cancer Epidemiol Biomark Prev 11:1550–1554, 2002, and Xu et al., Counterpoint: The myeloperoxidase (463)G → A polymorphism does not decrease lung cancer susceptibility in Caucasians. 11: I555–1559, 2002. Cancer Epidemiol Biomarkers Prev 12:683

Dally H, Edler L, Jäger B, Schmezer P, Spiegelhalder B, Drings P, Dienemann H, Schulz V, Kayser K, Bartsch H, Risch A (2003b) The CYP3A4*1B allele increases risk for small cell lung cancer: effect of gender and smoking dose. Pharmacogenetics 13:607–618

Dresler CM, Fratelli C, Babb J, Everley L, Evans AA, Clapper ML (2000) Gender differences in genetic susceptibility for lung cancer. Lung Cancer 30:153–160

Efferth T, Volm M (2005) Pharmacogenetics for individualized cancer chemotherapy. Pharmacol Ther 107:155–176

Eichelbaum M, Ingelman-Sundberg M, Evans WE (2006) Pharmacogenomics and individualized drug therapy. Annu Rev Med 57:119–137

Evans WE, Relling MV (2004) Moving towards individualized medicine with pharmacogenomics. Nature 429:464–468

Fijneman RJA (2005) Genetic predisposition to sporadic cancer: how to handle major effects of minor genes? Cellular Oncology 27:281–292

Fischer JR, Lahm H (2004) Validation of molecular and immunological factors with predictive importance in lung cancer. Lung Cancer 45:S5151–S1617

Gautschi O, Hugli B, Ziegler A, Bigosch C, Bowers NL, Daniel Ratschiller D, Jermann M, Stahel RA, Heighway J, Betticher DC (2006) Cyclin Dl (CCND1) A870G gene polymorphism modulates smoking-induced lung cancer risk and response to platinum-based chemotherapy in non-small cell lung cancer (NSCLC) patients. Lung Cancer 51:303–311

Grattendick K, Stuart R, Roberts E, Lincoln J, Lefkowitz SS, Bollen A, Moguilevsky N, Friedman H, Lefkowitz DL (2002) Alveolar macrophage activation by myeloperoxidase: a model for exacerbation of lung inflammation. Am J Respir Cell Mol Biol 26:716–722

Hoeijmakers JH (2001) Genome maintenance mechanisms for preventing cancer. Nature 411:366–374

Hu JJ, Roush GC, Dubin N, Berwick M, Roses DF, Harris MN (1997) Poly(ADP-ribose) polymerase in human breast cancer: a case-control analysis. Pharmacogenetics 7:309–316

Huang Z, Guengerich FP, Kaminsky LS (1998) 16Alpha-hydroxylation of estrone by human cytochrome P4503A4/5. Carcinogenesis 19:867–872

Hümmerich J, Werle-Schneider G, Popanda O, Celebi O, Chang-Claude J, Kropp S, Mayer C, Debus J, Bartsch H, Schmezer P (2006) Constitutive mRNA expression of DNA repair-related genes as a biomarker for clinical radiosensitivity: a pilot study in prostate cancer patients receiving radiotherapy Int J Radiat Biol 82:593-604

Iwakawa M, Goto M, Noda S, Sagara M, Yamada S, Yamamoto N, Kawakami Y, Matsui Y, Miyazawa Y, Yamazaki H, Tsuji H, Ohno T (2005) DNA repair capacity measured by high throughput alkaline comet assays in EBV-transformed cell lines and peripheral blood cells from cancer patients and healthy volunteers. Mutat Res 588:1–6

Jassem J (1999) Chemotherapy of advanced non-small cell lung cancer. Ann Oncol 10 [Suppl 6]:77–82

Kayser K (1992) Analytical lung pathology. Springer, Berlin Heidelberg New York

Larsen JE, Colosimo ML, Yang LA, Bowman R, Zimmerman PV, Fong KM (2006) CYP1A1 I1e462Val and MPO G-46 3A interact to increase risk of adenocarcinoma but not squamous cell carcinoma of the lung. Carcinogenesis 27:525–532

Lee W, Lockhart AC, Kim RB, Rothenberg ML (2005) Cancer pharmacogenomics: powerful tools in cancer chemotherapy and drug development. Oncologist 10:104–111

Lipshutz R (2005) Using microarrays to detect disease and tailor therapy. Pharmaceut Discov 5:28–37

Lockett KL, Hall MC, Xu J, Zheng SL, Berwick M, Chuang SC, Clark PE, Cramer SD, Lohman K, Hu JJ (2004) The ADPRT V762A genetic variant contributes to prostate cancer susceptibility and deficient enzyme function. Cancer Res 64:6344–6348

Matullo G, Peluso M, Polidoro S, Guarrera S, Munnia S, Krogh V, Masala G, Berrino F, Panico S, Tumino R, Vineis P, Palli D (2003) Combination of DNA repair gene single nucleotide polymorphisms and increased levels of DNA adducts in a population-based study. Cancer Epidemiol Biomarkers Prev 12:674–677

Matsuzaki H, Dong S, Loi H, Di X, Liu G, Hubbell E, Law J, Berntsen T, Chadha H, Hui H, Yang G, Kennedy GC, Webster TA, Cawley S, Walsh PS, Jones KW, Fodor SP, Mei R (2004) Genotyping over 100,000 SNPs on a pair of oligonucleotide arrays. Nat Methods 1:109–111

Mayer C, Popanda O, Zelezny O, von Brevern M-C, Bach A, Bartsch H, Schmezer P (2002) DNA repair capacity after gamma-irradiation and expression profiles of DNA repair genes in resting and proliferating human peripheral blood lymphocytes. DNA Repair (Amst) 1:237–250

Mayne ST, Buenconsejo J, Janerich DT (1999) Previous lung disease and risk of lung cancer among men and women nonsmokers. Am J Epidemiol 149:13–20

Mohrenweiser HW, Wilson DM III, Jones IM (2003) Challenges and complexities in estimating both the functional impact and the disease risk associated with the extensive genetic variation in human DNA repair genes. Mutat Res 526:93–125

Muscat JE, Wynder EL (1995) Lung cancer pathology in smokers, ex-smokers and never smokers. Cancer Lett 88:1–5

Nebert DW, Vesell ES (2004) Advances in pharmacogenomics and individualized drug therapy: exciting challenges that lie ahead. Eur J Pharmacol 500:267–280

Pauk N, Kubik A, Zatloukal P, Krepela E (2005) Lung cancer in women. Lung Cancer 18:1–9

Peters L, McKay M (2001) Predictive assays: will they ever have a role in the clinic? Int J Radiat Oncol Biol Phys 49:501–504

Popanda O, Ebbeler R, Twardella D, Helmbold I, Gotzes F, Schmezer P, Thielmann HW, von Fournier D, Haase W, Sautter-Bihl ML, Wenz F, Bartsch H, Chang-Claude J (2003) Radiation-induced DNA damage and repair in lymphocytes from breast cancer patients and their correlation with acute skin reactions to radiotherapy. Int J Radiat Oncol Biol Phys 55:1216–1225

Popanda O, Schattenberg T, Phong CT, Butkiewicz D, Risch A, Edler L, Kayser K, Dienemann H, Schulz V, Drings P, Bartsch H, Schmezer P (2004) Specific combinations of DNA repair gene variants and increased risk for non-small cell lung cancer. Carcinogenesis 25:2433–2441

Rajaee-Behbahani N, Schmezer P, Risch A, Rittgen W, Kayser KW, Dienemann H, Schulz V, Drings P, Thiel S, Bartsch H (2001) Altered DNA repair capacity and bleomycin sensitivity as risk markers for non-small cell lung cancer. Int J Cancer 95:86–91

Rajaee-Behbahani N, Schmezer P, Ramroth H, Bürkle A, Bartsch H, Dietz A, Becher H (2002) Reduced poly(ADP-ribosyl)ation in lymphocytes of laryngeal cancer patients: results of a case–control study. Int J Cancer 98:780–784

Raunio H, Hakkola J, Pelkonen O (2005) Regulation of CYP3A genes in the human respiratory tract. Chem Biol Interact 151:53–62

Relling MV, Dervieux T (2001) Pharmacogenetics and cancer therapy. Nat Rev Cancer 1:99–108

Relling MV, Hancock ML, Boyett JM, Pui CH, Evans WE (1999) Prognostic importance of 6-mercaptopurine dose intensity in acute lymphoblastic leukemia. Blood 93:2817–2823

Risch HA, Howe GR, Jain M, Burch JD, Holowaty EJ, Miller AB (1993) Are female smokers at higher risk for lung cancer than male smokers? A case–control analysis by histologic type. Am J Epidemiol 138:281–293

Risch A, Wikman H, Thiel S, Schmezer P, Edler L, Drings P, Dienemann H, Kayser K, Schulz V, Spiegelhalder B, Bartsch H (2001) Glutathione-S-transferase M1, M3, T1 and P1 polymorphisms and susceptibility to non-small-cell lung cancer subtypes and hamartomas. Pharmacogenetics 11:757–764

Rosell R, Taron M, Ariza A, Barnadas A, Mate JL, Reguart N, Margel M, Felip E, Mendez P, Garcia-Campelo R (2004) Molecular predictors of response to chemotherapy in lung cancer. Semin Oncol 31:20–27

Schmezer P, Rajaee-Behbahani N, Risch A, Thiel S, Rittgen W, Drings P, Dienemann H, Kayser KW, Schulz V, Bartsch H (2001) Rapid screening assay for mutagen sensitivity and DNA repair capacity in human peripheral blood lymphocytes. Mutagenesis 16:25–30

Schunck C, Johannes T, Varga D, Lorch T, Plesch A (2004) New developments in automated cytogenetic imaging: unattended scoring of dicentric chromosomes, micronuclei, single cell gel electrophoresis, and fluorescence signals. Cytogenet Genome Res 104:383–389

Scripture CD, Sparreboom A, Figg WD (2005) Modulation of cytochrome P450 activity: implications for cancer therapy. Lancet Oncol 6:780–789

Spitz MR, Wei Q, Dong Q, Amos CI, Wu X (2003) Genetic susceptibility to lung cancer: the role of DNA damage and repair. Cancer Epidemiol Biomarkers Prev 12:689–698

Spitz MR, Wu X, Mills G (2005) Integrative epidemiology: from risk assessment to outcome prediction. J Clin Oncol 23:267–275

Tan XL, Popanda O, Ambrosone CB, Kropp S, Helmbold I, von Foumier D, Haase W, Sautter-Bihl ML, Wenz F, Schmezer P, Chang-Claude J (2005) Association between TP53 and p21 genetic polymorphisms and acute side effects of radiotherapy in breast cancer patients. Breast Cancer Res Treat 97:255–262

Thomas M, Baumann M, Deppermann M, Freitag L, Gatzemeier U, Huber R, Passlick B, Serke M, Ukena D (2002) Recommendations on the therapy of bronchial carcinoma. Pneumologie 56:113–131

Toyooka S, Tokumo M, Shigematsu H, Matsuo K, Asano H, Tomii K, Ichihara S, Suzuki M, Aoe M, Date H, Gazdar AF, Shimizu N (2006) Mutational and epigenetic evidence for independent pathways for lung adenocarcinomas arising in smokers and never smokers. Cancer Res 66:1371–1375

Twardella D, Popanda O, Helmbold I, Ebbeler R, Benner A, von Fournier D, Haase W, Sautter-Bihl ML, Wenz F, Schmezer P, Chang-Claude J (2003) Personal characteristics, therapy modalities and individual DNA repair capacity as predictive factors of acute skin toxicity in an unselected cohort of breast cancer patients receiving radiotherapy. Radiother Oncol 69:145–153

US NIH Cancer Therapy Evaluation Program (1999) Common Toxicity Criteria; Available from: http://ctep.cancer.gov/reporting/ctc.html. Cited 4 August 2006

Villafranca E, Okruzhnov Y, Dominguez MA, Garcia-Foncillas J, Azinovic L, Martinez E, Illarramendi JJ, Arias F, Martinez MR, Salgado E, Angeletti S, Brugarolas A (2001) Polymorphisms of the repeated sequences in the enhancer region of the thymidylate synthase gene promoter may predict downstaging after preoperative chemoradiation in rectal cancer. J Clin Oncol 19:1779–1786

Vineis P (2004) Individual susceptibility to carcinogens. Oncogene 23:6477–6483

Vineis P, Bartsch H, Caporaso N, Harrington AM, Kadlubar FF, Landi MT, Malaveille C, Shields PG, Skipper P, Talaska G, Tannenbaum SR (1994) Genetically based N-acetyltransferase metabolic polymorphism and low-level environmental exposure to carcinogens. Nature 369:154–156

Wikman H, Thiel S, Jäger B, Schmezer P, Spiegelhalder B, Edler L, Dienemann H, Kayser K, Schulz V, Drings P, Bartsch H, Risch A (2001) Relevance of N-acetyltransferases 1 and 2 (NAT1, NAT2) genetic polymorphisms in non-small cell lung cancer susceptibility. Pharmacogenetics 11:157–168

Wild CP (2005) Complementing the genome with an "exposome": the outstanding challenge of environmental exposure measurement in molecular epidemiology. Cancer Epidemiol Biomarkers Prev 14:1847–1850

Zochbauer-Muller S, Pirker R, Huber H (1999) Treatment of small cell lung cancer patients. Ann Oncol 10 [Suppl 6]:83–91

3 Tumor Promotion as a Target of Cancer Prevention

Friedrich Marks, Gerhard Fürstenberger, Karin Müller-Decker

Recent Results in Cancer Research, Vol. 174
© Springer-Verlag Berlin Heidelberg 2007

Abstract

Tumor promotion is an essential process in multistage cancer development providing the conditions for clonal expansion and genetic instability of preneoplastic and premalignant cells. It is caused by a continuous disturbance of cellular signal transduction that results in an overstimulation of metabolic pathways along which mediators of cell proliferation and inflammation as well as genotoxic by-products are generated. Among such pathways the oxidative metabolism of arachidonic acid has turned out to be of utmost importance in tumor promotion. The aberrant overexpression of cyclooxygenase-2, an inducible enzyme of prostanoid synthesis and lipid peroxidation, is a characteristic feature of more than two-thirds of all human neoplasias, and the specific inhibition of this enzyme has been found to have a substantial chemopreventive effect in both animal models and man. The prostaglandins produced by COX-2 promote tumor development by stimulating cell proliferation and angiogenesis and by suppressing programmed cell death and immune defense. In mice, a COX-2 transgene fused with the keratin 5 promoter, which is constitutively active in the basal (proliferative) compartment of stratified and simple epithelia, causes a preneoplastic and premalignant phenotype in several organs. Among these organs, skin, mammary gland, urinary bladder, and pancreas have been investigated in more detail. Histologically and biochemically, the COX-2-dependent alterations resemble an autopromoted state that – as shown for skin and urinary bladder – strongly sensitizes the tissue for carcinogenesis. In transgenic animals COX-2 expression is not restricted to keratin 5-positive cells but is seen also in adjacent keratin 5-negative cells. This spreading of the COX-2 signal indicates a paracrine mechanism of autoamplification. While cancer chemoprevention by COX-2 inhibition is a rapidly developing field, much less is known about other pathways of unsaturated fatty acid metabolism, although some of them may play a role in carcinogenesis rivaling that of prostaglandin formation. Here an urgent demand for systematic research exists.

Introduction

Tumor promotion means acceleration of tumor development by nongenotoxic stimuli. The theoretical concept is based on the fact that cancer generally develops via several – let us say half a dozen or so – stages that represent a stepwise accumulation of genetic defects frequently becoming visible as clinical manifestations.

The initial genetic change is thought to be due mainly to a single hit of an environmental agent (such as chemicals, UV light, ionizing radiation, and certain viruses). Indeed, most tumors are monoclonal, i.e., start with a single genetic mutation in a single cell. Apart from extreme conditions, the probability of the additional changes to occur accidentally in just this particular cell is practically zero.

This probability is dramatically increased by tumor promotion, mainly along two routes:

1. Clonal expansion of the mutated preneoplastic or premalignant cell due to a continuous stimulation of cell proliferation

2. Generation of genetic instability by an activation of metabolic pathways yielding genotoxic products (such as organic free radicals, reactive oxygen species, etc.), and perhaps by an impairment of DNA repair, thus rendering tumor development more and more independent of the environment.

It is easily conceivable that cancer development must depend critically on tumor promotion.

The other side of this coin is, of course, cancer prevention: even when there is no chance to avoid the contact with genotoxic carcinogens, we should seriously consider the possibility of interrupting cancer development (i.e., to bring it to a halt at a still harmless stage) by interfering with the cellular events tumor promotion is based upon. To this end we have to know the molecular mechanisms involved.

Molecular Mechanisms of Tumor Promotion

Our knowledge of the cellular and molecular mode of action of tumor promoters is almost exclusively based on animal models. A common theme arising from such studies is that tumor promotion is caused by a long-lasting and continuously repeated disturbance of cellular signal transduction.

The classical animal model of multistage carcinogenesis is mouse skin, which was introduced in the first half of the last century (for reviews see DiGiovanni 1992; Marks and Fürstenberger 1995). In this model, tumor development is initiated by a single local application of a genotoxic carcinogen (such as, for instance, dimethylbenzanthracene, DMBA) in a dose that does not cause tumorigenesis by its own, i.e., without subsequent promoter treatment. As skin tumor promoters, natural and industrial products have become employed with the phorbol ester TPA (tetradecanoyl-phorbol acetate, alias PMA, phorbol myristate acetate), derived from the Euphorbia plant Croton tiglium being the most potent and the most prominent one.

As far as mouse skin tumor promotion is concerned, these studies have led to the following conclusions:

1. Without promotion no tumors arise, provided the concentration of genotoxic carcinogens is low (resembling the environmental situation).
2. Up to the stage of autonomous benign tumors promotion is reversible.
3. Promotion is caused by a repeated disturbance of signal transduction, in this case of protein kinase C (PKC) -dependent signaling, since TPA specifically mimics the effects of diacylglycerol, the endogenous PKC activator.
4. Promotion proceeds along pathways normally reserved for wound repair and tissue regeneration.
5. A key event in promotion is an overstimulation of arachidonic acid metabolism resulting in the formation of prostaglandins, which have been identified as endogenous mediators of tumor promotion.

Figure 1 summarizes the present mechanistic concept of skin tumor promotion with DMBA as a tumor initiator and TPA as a promoter (see also Marks et al. 2000). The key message is that by positive feedback in combination with a genetic defect (in the case of DMBA treatment an oncogenic mutation of H-Ras), signaling cascades become overstimulated, leading to excessive cell proliferation and to genotoxic metabolites that are generated, in particular, by lipid peroxidation in the course of arachidonic acid metabolism. A central point for an understanding tumor promotion is that while normal cells rapidly adapt to a continuous promoter treatment, initiated cells do not do so, thus gaining a selective advantage over their nonmutated neighbors. The molecular mechanism of adaptation is still unknown.

Of course, in other models and tissues tumor initiation may not be restricted to a Ras mutation and – considering the variability and versatility of mitogenic and oxidative signal processing – tumor promoters may interfere with targets other than protein kinase C, though the mechanistic principles may remain untouched. Consequently, intestinal carcinogenesis is initiated most frequently by a loss-of-function mutation of the APC tumor suppressor protein, a component of the mitogenic Wnt-β-catenin signaling cascade, and tumor development is thought to be promoted by bile acid metabolites and food con-

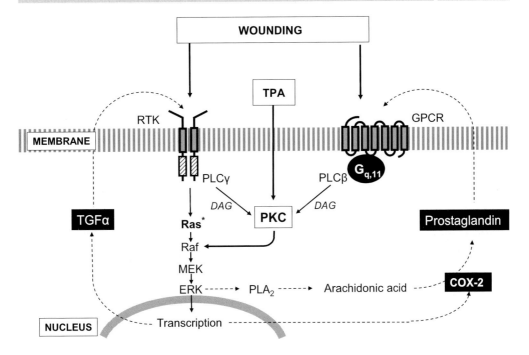

Fig. 1 A mechanism of tumor promotion in mouse skin. In the mouse skin model of carcinogenesis tumor development is promoted by either repeated wounding or phorbol ester application. Upon wounding, endogenous factors are released such as growth factors interacting with receptor tyrosine kinases (RTK, left) and pro-inflammatory mediators interacting with G-protein-coupled receptors (right). As a result, intracellular signaling pathways such as the phospholipase C (PLC)-diacylglycerol (DAG) protein kinase C (PKC) cascade and the RAS-RAF-MAPkinase cascade are activated. The phorbol ester tumor promoter TPA makes a short-cut by mimicking the stimulatory effect of diacylglycerol on protein kinase C, which in turn stimulates the protein kinase Raf. Via the Raf-MEK-ERK (MAPkinase) module, the release of arachidonic acid by phospholipase A_2 (PLA$_2$) and the transcription of numerous genes are upregulated, including those of TGFα and cyclooxygenase-2 (COX-2). As a result, two positive feedback loops that synergize with each other become established, resulting in an auto/paracrine overstimulation. In one of those loops (shown to the left), TGFα acts back on the EGF receptor, whereas in the other one (shown to the right), COX-2 transforms arachidonic acid into prostaglandin. By interacting with the corresponding Gq,11-protein-coupled receptor, the latter induces DAG release by phospholipase Cβ (PLCβ), thus augmenting the effect of the tumor promoter, in addition to other effects (see Fig. 2). In epidermal cells initiated by DMBA, the Ras-Raf-ERK cascade is out of control because of a point-mutated hyperactive Ras protein. In contrast to normal cells, these cells cannot fully adopt to a repeated promoter treatment and gain a selective advantage, leading to clonal expansion

stituents (reviewed by Marks and Fürstenberger 2000). Nevertheless, in the skin as well as in intestinal epithelium (Dannenberg et al. 2005), a synergism between autoamplifying signaling cascades activated by growth factors (such as EGF and its relatives) and prostaglandins seems to play a key role in tumor promotion.

Prostaglandins are Endogenous Tumor Promoters

In the animal models of skin and intestinal carcinogenesis, tumor development can be interrupted almost completely by nonsteroidal anti-inflammatory drugs (NSAIDs).

This effect could be traced back to an inhibition of prostaglandin synthesis. In fact, prostaglandins exhibit exactly those effects that are thought to promote tumor development including a stimulation of cell proliferation, inflammation, and angiogenesis, and an inhibition of differentiation, apoptosis, and immune defense. Moreover, in the course of prostaglandin synthesis (being a type of enzymatic lipid peroxidation) reactive oxygen species and other genotoxic agents (such as malondialdehyde) are formed as intermediates and by-products.

In the skin model using NMRI mice, prostaglandin $F_{2\alpha}$ ($PGF_{2\alpha}$) has been shown to mediate tumor promotion (Fürstenberger et al. 1989; Müller-Decker et al. 1998; Marks et al. 2002), whereas in other mouse strains and in intestinal carcinogenesis, E-type prostaglandins play this role (Wang and DuBois 2006). This difference becomes more or less irrelevant at the level of signal transduction exhibiting a high degree of cross-talk (Fig. 2). The cellular $PGF_{2\alpha}$ receptor FP seems to couple exclusively with a $G_{q,11}$-protein (Alexander et al. 2001), thus activating the diacylglycerol / inositol 1,4,5-trisphosphate cascades of signaling that are known to stimulate cell proliferation and angiogenesis while inhibiting apoptosis. E-type prostaglandins interact with four different receptor isoforms (EP_1 to EP_4) that couple with Gs-, $G_{q,11}$- or $G_{i,o}$-proteins (Alexander et al. 2001). For intestinal carcinogenesis, the Gs-coupled receptor EP_2 has been found to be of particular relevance. There is experimental evidence that in colon cancer cells this receptor activates several signaling cascades. Thus, the major effect of the α-subunit of the Gs-protein is to stimulate adenylate cyclase. Along this pathway, a wide variety of cAMP-dependent downstream events become modulated, including the activation of numerous genes that may be involved in colon tumorigenesis (Holla et al. 2005; Dannenberg et al. 2005). Recently, the α-subunit of the EP_2 receptor-coupled Gs-protein has been shown to activate the pro-mitogenic axin-β-catenin signaling pathway also, whereas the βγ-subunit stimulates phosphoinositide 3-kinase, leading in turn to an activation of protein kinase B/Akt and – as a consequence – to an inhibition of programmed cell death (Castellone et al. 2005). Since Gβγ-subunits are also released from $G_{q,11}$- (and $G_{i,o}$-) proteins, the anti-apoptotic PI3 kinase-PKB/Akt pathway is most prob-

ably activated by other prostaglandin receptors as well (Fig. 2).

Moreover, G-protein-coupled receptors such as the prostaglandin receptors may transactivate signaling cascades that hitherto were thought to be stimulated by growth factors leading to an activation of MAP-kinases (Shenoy and Lefkowitz 2003). Among many other effects, the expression of growth factors and cyclooxygenase-2, the key enzyme of prostaglandin synthesis, becomes upregulated along these and the above-mentioned pathways, resulting in a dramatic amplification due to positive feedback (Fig. 1).

The rate-limiting step of prostaglandin synthesis is the twofold oxygenation of arachidonic acid catalyzed by cyclooxygenases. In human and murine tissues, these enzymes are expressed in two isoforms, COX-1 and COX-2.

While COX-1 is a constitutive housekeeping enzyme supplying the everyday needs of prostaglandins, COX-2 is an emergency enzyme expressed in most tissues only on demand, i.e., when there is an increased requirement for prostanoids, as, for instance, in stress situations such as inflammation, wound repair and – being the reverse side of the coin – neoplastic growth (since a constitutive COX-2 expression is also observed in embryonic tissues, the stress-induced transient COX-2 expression in adult tissues may be considered to represent a re-activation of an embryonic process of signaling). The COX-2 gene promoter contains binding sites for several transcription factors (including CREB, SP1, NFκB, C/EBP, and Ets). Therefore, COX-2 expression is initiated by a wide variety of mitogenic hormones, growth factors, and cytokines and perpetuated by prostaglandins through positive feedback. In addition to endogenous factors, chemical carcinogens and skin and intestinal tumor promoters induce an expression of COX-2. In fact, in the animal models mentioned above, tumor-promoting prostaglandin synthesis is mainly catalyzed by COX-2, and studies on COX-2 knockout animals have revealed a causal relationship between COX-2 expression and intestinal and skin cancer development (Oshima et al. 1996; Tiano et al. 2002).

The animal experiments are mirrored by clinical observations. Aberrant COX-2 expression has been found to be a consistent feature of at least

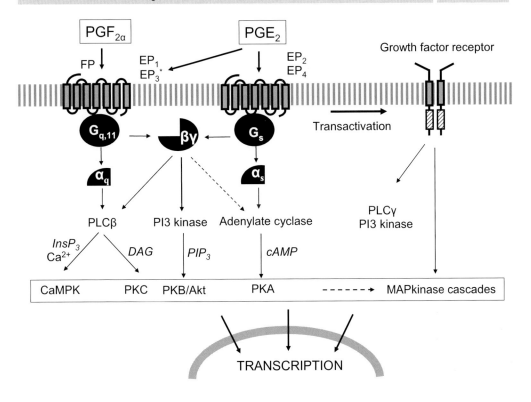

Fig. 2 Prostaglandin signaling. The major arachidonic acid-derived prostaglandins, PGE_2 and $PGF_2\alpha$, interact with G-protein-coupled receptors characterized by seven transmembrane domains. The $PGF_2\alpha$ receptor FP, as well as the PGE_2 receptors EP_1 and EP_3 couple with a $Gq_{,11}$-protein, the PGE_2 receptors EP_2 and EP_4 with a Gs-protein. Upon receptor activation, the G-proteins dissociate. The $G\alpha s$-subunit stimulates adenylate cyclase and the $G\alpha q_{,11}$-subunit phospholipase $C\beta$ ($PLC\beta$), while the $G\beta\gamma$-subunits released from both G-proteins may activate certain isoforms of $PLC\beta$, phosphoinositide 3-kinase (PI3 kinase) and adenylate cyclase. These enzymes catalyze the generation of the second messengers inositol 1,4-5-trisphosphate ($InsP_3$, leading to an elevation of cytoplasmic Ca^{2+}), diacylglycerol (DAG), phosphatidylinositol 3,4,5-trisphosphate (PIP_3) and cyclic AMP (cAMP) that specifically activate protein kinases such as Ca^{2+}/calmodulin-dependent kinases (CaMPK), protein kinase C (PKC), protein kinase B/Akt, and protein kinase A (PKA). Along pathways controlled by these kinases, the transcription of a wide variety of genes becomes stimulated. In addition, the G-protein-coupled prostaglandin receptors may transactivate signaling cascades originating from tyrosine kinase-coupled growth factor receptors (GFR) and leading to an upregulation of phospholipase $C\gamma$ (which like $PLC\beta$ catalyzes the release of $InsP_3$ and DAG) and PI 3-kinase as well as of MAPkinase cascades, inducing the transcription of additional genes. Alternatively, the EP_3 receptor may also interact with a $Gi_{,o}$-protein, resulting in an inhibition of adenylate cyclase and a particularly strong release of $G\beta\gamma$-subunits (not shown). The genes activated by prostaglandin signaling encode proteins stimulating cell proliferation, angiogenesis, and genotoxic metabolism, and inhibiting apoptosis, cell differentiation, and immune defense. Among these genes are those of COX-2 and $TGF\alpha$ (see Fig. 1)

75% of all human cancers and the corresponding premalignant states. Moreover, an anti-tumor effect of NSAIDs was detected by epidemiological and clinical evaluations and traced back mainly to an inhibition of COX-2-catalyzed prostaglandin synthesis (reviewed by Marks and Fürstenberger 2000; Turini and DuBois 2002; Thun et al. 2002; Dannenberg et al. 2005). Mechanistically, this presently represents one of the most clearcut examples of cancer chemoprevention with a particularly high potential for practical use (Gasparini et al. 2003; Steele et al. 2003; Subbaramaiah and Dannenberg 2003). As far as classical NSAIDs are concerned, such approaches are limited by side effects, in particular on the gastrointestinal tract, which result from COX-1 inhibition. Therefore, newly developed COX-2-specific inhibitors (Coxibs) were greeted with great enthusiasm. However, in the meantime, some of them have been discredited since the risk of thrombotic events such a myocardial infarction and stroke has been found to increase upon long-term application as it is required for cancer prevention (Bresalier et al. 2005; Nussmeier et al. 2005; Solomon et al. 2005). This does not devaluate arachidonic acid metabolism as a target of cancer chemoprevention but calls for additional in-depth studies of the cellular and molecular mechanisms involved.

Transgenic COX-2 Overexpression Creates a Preneoplastic Situation in Mouse Skin

To evaluate the role of COX-2 in mouse skin carcinogenesis, we have bred transgenic mouse lines carrying the cox-2 gene under the control of a keratin 5 (K5) promoter. This gene promoter is constitutively active in the proliferative compartment of stratified and simple epithelia, causing a continuous production of keratin 5 and – in transgenic animals – of COX-2.

COX-2 transgenic animals were viable but showed a particular skin phenotype characterized by a shaggy hair coat. In fact, a spatiotemporally controlled expression of COX-2 accompanies hair follicle development, and the effect of transgenic COX-2 overexpression was shown to be caused by a disturbance of hair follicle cycling resulting in alopecia (Müller-Decker et al. 2003). The skin of the transgenic animals exhibited a preneoplastic morphology. Characteristic signs were epidermal hyper- and dysplasia (due to a delayed terminal differentiation rather than to hyperproliferation) and increased angiogenesis. In parallel, a substantial rise in the prostaglandin level in both skin and blood plasma was seen. The development of the gross phenotype, including the histological alterations and the increase in the prostaglandin level was prevented by feeding the mice with Celebrex, a selective COX-2 inhibitor (Neufang et al. 2001; Müller-Decker et al. 2002; Müller-Decker et al. 2003). Most remarkably, upon tumor initiation with DMBA, the transgenic animals developed papillomas, carcinomas, and sebaceous gland adenomas without promoter treatment (Müller-Decker et al. 2002). In other words: the transgenic overexpression of COX-2 had rendered the skin "autopromoted."

These results show that in mouse skin COX-2 expression:

1. Provides a necessary and sufficient condition for the activation of endogenous tumor-promoting processes
2. Does not evoke tumorigenesis by its own but strongly sensitizes the tissue for the effects of genotoxic carcinogens.

Transgenic COX-2 Expression Induces Mammary Gland Hyperplasia

In K5.COX-2 transgenic mice, aberrant COX-2 expression was not restricted to the skin but also found in other epithelia expressing K5 such as mammary gland, exocrine pancreas, and urinary bladder.

Mammary gland epithelium consists of two compartments: luminal cells for milk secretion and contractile myoepithelial cells for milk ejection. Keratin 5 is expressed by myoepithelial cells rather than by luminal cells. Cancers of the myoepithelium are rare. Instead, the great majority of breast cancers develop in a multistage process from luminal cells.

Our COX-2 transgenic mice exhibited, nevertheless, a pronounced mammary phenotype in that the mammary glands became very enlarged concomitant with a fivefold increase in the prostaglandin tissue level (Müller-Decker et al. 2005). This effect did not depend on pregnancy and lactogenic hormones. Feeding the animals with the COX-2 inhibitor Celecoxib prevented the mammary gland hyperplasia.

Most remarkably, COX-2 was found both in the K5-positive myoepithelial cells and in adjacent K5-negative luminal cells. Probably the K5-positive cells expressing the k5 promotor. cox-2 transgene generated a paracrine signal that induced COX-2 expression in adjacent K5-negative cells. According to the mechanistic concept depicted in Fig. 1, this signal might be a growth factor or a prostaglandin species. By such an amplifying mechanism, even a locally restricted hot spot of COX-2 expression would spread within the tissue.

Although the rate of cell proliferation was strongly increased in both epithelial compartments, tumors did not arise. Whether or not the situation resembles that found in the skin, where cancer development requires tumor initiation in addition to constitutive COX-2 expression, is unknown.

COX-2 has been consistently found to be overexpressed in ductal carcinomas in situ and invasive adenocarcinomas of the human breast (Howe et al. 2001; Ristimäki et al. 2002; Half et al. 2002; Subbaramaiah et al. 2002). Consequently, COX-2 has been suggested to be a promising target of breast cancer chemoprevention (Howe et al. 2001, 2002; Singh-Ranger and Mokbel 2002). Moreover, transgenic overexpression of COX-2 under the control of the MMTV (mouse mammary tumor virus) promoter was sufficient to induce mammary carcinogenesis in multiparous, but not in virgin, mice (Liu et al. 2001).

Transgenic Overexpression of COX-2 Creates a Premalignant State in Pancreas

Our K5.COX-2 transgenic mouse lines developed a severe and fatal pancreatic phenotype characterized by a strongly enlarged polycystic pancreas (Müller-Decker et al. 2006). These alterations correlated with increased steady-state levels of COX-2, resulting in very high tissue levels of prostaglandins. In addition, the levels of the EGF receptor isoform HER and of Ras expression and activity were found to be elevated indicating an upregulation of growth-factor signaling as shown in Fig. 1. Histopathological analysis revealed a pronounced ductal hyperplasia and dysplasia accompanied by a high mitotic activity, inflammatory infiltration, and periductal fibrosis. The lesions exhibited a mixed pattern resembling benign pancreatic neoplasia in humans such as serous cystic adenomas, intraductal papillary mucinous neoplasms, and pancreatic intraepithelial neoplasia, which are thought to be premalignant states. However, carcinoma development was not observed, thus resembling the situation in skin.

The major cytokeratin produced by wild type pancreatic epithelium is K19, whereas K5 is found only duct in about 5% of the cells. However, in the transgenic animals, aberrant COX-2 expression was also observed in many K19-positive cells, again indicating a paracrine mechanism of amplification and spreading.

As in the skin and the mammary gland, in the pancreas the development of the transgenic phenotype was also prevented by feeding the animals with the COX-2 inhibitor Celebrex.

Specific COX-2 inhibitors have also been found to suppress chemically induced pancreatic tumorigenesis in hamsters (Nishikawa et al. 2004) and the growth of pancreatic tumor xenografts in mice (Raut et al. 2004). Moreover, aberrant COX-2 expression has been reported for benign and malignant pancreatic tumors of man (Molina et al. 1999; Okami et a.l 1999; Tucker at al 1999; Merati et al. 2001, 2002; Niijima et al. 2002; Kokawa et al. 2002; Franco et al. 2004; Müller-Decker et al. 2006).

Transgenic Overexpression of COX-2 Sensitizes Urinary Bladder for Carcinogenesis

Like skin epidermis, the bladder epithelium of wild type animals was almost devoid of COX-2 (expressing only COX-1), whereas the transgenic animals exhibited strong signals of both COX-2 mRNA and protein co-localizing with K5, and a fivefold elevation of the prostaglandin level, whereas COX-1 expression remained unchanged (Klein et al. 2005). Approximately 75% of the homozygous transgenic animals developed severe epithelial dysplasia starting with an inflammatory reaction and progressing to a transitional cell hyperplasia (caused by hyperproliferation) within 6 months. After 4–6 additional months approximately 10% of the animals had developed transitional cell carcinoma indicating an unidentified initiating (genotoxic) event to synergize with COX-2 hyperactivity.

As in the skin hyperplastic transformation of the epithelium was accompanied by vascular hyperproliferation paralleled by a strong increase in vascular endothelial growth factor (VEGF), the expression of which is known to be induced by prostaglandin E_2.

These symptoms were considerably weaker in heterozygous transgenic animals, indicating a causative role of COX-2 expression. Moreover, when the transgenic animals were fed with the COX-2 inhibitor Celebrex, the symptoms described above did not show up (unpublished data).

Our results are consistent with observations of other authors. Thus, a dramatic expression of COX-2 has been found in chemically induced bladder carcinomas in rats and dogs (Kitayama et al. 1999; Khan et al. 2000). Moreover, in animal models, tumorigenesis was suppressed by a specific COX-2 inhibitor or a nonspecific NSAID (Grubbs et al. 2000; Mohammed et al. 2002). Aberrant COX-2 expression has also been reported for urinary bladder carcinomas in humans where it correlated positively with the stage and the grade of tumor development (Komhoff et al. 2000; Shirahama et al. 2001; Kim et al. 2002; Shariat et al. 2003a, b). Based on such observations, urinary bladder has been proposed to provide a promising target of cancer chemoprevention by NSAIDs and COX-2 inhibitors, at least for high-risk groups (Sabichi and Lippman 2004). This proposal is supported by a clinical study (Castelao et al. 2000).

Polyunsaturated Fatty Acid Metabolism, Lipid Peroxidation, and Cancer: Two Sides of a Coin

In addition to cyclooxygenases, other enzymes catalyze the oxidation of polyunsaturated fatty acids (PUFAs) to products the (patho)physiological roles of which are only known fragmentarily (for a review see Marks 1999). Among those enzymes are at least six lipoxygenases (in man) differing in substrate and positional specificity, and several cytochrome P-450-containing monooxygenases. Both enzymatic pathways are known to be a source of reactive oxygen species and other genotoxic by-products.

In fact, in the mouse skin model, the oxygenation of arachidonic acid catalyzed by 8- and 12S-lipoxygenase has been shown to become activated in the course of tumor promotion. The accumulation of the corresponding arachidonic acid metabolites correlates with chromosomal aberrations and pro-mutagenic etheno-DNA adducts that may participate in tumorigenesis (see

Nair et al. 2000 and references therein). Moreover, polyunsaturated fatty acids are also prone to nonenzymatic autoxidation, yielding so-called iso-prostanoids and related compounds. The upregulation of these reactions in situations of oxidative cellular stress accompanying acute poisoning, heavy smoking, Alzheimer's dementia, and tumorigenesis is generally believed to be of considerable pathophysiological significance, which cannot yet be reliably estimated, however.

Indeed, compared with the cyclooxygenases, much less is known about the relationships between neoplastic growth and lipoxygenases, other PUFA-metabolizing enzymes and nonenzymatic fatty acid oxygenation. Nevertheless, a steadily increasing body of evidence indicates a role of these processes in carcinogenesis that may rival that of cyclooxygenases, and specific enzyme inhibitors resembling NSAIDs that may become applicable in cancer chemoprevention in the future are being developed (for reviews see Shureiqi and Lippman 2001; Steele et al. 2003; Catalano and Procopio 2005; Fürstenberger et al. 2006). However, even though the investigation of this field is impeded by the large variety of these enzymes (as compared with only two cyclooxygenases!), an important difference must be taken into account: while cyclooxygenases are specific for C_{20}-fatty acids such as arachidonic acid, lipoxygenases and other PUFA-metabolizing enzymes also accept C_{18} fatty acids such a linoleic and linolenic acid. The latter two are mostly plant-derived, whereas arachidonic acid is more or less restricted to animals. Some indirect evidence indicates that in contrast to the eicosanoids (C_{20}), derivatives of unsaturated C_{18}-fatty acids (octadecanoids) exhibit an anti- rather than a pro-carcinogenic effect, thus explaining – at least partially – the well-known cancer protection by a more vegetarian (or Mediterranean!) diet.

Considering the rapid progress that has been made in the cyclooxygenase field, this still somewhat neglected subject of research requires particular attention right now, since it gives great hopes for novel approaches of cancer chemoprevention.

References

Alexander SPH, Mathie A, Peters JA (2001) TIPS 2001. Nomenclature Supplement, 11th edn. Trends Pharmacol Sci 22:1

Bresalier RS, Sandler RS, Quan H et al (2005) Cardiovascular events associated with Celecoxib in a colorectal adenoma chemoprevention trial. N Engl J Med 352:1092–1102

Castelao JE, Yuan JM, Gago-Dominguez M et al (2000) Non-steroidal anti-inflammatory drugs and bladder cancer prevention. Br J Cancer 82:1364–1369

Castellone MD, Teramoto H, Williams BO et al (2005) Prostaglandin E$_2$ promotes colon cancer cell growth through a novel Gs-axin-β-catenin signalling axis. Science 310:1504–1510

Catalano A, Procopio A (2005) New aspects on the role of lipoxygenases in cancer progression. Hisol Histopathol 20:969–975

Dannenberg AJ, Lippman SM, Mann JR et al (2005) Cyclooxygenase-2 and epidermal growth factor receptor: pharmacologic targets for chemoprevention. J Clin Oncol 23:254–266

DiGiovanni J (1992) Multistage carcinogenesis in mouse skin. Pharmacol Ther 54:63–128

Franco L, Doria D, Betrazzoni E (2004) Increased expression of inducible nitic oxide synthase and cyclooxygenase-2 in pancreatic cancer. Prostagl Other Lipid Mediat 73:51–58

Fürstenberger G, Gross M, Marks F (1989) Eicosanoids and multistage carcinogenesis in NMRI mouse skin: role of prostaglandins E and F in conversion (first stage of tumor promotion) and promotion (second stage of tumor promotion). Carcinogenesis 10:91–96

Fürstenberger G, Krieg P, Müller-Decker K, Habenicht AJR (2006) What are cyclooxygenases and lipoxygenases doing in the drivers seat of carcinogenesis? Int J Cancer 119:2247–2254 (2006)

Gasparini G, Longo R, Sarmiento R et al (2003) Inhibitors of cyclooxygenase-2: a new class of anticancer agents? Lancet Oncol 4:605–615

Grubbs CJ, Lubet RA, Koki AT et al (2000) Celecoxib inhibits N-butyl-N-(4-hydroxybutyl) nitrosamine-induced urinary bladder cancers in male B6D2F1 mice and female Fischer-344 rats. Cancer Res 60:5599–5602

Gupta RA, DuBois RN (2001) Colorectal cancer prevention and treatment by inhibition of cyclooxygenase-2. Nature Rev Cancer 1:11–21

Half E, Tang XM, Gwyn K et al (2002) Cyclooxygenase-2 expression in human breast cancers and adjacent ductal carcinoma in situ. Cancer Res 62:1676–1681

Holla RV, Mann JR, Shi Q et al (2005) Prostaglandin E$_2$ regulates the nuclear receptor NR4A2 in colorectal cancer. J Biol Chem 281:2676–2682

Howe LR, Subbaramaiah K, Brown AMC et al (2001) Cyclooxygenase-2: a target for the prevention and treatment of breast cancer. Endocr Related Cancer 8:97–114

Howe LR, Subbaramaiah K, Patel J (2002) Celecoxib, a selective COX-2 inhibitor, protects against human epidermal growth factor receptor 2 (HER-2)neu-induced breast cancer. Cancer Res 62:5405–5407

Khan KN, Knapp DW, Denicola DB et al (2000) Expression of cyclooxygenase-2 in transitional cell carcinoma of the urinary bladder in dogs. Am J Vet Res 61:478–481

Kim SI, Kwon SM, Kim YS et al (2002) Association of cyclooxygenase-2 expression with prognosis of stage T1 grade 3 bladder cancer. Urology 60:816–821

Kitayama W, Denda A, Okajima E et al (1999) Increased expression of cyclooxygenase-2 in rat urinary bladder tumors induced by N-butyl-N(4-hdroxybutyl) nitrosamine. Carcinogenesis 20:2305–2310

Klein DR, van Pelt CS, Sabichi AL et al (2005) Transitional cell hyperplasia and carcinomas in urinary bladders of transgenic mice with keratin 5 promoter-driven cyclooxygenase-2 overexpression. Cancer Res 65:1808–1813

Kokawa A, Kondo H, Gotoda T et al (2001) Increased expression of cyclooxygenase-2 in human pancreatic neoplasms and potential for chemoprevention by cyclooxygenase inhibitors. Cancer 15:333–338

Komhoff M, Guan Y, Shappell HW et al (2000) Enhanced expression of cyclooxygenase-2 in high grade human transitional cell bladder carcinomas. Am J Pathol 157:29–35

Liu CH, Chang SH, Narko K et al (2001) Overexpression of cyclooxygenase-2 is sufficient to induce tumorigenesis in transgenic mice. J Biol Chem 276:18563–18569

Maitra A, Ashfaq R, Gunn CR et al (2002) Cyclooxygenase-2 expression in pancreatic adenocarcinoma and pancreatic intraepithelial neoplasia: an immunohistological analysis with automated cellular imaging. Am J Clin Pathol 118:194–201

Marks F (1999) Arachidonic acid and companions: an abundant source of biological signals. In: Marks F, Fürstenberger G (eds) Prostaglandins, leukotrienes, and other eicosanoids: Wiley, Weinheim, pp 1–46

Marks F, Fürstenberger G (1995) Tumor promotion in the skin. In: Arcos CE, Arcos MF, Woo YT (eds). Chemical induction of cancer. Birkhäuser, Boston, pp 125–160

Marks F, Fürstenberger G (2000) Cancer chemoprevention through interruption of multistage carcinogenesis: the lessons learnt by comparing mouse skin carcinogenesis with human large bowel cancer. Eur J Cancer 36:314–329

Marks F, Müller-Decker K, Fürstenberger G (2000) A causal relationship between unscheduled eicosanoid signaling and tumor development: cancer chemoprevention by inhibitors of arachidonic acid metabolism. Toxicol 153:11–26

Marks F, Fürstenberger G, Neufang G et al (2003) Mouse skin as a model for cancer chemoprevention by nonsteroidal anti-inflammatory drugs. Rec Results Cancer Res 163:46–57

Merati K, Said Siadaty M, Andrea A et al (2001) Expression of inflammatory modulator COX-2 in pancreatic ductal adenocarcinoma and its relationship to pathologic and clinical parameters. Am J Clin Oncol 24:447–452

Mohammed SI, Bennett PF, Craig BA et al (2002) Effects of the cyclooxygenase inhibitor, piroxicam, on tumor response, apoptosis, and angiogenesis in a canine model of human invasive urinary bladder cancer. Cancer Res 62:356–358

Molina MA, Sitja-Arnau M, LeMoine MG et al (1999) Increased cyclooxygenase-2 expression in human pancreatic carcinomas and cell lines: growth inhibition by nonsteroidal anti-inflammatory drugs. Cancer Res 59:4356–4362

Müller-Decker K, Kopp-Schneider A, Marks F et al (1998) Localization of prostaglandin H synthase isoenzymes in murine epidermal tumors: suppression of skin tumor promotion by inhibition of prostaglandin H synthase-2. Molec Carcinogenesis 23:36–44

Müller-Decker K, Neufang G, Berger I et al (2002) Transgenic cyclooxygenase-2 overexpression sensitizes mouse skin for carcinogenesis. Proc Natl Acad Sci U S A 99:12483–12488

Müller-Decker K, Leder C, Neumann M et al (2003) Expression of cyclooxygenase isoenzymes during morphogenesis and cycling of pelage hair follicles in mouse skin: disturbed hair follicle cycling and alopecia upon cyclooxygenase-2 overexpression. J Invest Dermatol 121:661–668

Müller-Decker K, Berger I, Ackermann K et al (2005) Cystic duct dilatations and proliferative epithelial lesions in mouse mammary glands upon keratin 5 promoter-driven overexpression of cyclooxygenase-2. Am J Pathol 166:575–584

Müller-Decker K, Fürstenberger G, Annan N et al (2006) Preinvasive duct-derived neoplasms in pancreas of keratin 5 promoter cyclooxygenase-2 transgenic mice. Gastroenterology 130:2165–2178

Nair J, Fürstenberger G, Bürger F et al (2000) Promutagenic etheno-DNA adducts in multistage mouse skin carcinogenesis: correlation with lipoxygenase-catalyzed arachidonic acid metabolism. Chem Res Toxicol 13:703–709

Neufang G, Fürstenberger G, Heidt M et al (2001) Abnormal differentiation of epidermis in transgenic mice constitutively expressing cyclooxygenase-2 in skin. Proc Natl Acad Sci U S A 98:7629–7634

Niijima M, Yamaguchi T, Ishihara T et al (2002) Immunohistochemical analysis and in situ hybridization of cyclooxygenase-2 expression in intraductal papillary-mucinous tumors of the pancreas. Cancer 94:1565–1573

Nishikawa A, Furukawa F, Lee IS et al (2004) Potent chemopreventive agabts against pancreatic cancer. Curr Cancer Drug Targets 4:373–384

Nussmeier NA, Whelton AA, Brown MT et al (2005) Complications of the COX-2 inhbitors Parecoxib and Valdecoxib after cardiac surgery. N Engl J Med 352:1081–1091

Okami J, Yamamoto H, Fujiwara Y et al (1999) Overexpression of cyclooxygenase-2 in carcinoma of pancreas. Clin Cancer Res 5:2018–2014

Oshima M, Dinchuk JE Kargman SL et al (1996) Suppression of intestinal polyposis in APCΔ^{717} knockout mice by inhibition of cyclooxygenase 2 (COX-2). Cell 67:803–809

Raut CP, Nawrocki S, Lashinger LM (2004) Celecoxib inhibits angiogenesis by inducing endothelial cell apoptosis in human pancreatic tumor xenografts. Cancer Biol Therap 3:1217–1224

Ristimäki A, Sivula A, Lundin J et al (2002) Prognostic significance of elevated cyclooxygenase-2 expression in breast cancer. Cancer Res 62:632–635

Sabichi AL, Lippman SM (2004) COX-2 inhibitors and other nonsteroidal anti-inflammatory drugs in genitourinary cancer. Semin Oncol 31:36–44

Shariat SF, Kim JH, Ayala GE et al (2003a) Cyclooxygenase-2 is highly expressed in carcinoma in situ and T1 transitional cell carcinoma of the bladder. J Urol 169:938–942

Shariat SF, Matsumoto K, Kim J et al (2003b) Correlation of cyclooxygenase-2 expression with molecular markers, pathological features and clinical outcome of transitional cell carcinoma of the bladder. J Urol 170:985–989

Shenoy SK, Lefkowitz RJ (2003) Multifaceted roles of β-arrestins in the regulation of seven-membrane-spanning receptor trafficking and signalling. Biochem J 375:503–515

Shirahama T, Arima J, Akiba S et al (2001) Relation between cyclooxygenase-2 expression and tumor invasiveness and patient survival in transitional cell carcinoma of the urinary bladder. Cancer 92:188–193

Shureiqi I, Lippman SM (2001) Lipoxygenase modulation to reverse carcinogenesis. Cancer Res 61:6307–6312

Singh-Ranger G, Mokbel K (2002) Role of cyclo-oxygenase-2 (COX-2) in breast cancer, and implications of COX-2 inhibition. Eur J Surg Oncol 28:729–737

Solomon SD, McMurray JJ, Pfeffer MA et al (2005) Cardiovascular risk associated with Celecoxib in a clinical trial for colorectal adenoma prevention. N Engl J Med 352:1071–1080

Steele VE, Hawk ET, Viner JL et al (2003) Mechanisms and applications of non-steroidal anti-inflammatory drugs in the chemoprevention of cancer. Mutation Res 523/524:137–144

Suibbaramaiah K, Dannenberg AJ (2003) Caclooxygenase-2: a molecular target for cancer prevention and treatment. Trends Pharmacol Sci 24:96–102

Thun MJ, Henley SJ, Patrono C (2002) Nonsteroidal anti-inflammatory drugs as anticancer agents: mechanistic, pharmacologic, and clinical issues. J Natl Cancer Inst 94:252–299

Tiano HF, Loftin CD, Akunda J et al (2002) Deficiency of either cyclooxygenase (COX)-1 or COX-2 alters epidermal differentiation and reduces mouse skin carcinogenesis. Cancer Res 62:3395–3401

Tucker MJ, Dannenberg AJ, Yang EK et al (1999) Cyclooxygenase-2 expression is up-regulated in human pancreatic cancer. Cancer Res 59:987–990

Turini ME, DuBois RN (2002) Cyclooxygenase-2: a therapeutic target. Annu Rev Med 53:35–57

Wang D, DuBois RN (2006) Prostaglandins and cancer. Gut 55:115–122

4 Insulin-Like Growth Factor-Related Signaling and Cancer Development

Michael Pollak

Recent Results in Cancer Research, Vol. 174
© Springer-Verlag Berlin Heidelberg 2007

Abstract

In this review, selected examples of recent research developments concerning insulin-like growth factors (IGFs) and insulin in the context of cancer risk assessment and prevention will be discussed. We reviewed background information related to IGF physiology at the cellular and whole-organism levels, together with prior work concerning IGF-I levels and risk of a variety of cancers, including breast, prostate, colon, and lung in 2004 (Pollak et al. 2004). A comprehensive update to that general review (Pollak et al. 2004) is scheduled for Nature Reviews Cancer in early 2007.

General Background Issues Concerning Cancer Risk Assessment

Individuals are distinct from each other not only regarding their level of cancer risk, but also with respect to the dominant mechanism underlying their risk. As an example related to breast cancer, consider five women: a carrier of a BRCA1 mutation, a woman who started to menstruate at age 9, a woman with high birthweight, a woman with high mammographic density, and a woman with radiation exposure at puberty. All are at increased risk relative to women without identified risk factors, but because the mechanism responsible for increased risk is distinct in each case, one cannot presume that any specific risk reduction strategy will benefit each woman to the same degree. A panel of ideal serum or DNA markers of risk would not only quantify magnitude of risk, but would also provide information regarding the mechanism underlying the increased risk; this would be useful in selecting a particular risk reduction strategy that is effective for the risk mechanism involved.

At present, markers of risk fall short of this ideal. For example, mammographic breast density is known to be associated with increased risk, but because the mechanisms that link density to risk are poorly understood, there is no standard risk reduction strategy recognized as particularly appropriate for these women. Risk reduction strategies that have been studied in major clinical prevention trials, such as tamoxifen, are known to reduce breast cancer risk, but we do not understand clearly for which women such interventions are most effective. While risk reduction on the order of 40% has been reported for women taking tamoxifen as a chemopreventive, it is unlikely that all women in tamoxifen prevention trials derived a similar degree of protection: based on the varying molecular pathology that is responsible for risk in individual women, some may have enjoyed a 90% risk reduction with tamoxifen, while others may have derived no benefit. An important research goal is to develop markers of risk that would both quantitate risk and allow rational selection of an appropriate intervention for an individual woman.

Another general issue concerns definition of cancer prevention. Recent work (Thompson et al. 2003, 2004) supports prior studies that suggested that early steps of malignant transformation are common by middle age, particularly in organs such as breast and prostate. In the case of prostate, even histologically invasive cancer that is clinically silent is common (Thompson et al. 2003, 2004). Obviously, prevention interventions that are clinically useful are those that prevent clinically important disease. Such prevention interventions may not have to act to limit early carcinogenesis in all cases (this would imply the need for interventions relatively early in life), but rather may act to inhibit neoplastic progression of early lesions. This point has implications for development of markers of risk: for a disease such as prostate cancer, which is now recognized to be present in a large proportion of the adult male population (Thompson et al. 2003, 2004), prevention of clinically important disease may be aided more by discovery of markers of probability of progression than markers that indicate the presence of early disease or markers that indicate risk of developing early disease.

IGF-Related Serum Markers and Prostate Cancer

The first prospective study (Chan et al. 1998) that linked circulating IGF-I levels to risk of prostate cancer was reported in Science in 1998, and generated considerable interest in the field, both in terms of population and laboratory (e.g., Majeed et al. 2005) studies. However, the study was small (only 152 cases and 152 controls), and there was little information regarding the nature of the prostate cancers that were found at increased frequency among those men with higher IGF-I levels (especially if these levels were associated with a relatively low level of IGFBP-3, the major serum IGF-binding protein). Subsequent studies and a meta-analysis (Renehan et al. 2004) confirmed the association of IGF-I levels with increased risk of a subsequent diagnosis of prostate cancer. It should be emphasized that these studies did not establish IGF-I as a tumor marker for prostate cancer: to use an analogy from cardiology, higher levels of IGF-I were found to be indicative of increased risk of a later diagnosis of prostate cancer, as elevated cholesterol indicates increased risk of a subsequent myocardial infarction. However, cardiologists do not measure cholesterol to make a diagnosis of myocardial infarction in a patient with chest pain, and a measurement of a high IGF-I level does not indicate the presence of prostate cancer.

Ongoing work (e.g., Ma et al. 2005), is seeking to extend earlier results concerning the relationship between IGF-I and prostate cancer risk by studying larger numbers of cases and controls, in order to determine if men with higher IGF-I levels are at risk for any particular subtype of prostate cancer. This work is complicated by changes in patterns of PSA screening in study populations. In older work, many cases were not detected by screening, but rather were men who presented with symptoms of prostate cancer; these men obviously had more advanced disease as a group than men with prostate cancer detected by screening. In later series, particularly those from North America, many subjects classified as prostate cancer cases had relatively early prostate cancer detected by screening. There is now emerging evidence from prospective study populations that higher levels of IGF-I (particularly when associated with relatively low levels of IGFBP-3) may in fact be specifically related to risk of a subsequent diagnosis of advanced or poor prognosis prostate cancer, while IGF-I (and IGFBP-3) levels are not associated with risk of a subsequent diagnosis of localized, good-prognosis disease.

This area of research clearly deserves further attention, because of two important unmet clinical needs. In a screening context, a marker associated with probability of developing advanced disease would aid in clinical decision-making when a screening exercise detects an early cancer – together with currently used criteria such as the Gleason score, such a marker might aid in making decisions for (or against) watchful waiting in individual cases. In a prevention context, subtly distinct from the screening context, given the very common presence of early prostate cancer lesions in adult males, a case could be made that all men with a high probability of developing more advanced prostate cancer (regardless of whether they have a current prostate cancer diagnosis) could be considered candidates for a prevention strategy that acts by reducing likelihood of progression of early cancers.

IGF-Related Markers and Breast Cancer Risk

One of the earliest prospective studies concerning IGF-I serum levels and subsequent risk of breast cancer (Hankison et al. 1998) reported that IGF-I levels were strongly related to risk of premenopausal, but not postmenopausal breast cancer. Several subsequent studies (e.g., Toniolo et al. 2000) reached similar conclusions, but there has been inconsistency in the literature, with some recent negative studies (e.g., Rinaldi et al. 2005; Schernhammer et al. 2006). The reason for this inconsistency is under investigation. The initial positive studies may simply have been chance findings, but it is also possible that there is an undiscovered modifying factor that influences the relationship between IGF-I level and risk. For example, cohorts or subcohorts with higher BMI or insulin levels might show a higher overall risk level than other cohorts, and such increased risk might well obscure any effect of IGF-I. While this explanation is plausible and deserves exploration, to date no data explain the inconsistencies that have been presented.

It is also possible that IGF-I levels sampled at younger ages are more related to later risk of breast cancer (Rollinson et al. 2005) than levels in samples obtained later in life. This is plausible because there is precedent for breast cancer risk factors that act mainly during a vulnerable period around the time of puberty to influence lifetime breast cancer risk. Although it has been assumed that individuals stay true to their centile of breast cancer throughout life (i.e., being in the top decile of the population at age 45 implies one was at the top decile at age 15), this has never been verified, as sample sets obtained from subjects repetitively sampled over decades are rare.

There is reasonably strong laboratory evidence (e.g., Pollak et al. 2001) that is consistent with the original reports of a positive association with risk. Furthermore, there is interesting circumstantial evidence consistent with the original observations from several reports linking mammographic breast density, a known strong breast cancer risk factor, to IGF-I and IGFBP-3 levels (Diorio et al. 2005, 2006; Byrne et al. 2000; Maskarinec et al. 2003). Additional circumstantial evidence comes from work relating birth weight and preadult growth patterns (both known to be influenced by IGF physiology) to breast cancer risk (Ahlgren et al. 2004).

Finally, a recent report on one of the largest sample sets studied to date (Al-Zahrani et al. 2006) did reveal a modest positive association between IGF-I levels and risk, and also extended prior work (Deal et al. 2001) by providing data showing that specific polymorphisms in genes encoding proteins involved in IGF-I physiology were related to both circulating levels and to risk of breast cancer.

Obesity, Insulin, Risk of Cancer, and Risk of Aggressive Cancer

Metabolic host risk factors or host prognostic factors (as distinct from better described tumor factors such as PTEN deletion or HER2 amplification) can influence the natural history of cancer. There is increasing evidence that obesity is related to increased risk of and/or worsened prognosis of many common kinds of cancer (Calle et al. 2003). The molecular and endocrinologic mechanism(s) underlying this relationship are the subject of ongoing research in many laboratories. This research is important because in view of the fact that obesity is becoming increasingly common around the world, there is concern that there may be a secondary effect of increased frequency of cancer diagnosis, and/or more aggressive behavior of cancers in populations.

Obesity and excess caloric intake are associated with many metabolic changes, including, for example, elevations of circulating insulin and leptin levels. Elevated insulin levels can increase IGF bioactivity by suppressing expression of certain IGF-binding proteins, particularly IGFBP-1. Elevated insulin levels might also directly stimulate neoplastic cell proliferation and survival by activating receptors on cancer cells that are upstream from the AKT survival signaling pathway. More studies are needed, however, to clarify with precision the receptors involved. Physiological levels of insulin, even if elevated in the context of obesity, are likely insufficient to activate IGF-I receptors directly. It is possible that certain neoplastic cells exhibit insulin receptors and/or hybrid insulin-IGF receptors that could respond to levels of insulin found in obese patients. At present, the possibility that the adverse influence of obesity could involve increased signaling downstream of insulin and/or insulin receptors is a plausible but unproven hypothesis. Advances in our understanding will require both laboratory models and clinical research. Early clinical results are consistent with the hypothesis (Wei et al. 2005; Ma et al. 2004; Schairer et al. 2004).

An interesting related point concerns the drug metformin, which has been in extensive use in the management of type II diabetes for many years. This drug is known to lower the elevated insulin levels found in type II diabetes, but to have little effect when given to people with normal insulin levels. Although there was a prior hypothesis that metformin acted as a sensitizer of cells to insulin action, and that this accounted for the drop in insulin level, recent evidence suggests that the drug acts primarily in vivo by reducing glucose output by the liver (gluconeogenesis) and that the fall in circulating insulin level is secondary to the fall in glucose (Shaw et al. 2005). Interestingly, the molecular pathways involved in this action of metformin in the liver involve activation of the amp-kinase/lkb1 tumor suppressor pathway. Specifically in hepatocytes, this pathway shuts off glucose output (Shaw et al. 2005). However, we have shown in ongoing laboratory studies that for some cancer cell lines, metformin acts as a growth inhibitor specifically by activating the same ampk/lkb1 tumor suppressor pathway. In these cell lines, as expected on the basis of studies of the LKB1/ampk pathway, metformin-induced ampk activation results in growth inhibition at the level of m-tor. In a sense, metformin may act by simulating low cellular energy supply, and thereby activating the physiologic control systems that presumably have evolved to block or at least dampen the action of mitogenic signals if there is not sufficient energy available for cell division.

Thus on theoretical grounds, metformin might act in two ways to constrain abnormal cell growth: (a) in vivo, it could reduce direct action of insulin or insulin-dependent mitogenic signals through its action as an insulin-lowering agent, and (b) it might have a direct growth inhibitory role by stimulating the lkb1/ampkinase tumor suppressor pathway. These mechanisms are not mutually exclusive, but research in this area is in its infancy, and much more work is needed to evaluate the actions of metformin. Nevertheless, it is tempting to speculate that this old drug or new derivatives might find new uses in the context of cancer prevention, particularly among obese individuals. Two recent studies provide further motivation for studies in this area: one report provides early evidence that the death rate from cancer is lower among diabetics taking metformin than diabetics on other treatments (Bowker et al. 2006), while the other reports that a cancer diagnosis is less common among metformin users than other diabetics (Evans et al; 2005).

Conclusion

The field of IGF and insulin signaling in relation to cancer risk and prevention remains an active research area for laboratory scientists, clinicians, and population scientists. While interesting new experimental and population studies have been reported, substantial gaps in basic knowledge remain to be filled before the possibility of potential clinical applications can be addressed.

References

Ahlgren M, Melbye M, Wohlfahrt J, Sorensen TI (2004) Growth patterns and the risk of breast cancer in women. N Engl J Med 351:1619–1626

Al-Zahrani A, Sandhu M, Luben R, Thompson B, Baynes C, Pooley K, Lucarini C, Munday H, Perkins B, Smith P, Pharaoh P, Wareham N, Easton D, Ponder BA, Dunning AM (2006) IGF-I and IGFBP3 tagging polymorphisms are associated with circulating levels of IGF-I, IGFBP-3, and risk of breast cancer. Hum Mol Genet 15:1–10

Bowker SL, Majumdar SR, Veugelers P, Johnson JA (2006) Increased cancer-related mortality for patients with type 2 diabetes who use sulfonylureas or insulin. Diabetes Care 29:254–258

Byrne C, Colditz G, Willett W, Speizer F, Pollak M, Hankinson S (2000) Plasma insulin-like growth factor (IGF) I, IGF-binding protein 3, and mammographic density. Cancer Research 60:3744–3748

Calle EE, Kaaks R (2004) Overweight, obesity and cancer: epidemiological evidence and proposed mechanisms. Nat Rev Cancer 4:579–591

Calle EE, Rodriguez C, Walker-Thurmond K, Thun MJ (2003) Overweight, obesity, and mortality from cancer in a prospectively studied cohort of US adults. N Engl J Med 348:1625–1638

Chan J, Stampfer M, Giovannucci E, Gann P, Ma J, Wilkinson P, Hennekens C, Pollak M (1998) Plasma insulin-like growth factor-I and prostate cancer risk: a prospective study. Science 279:563–566

Deal C, Ma J, Wilkin F, Paquette J, Rozen F, Ge B, Hudson T, Stampfer M, Pollak M (2001) Novel promoter polymorphism in IGFBP3: correlation with serum levels and interaction with known regulators. J Clin Endocrinol Metabol 86:1274–1280

Diorio C, Pollak M, Byrne C, Masse B, Hebert-Croteau N, Yaffe M, Cote G, Berube S, Morin C, Brisson J (2005) Insulin-like growth factor-I, IGF-binding protein-3, and mammographic breast density. Cancer Epidemiol Biomarkers Prev 14:1065–1073

Diorio C, Berube S, Byrne C, Masse B, Hebert-Croteau N, Yaffe M, Cote G, Pollak M, Brisson J (2006) Influence of insulin-like growth factors on the strength of the relation of vitamin D and calcium intakes to mammographic breast density. Cancer Res 66:588–597

Evans JM, Donnelly LA, Emslie-Smith AM, Alessi DR, Morris AD (2005) Metformin and reduced risk of cancer in diabetic patients. BMJ 330(7503):1304–1305

Hankinson S, Willett W, Colditz G, Hunter D, Michaud D, Deroo B, Rosner B, Speizer F, Pollak M (1998) Circulating concentrations of insulin-like growth factor I and risk of breast cancer. Lancet 351:1393–1396

Ma J, Giovannucci E, Pollak M, Leavitt A, Tao Y, Gaziano JM, Stampfer MJ (2004) A prospective study of plasma C-peptide and colorectal cancer risk in men. J Natl Cancer Inst 96:546–553

Ma J, Pollak M et al (2005) Presentaion at Prostate Cancer Biomarker Meeting Denver, Dec 2005

Majeed N, Blouin M-J, Kaplan-Lefko PJ, Barry-Shaw J, Greenberg NM, Gaudreau P, Bismar TA, Pollak M (2005) A germ line mutation that delays prostate cancer progression and prolongs survival in a murine prostate cancer model. Oncogene 24:4736–4740

Maskarinec G, Williams AE, Kaaks R (2003) A cross-sectional investigation of breast density and insulin-like growth factor I. Int J Cancer 107:991–996

Pollak M, Blouin M-J, Jian-Chun Z, Kopchick JJ (2001) Reduced mammary gland carcinogenesis in transgenic mice expressing a growth hormone antagonist. Br J Cancer 85:428–430

Pollak MN, Schernhammer ES, Hankinson SE (2004) Insulin-like growth factors and neoplasia. Nat Rev Cancer 4:505–518

Renehan AG, Zwahlen M, Minder C, O'Dwyer ST, Shalet SM, Egger M (2004) Insulin-like growth factor (IGF)-I, IGF binding protein-3, and cancer risk: systematic review and meta-regression analysis. Lancet 363(9418):1346–1353

Rinaldi S, Toniolo P, Muti P, Lundin E, Zeleniuch-Jacquotte A, Arslan A, Micheli A, Lenner P, Dossus L, Krogh V, Shore RE, Koenig KL, Riboli E, Stattin P, Berrino F, Hallmans G, Lukanova A, Kaaks R (2005) IGF-I, IGFBP-3 and breast cancer in young women: a pooled re-analysis of three prospective studies. Eur J Cancer Prev 14:493–496

Rollison DE, Newschaffer CJ, Tao Y, Pollak M, Helzlsouer KJ (2005) Premenopausal levels of circulating insulin-like growth factor I and the risk of postmenopausal breast cancer. Int J Cancer. 118:1279–1284

Schairer C, Hill D, Sturgeon SR, Fears T, Pollak M, Mies C, Ziegler RG, Hoover RN, Sherman ME (2004) Serum concentrations of IGF-I, IGFBP-3 and c-peptide and risk of hyperplasia and cancer of the breast in postmenopausal women. Int J Cancer 108:773–779

Schernhammer ES, Pollak M, Hankinson SE et al (2006) Endocr-related cancer. in press, 2006

Shaw RJ, Lamia KA, Vasquez D, Koo SH, Bardeesy N, Depinho RA, Montminy M, Cantley LC (2005) The kinase LKB1 mediates glucose homeostasis in liver and therapeutic effects of metformin. Science 310:1642–1646

Thompson IM, Goodman PJ, Tangen CM, Lucia MS, Miller GJ, Ford LG, Lieber MM, Cespedes RD, Atkins JN, Lippman SM, Carlin SM, Ryan A, Szczepanek CM, Crowley JJ, Coltman CA Jr (2003) The influence of finasteride on the development of prostate cancer. N Engl J Med 349:215–224

Thompson IM, Pauler DK, Goodman PJ, Tangen CM, Lucia MS, Parnes HL, Minasian LM, Ford LG, Lippman SM, Crawford ED, Crowley JJ, Coltman CA Jr (2004) Prevalence of prostate cancer among men with a prostate-specific antigen level <or =4.0 ng per milliliter. N Engl J Med 350:2239–2246

Toniolo P, Bruning PF, Akhmedkhanov A, Bonfrer JM, Koenig KL, Lukanova A, Shore RE, Zeleniuch-Jacquotte A (2000) Serum insulin-like growth factor-I and breast cancer. Int J Cancer 88:828–832

Wei EK, Ma J, Pollak MN, Rifai N, Fuchs CS, Hankinson SE, Giovannucci E (2005) A prospective study of C-peptide, insulin-like growth factor-I, insulin-like growth factor binding protein-1, and the risk of colorectal cancer in women. Cancer Epidemiol Biomarkers Prev 14:850–855

Part II Inflammation, Infection, and Cancer Prevention

5 Cytokines Are a Therapeutic Target for the Prevention of Inflammation-Induced Cancers

Stefan Rose-John, Heidi Schooltink

Recent Results in Cancer Research, Vol. 174
© Springer-Verlag Berlin Heidelberg 2007

Abstract

Interleukin-6 (IL-6) is an inflammatory cytokine with a well-documented role in cancer. The cytokine binds to a membrane-bound IL-6 receptor (IL-6R) and this complex associates with two molecules of the signal transducing protein gp130, initiating intracellular signaling. Whereas gp130 is expressed on all cells of the body, the IL-6R is only found on some cells, mainly hepatocytes and several leukocytes. Cells, which only express gp130 and no IL-6R, cannot respond to IL-6. We have shown that the IL-6R exists as a soluble protein generated by limited proteolysis of the membrane-bound receptor or by translation from an alternatively spliced mRNA. The complex of soluble IL-6R (sIL-6R) and IL-6 can bind to gp130 on cells that lack the membrane-bound IL-6R and trigger gp130 signaling. We have named this process trans-signaling. We review data that show that IL-6 uses classical signaling via the membrane-bound receptor and trans-signaling via the soluble receptor in physiological and pathophysiological situations. We have developed designer cytokines, which specifically enhance or inhibit IL-6 trans-signaling. These designer cytokines have been shown to be extremely useful in therapeutic applications such as blockade of chronic inflammation and cancer

Cytokines

Cytokines are small soluble proteins, which are secreted by and act on a variety of different cell types. Because of structural features, cytokines can be grouped into different families. One of them, named after the first discovered member of the family is the interleukin 6 (IL-6) family (Taga and Kishimoto 1997). This family further comprises IL-11, ciliary neurotrophic factor (CNTF), cardiotrophin-1 (CT-1), cardiotrophin like cytokine (CLC), leukemia inhibitory factor (LIF), neuropoietin (NPN) and oncostatin M (OSM). Recently two new cytokines also belonging to the IL-6 family, named IL-27 and IL-31, have been found (Dillon et al. 2004; Pflanz et al. 2004). Each of the cytokines of the IL-6 family seem to have specific activities in different compartments but interestingly, in some cases the cytokines of the family can substitute each other. This phenomenon has been called redundancy.

Recent advances have documented a series of IL-6 activities that are critical for resolving innate immunity and promoting acquired immunity (Jones 2005; Jones et al. 2005). The transition between innate and acquired immunity is a central event in the resolution of any inflammatory condition, and disruption of this immunological switch may potentially distort the immune response and affect the onset of autoimmune or chronic inflammatory disorders (Hoebe et al. 2004).

Receptor Complexes

The structural basis of redundancy in the IL-6 family is the composition of the receptor complexes, via which the members of the IL-6 family transduce their signals into the target cells. The central protein of the receptor complexes is the ubiquitously expressed glycoprotein gp130 (Taga and Kishimoto 1997). All receptor complexes use this protein as a signal transducing receptor subunit. Besides gp130, the receptor complexes may contain different ligand-binding proteins, which are specific for one cytokine, for example the receptors for IL-6, CNTF, and IL-11. Moreover, the receptor complexes for CNTF, CLC, CT-1, LIF, NPN, and OSM contain the LIF-receptor (LIF-R) protein, a signal-transducing receptor subunit which is homologous to gp130 (Taga and Kishimoto 1997).

Soluble Receptor Paradigm

When making contact with a target cell, IL-6 first binds to the specific IL-6 receptor (IL-6R). In a second step, this complex associates with two molecules of gp130, thereby initiating intracellular signaling (Taga and Kishimoto 1997; Rose-John 2001). Whereas gp130 is expressed on most if not all cells of the body, the expression of the IL-6R is restricted to hepatocytes, neutrophils, monocytes/macrophages, and some lymphocytes. Interestingly, cells that do not express the IL-6R on the cell surface can respond to IL-6 if a soluble form of the IL-6R (sIL-6R) is present (Mackiewicz et al. 1992; Taga et al. 1989) (Fig. 1a). Such a soluble IL-6R has been found in various body fluids. It turned out that the sIL-6R can be generated by two different mechanisms: limited proteolysis of the membrane protein and translation from an alternatively spliced mRNA (Lust et al. 1992; Rose-John and Heinrich 1994; Müllberg et al. 2000; Althoff et al. 2000, 2001; Hundhausen et al. 2003; Matthews et al. 2003; Abel et al. 2004). The stimulation of cells by the complex of IL-6 and sIL-6R has been termed trans-signaling (Rose-John and Heinrich 1994; Jones 2005; Jones et al. 2005). Because they lack a functional IL-6R on their surface, early hematopoietic progenitor cells (Peters et al. 1997, 1998; Audet et al. 2001; Hacker et al. 2003; Campard et al. 2006), embryonic stem cells (Rose-John 2002; Humphrey et al. 2004), endothelial cells (Romano et al. 1997), mesothelial cells (Hurst et al. 2001; McLoughlin et al. 2003), neural cells (März et al. 1998, 1999), smooth muscle cells (Klouche et al. 1999), and T

cells (Atreya et al. 2000; Becker et al. 2004, 2005) only respond to IL-6 in the presence of the sIL-6R.

Designer Cytokines

Construction of chimeric proteins containing modules of different proteins belonging to the IL-6R family helped us to identify cytokine binding motives on receptor proteins (Kallen et al. 1999 2000; Aasland et al. 2002, 2003). On the basis of these experiments together with other structural information available on membrane bound and soluble cytokine receptors, we designed several cytokine–cytokine receptor molecules.

Covalent linkage of the domains of the IL-6 and sIL-6R that are necessary for biological activity via a flexible polypeptide linker resulted in a recombinant fusion protein, that was found to be 100–1,000 times more active than the native IL-6/sIL-6R complex. Because of this enhanced activity, we termed this cytokine Hyper-IL-6 (Fischer et al. 1997). Cells lacking the IL-6R, which as a consequence do not respond to IL-6 alone, such as embryonic stem cells, endothelial cells, hematopoietic progenitor cells, neuronal cells, and smooth muscle cells, show a remarkable biologic response to Hyper-IL-6. Adoption of this approach led to the construction of fusion proteins between IL-11 and the soluble IL-11R (Pflanz et al. 1999) Furthermore, proteins consisting of CNTF fused to the soluble CNTF-R have been constructed. These proteins show high neurotrophic activity on neural cells lacking a surface CNTF-R (Guillet et al. 2002; Sun et al. 2002).

By fusing the entire extracellular domain of gp130 protein to the Fc region of human IgG1, we constructed a soluble form of gp130 (sgp130Fc). Surprisingly, in HepG2 cells this protein inhibited only the production of the acute-phase protein antichymotrypsin (ACT) induced by Hyper-IL-6, whereas the response to IL-6 alone remained unaffected (Jostock et al. 2001). We concluded that sgp130Fc does not interfere with responses mediated by the membrane bound IL-6R but exclusively inhibits IL-6 trans-signaling via the soluble IL-6R (Fig. 1b).

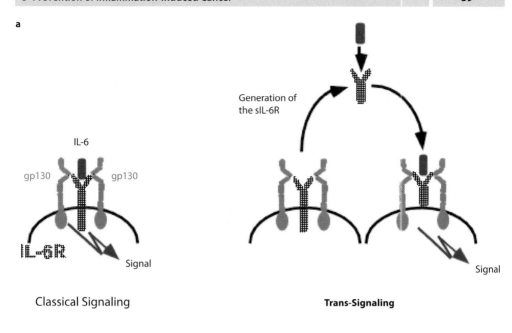

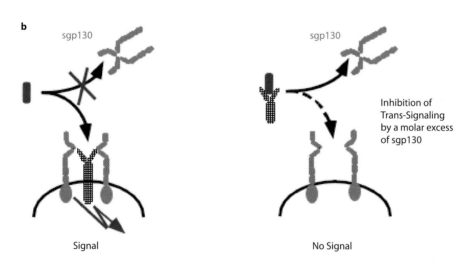

Fig. 1a, b Classical and trans-signaling of IL-6 and the inhibitory mechanism of sgp130. **a** The two modes of IL-6 activation: classical IL-6 activation via the membrane-bound IL-6R and trans-signaling via a soluble form of the IL-6R. In both cases, signals are transmitted by membrane-bound gp130. **b** Sgp130 binds the IL-6/sIL-6R complex to antagonize IL-6 trans-signaling, whereas classical signaling remains unaffected

Since gp130 is part of the receptors of the cytokines IL-6, IL-11, IL-27, CLC, CNTF, CT-1, LIF, OSM, and NPN, we asked whether the sgp130 inhibition was specific for the IL-6/sIL-6R complex or whether sgp130Fc also effected the biologic activity of the other IL-6-family cytokines (Jostock et al. 2001; Scheller et al. 2005). Our experiments showed that CNTF-mediated activities were unaffected by the sgp130Fc protein. To inhibit the proliferative activity of LIF and OSM on BAF/3 cells stably transfected with gp130 and LIF-R cDNAs, more than 100-fold higher sgp130Fc concentrations were needed than for the inhibition of Hyper-IL-6. These findings are in agreement with surface plasmon resonance experiments showing that Hyper-IL-6 and OSM bind to sgp130 with KD values of 6.9×10^{-9} M and 1.6×10^{-7} M, respectively (Richards et al. 2006). Because the recently found cytokine IL-27 also acts via a receptor complex consisting of gp130 and the related receptor protein WSX-1 (Pflanz et al. 2004), we examined whether sgp130Fc inhibited the biologic activity of IL-27 (Scheller et al. 2005). Our results clearly indicated that the sgp130Fc protein did not affect the IL-27-mediated STAT3 phosphorylation and proliferation of BAF/3 cells expressing gp130 and WSX-1. As a conclusion of these results, we postulated that the sgp130Fc protein is a specific inhibitor of the IL-6/sIL-6R trans-signaling complex.

Physiological Role of Soluble gp130

In experimental arthritis, colitis, and colon cancer, sgp130 has been shown to influence leukocyte trafficking and to reduce the severity of the diseases. Moreover, the phenotype of sgp130 transgenic mice resembles the phenotype of mice treated with sgp130 in vivo. Together these findings led us to the conclusion that sgp130 acts as the natural inhibitor only of IL-6/sIL-6R complexes. IL-6 does not directly bind sgp130, and as a consequence the classical IL-6 signal via the membrane forms of the IL-6R and gp130 remains unaffected. Figure 1b shows our concept of the molecular mechanism, by which soluble gp130 exerts selective inhibition of the IL-6/sIL-6R complex. The IL-6/sIL-6R complex shows equal affinity for the soluble and membrane-bound variants of sgp130, and a molar excess of sgp130 inhibits IL-6 trans-signaling. The selective inhibition of IL-6 trans-signaling appears to be an important pathophysiological regulation mechanism in inflammatory diseases.

IL-6 Trans-signaling and Inflammation

Many investigations have shown that IL-6 plays an important role in the transition from innate immunity to acquired immunity, a crucial event in the controlling of any inflammatory states (Hurst et al. 2001; Jones 2005; Jones et al. 2005). Disruption of this essential switch leads to an inappropriate immune response and might cause the onset of autoimmune or chronic inflammatory disorders (Hoebe et al. 2004). The discovery of the IL-6 trans-signaling mechanism may help to understand the contradictory role of IL-6 in acute and chronic inflammatory states (Kallen 2002). In acute inflammation such as septic shock (Ulich et al. 1991; Barton and Jackson 1993; Diao and Kohanawa 2005), IL-6 shows favorable effects, whereas under chronic inflammatory conditions, IL-6 seems to maintain the disease state. The contribution of IL-6 trans-signaling and the interference of IL-6 signaling with STAT1, IFN-γ, TGF-β, GATA-3, and NF-κB remarkably influence disease outcome (Becker et al. 2004; Doganci et al. 2005; Hegde et al. 2004; McLoughlin et al. 2005). Studies have been conducted to examine the role of IL-6 trans-signaling in acute inflammation, asthma, tumor expansion, and the inflammatory response associated with tumor progression. The common role of IL-6 trans-signaling in these various disease states was an orchestration of leukocyte recruitment and activation and control of apoptotic processes (Jones 2005; Jones et al. 2005). In this context, IL-6 suppresses neutrophil infiltration while promoting attraction and activation of mononuclear leukocytes, leading to a switch from the innate to the acquired immune system (Atreya et al. 2000; Becker et al. 2004; Hurst et al. 2001; McLoughlin et al. 2005). Interrupting IL-6 trans-signaling in experimental models of colitis and rheumatoid arthritis improved disease outcome (Atreya 2000; Nowell et al. 2003). This effect is caused by either inhibiting the recruitment or increasing the apoptotic clearance of mononuclear cells. Both effects lead to a diminished mononuclear cell concentration which are at least partly responsible for the chronic disease progression in inflamed tissue. The observation that IL-6 trans-signaling is a contributor to chronic disease progression is underlined by several in vitro and in vivo studies in which IL-6 inhibited apoptosis by inducing anti-apoptotic regulators via the STAT3 signal transduction pathway (Atreya et al. 2000; Teague et al. 2000; Curnow et al. 2004). The understanding of IL-6 mediated control of activated mononuclear cell populations is therefore a hallmark in understanding of chronic disease progression (Jones 2005; Jones et al. 2005).

Results from studies with IL-6 knockout mice show that IL-6 influences T cell recruitment via the local secretion of chemokines (CXCL10, CCL2, CCL4, CCL5, CCL11, CCL17) and the expression of chemokine receptors (CCR3, CCR4, CCR5, CXCR3) on CD3+ cells (Hurst et al. 2001; McLoughlin et al. 2005). Since sgp130 selectively antagonizes IL-6 trans-signaling in vivo without affecting the classical pathway via the membrane receptor, it is possible to distinguish between both mechanisms. Interestingly, sgp130 only blocked chemokine expression, whereas T cell chemokine receptor expression remained unaffected (McLoughlin et al. 2005). Differential activities for IL-6 classical and trans-signaling were also defined using a murine asthma model. In this case, IL-6 alone directed the T cell population toward the Th-2 subtype, whereas for the activation of this Th2 population IL-6 trans-signaling is necessary (Doganci et al. 2005).

In summary, T cell responses are differentially regulated by IL-6 alone and by the IL-6/sIL-6R complex. In this context, it is interesting to address the question whether T cells universally express IL-6R protein on their surface, or whether the expression of IL-6R is restricted to specific subsets of T cells. Of CD3+ T-cells from the circulation, 35%–45% express IL-6R, whereas only 2%–5% of CD3+ cells infiltrating an inflammatory tissue are IL-6R-positive (Atreya et al. 2000; Becker et al. 2004; Curnow et al. 2004). Thus under inflammatory conditions, the expression of the IL-6R or the homing of a CD3+IL-6R– T cell subset to inflammatory foci is dramatically downregulated. T cells treated in vivo with superantigen also show significantly lower levels of IL-6R (Teague et al. 2000). Thus, the loss of the IL-6R on the surface of T cells might be a marker for a less activated status of these cells.

Furthermore, IL-6-mediated control of cellular differentiation also takes place in the polarization of monocytic cells. The major observed effect is the inhibition of differentiation of monocytic cells toward dendritic cells, thus favoring the development of a macrophage phenotype (Chomarat et al. 2000; Mitani et al. 2000). The shifting of the differentiation of human monocytes can also be seen in IL-6–/– mice in vivo, where the expansion of bone marrow cells resulted in a tenfold higher number of CD11c+ dendritic cells as compared with wild type mice (Bleier et al. 2004). Interestingly, the activity of dendritic cells in IL-6–/– mice is impaired, implicating that IL-6 is also necessary for their activity. In this context, IL-6 has been shown to inhibit NF-κB activity and suppress the expression of the chemokine receptor CCR7 in dendritic cells (Hegde et al. 2004). Furthermore, IL-6 secretion by dendritic cells following toll-like receptor activation blocks the immunosuppressive activities of regulatory T cells (Pasare and Medzhitov 2003). Thus IL-6 not only seems to be responsible for the recruitment of dendritic cells, but also modulates the activity of dendritic cells in advancing adaptive immune reactions.

In summary, these studies highlight the central role of IL-6 in both innate and acquired immune responses. Changes in IL-6 production and in the expression of IL-6R on the surface of target cells may support the development of chronic inflammatory diseases. The finding that the IL-6 trans-signaling pathway has specific functions in chronic disease progression and the fact that a selective inhibitor for this pathway is available opens new promising perspectives for therapeutic intervention.

Colon Cancer as an Example of Inflammatory Induced Cancer

In earlier studies, we demonstrated the importance of the IL-6 trans-signaling pathway for the maintenance of chronic inflammatory bowl disease (Crohn disease) (Atreya et al. 2000).

Interestingly, our studies showed that in Crohn disease patients the T cells from gastric tissue are extremely resistant to apoptosis. Biochemical examinations showed that these T cells produced large amounts of IL-6 and that the intracellular JAK-STAT signal transduction pathway was activated. Surprisingly, treatment of these cells with a neutralizing monoclonal antibody to IL-6R induced apoptosis, although the cells lacked a membrane form of the IL-6R. As the treatment of the cells with sgp130 also induced apoptosis, this effect must have been mediated via the IL-6 trans-signaling pathway (Fig. 2). This finding showed that IL-6 trans-signaling is responsible for the surveillance of activated T cells within gastric tissue from Crohn disease patients by inhibiting apoptotic processes. The sIL-6R needed for IL-6 trans-signaling is most likely provided by shedding of the membrane IL-6R from lamina propria macrophages or infiltrating neutrophils (Atreya et al. 2000; Jostock et al. 2001). Interestingly, it was recently found that in addition to the levels of IL-6, the levels of sIL-6R and sgp130 are also elevated in chronic inflammatory bowel diseases, and that the IL-6 found in the circulation was preferentially complexed to sIL-6R and sgp130 (Mitsuyama et al. 2005).

Moreover, the production of sIL-6R as well as IL-6 trans-signaling processes play a dominant role in tumor cell growth. Interestingly, crosstalk between the TGFβ and IL-6 pathway was demonstrated (Fig. 3). Inhibition of TGFβ production resulted in an increased IL-6 production in mice. Surprisingly, the IL-6 overproduction is accompanied by a loss of membrane bound IL-6R from the cell surface of epithelial cells within tumor lesions. This loss of membrane bound IL-6R was most likely due to an increase of the cell surface expression of the protease ADAM17, which is responsible for cleavage of the IL-6R (Matthews et al. 2003). As the epithelial tumor growth could be inhibited either by a neutralizing antibody directed against the IL-6R or by sgp130Fc, we concluded that the growth of the tumor was promoted by IL-6 trans-signaling but not by the classic signaling via the membrane-bound IL-6R (Becker et al. 2004, 2005). The same observations of downregulation of the IL-6R on the surface of tumor epithelial cells and the upregulation of ADAM17 were made in human colon cancer patients, implying that a similar mechanism operates in human and mouse colon cancer development (Becker et al. 2005). These findings show that interrupting IL-6 trans-signaling with sgp130Fc in colon cancer patients will be a promising new therapeutical strategy.

Conclusions

The alternative signaling pathway of IL-6 via the sIL-6R/IL-6 complex seem to be an important mechanism for the development of chronic inflammatory diseases and inflammation-associated tumor growth. The ability of selective inhibition of sIL-6R-dependent IL-6 responses with sgp130 can be used in vivo to distinguish between classical IL-6 signaling and IL-6 trans-signaling (Fig. 4). There is now clear evidence that chronic inflammatory states often lead to neoplastic lesions. Sgp130 can be used to effectively block immunological processes that promote inflammatory disease progression. One clear advantage of selectively blocking IL-6 trans-signaling is the fact that classic IL-6 responses remain unaffected. These include the hepatic acute-phase response, which plays an important role in the defense of the body against infections and trauma. These

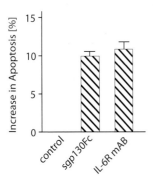

Fig. 2 Apoptosis of lamina propria mononuclear cells (LPMC) of Crohn disease patients upon treatment with sgp130. LPMCs were isolated and cultured for 48 h in the presence or absence of 10 µg/ml of a neutralizing mAB-specific for human IL-6R or 10 µg/ml sgp130Fc. Cells were stained for annexin V and propidiumiodide and analyzed by FACS. The increase in apoptotic (annexin V-positive and propidiumiodide-negative) cells is shown. The data presented are means of triplicate measurements with standard errors shown as vertical bars

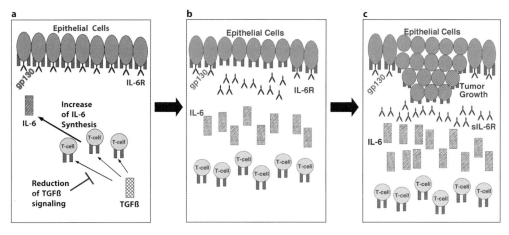

Fig. 3a–c Schematic model of TGF-β-regulated IL-6 trans-signaling in experimental colon cancer. **a** A reduction of TGFβ signaling results in increased IL-6 secretion. **b** The observed upregulation of the ADAM17 metalloproteinase on epithelial cells results in shedding of the IL-6R. Upon stimulation with the IL-6/sIL-6R complex, T cells become resistant to apoptosis and therefore the number of T cells increases. **c** Growth of epithelial cells in tumor lesions is observed upon stimulation with the IL-6/sIL-6R complex. Tumor growth can be inhibited by blocking the IL-6R using a monoclonal antibody or by inhibiting IL-6 trans-signaling with the sgp130Fc protein. Dark grey symbols, gp130; black symbols, membraned bound IL-6R and soluble IL-6R; light grey symbols, epithelial cells

Therapeutic Strategies for IL-6 Neutralization

IL-6 neutralizing Antibody (MRA)

Soluble gp130Fc Protein

Global IL-6 Neutralization

Selective blockade of IL-6 trans-signaling

Applications (positive clinical trial data)

Blocks effector T-cell functions

Rheumatoid arthritis

Regulates leukocyte recruitment

Juvenile rheumatoid arthritis

Governs leukocyte apoptosis

Castleman's disease

Modulates inflammatory chemokines

Crohn's disease

Some evidence of dual regulation of T-cell responses by IL-6 and IL-6 trans-signaling

Fig. 4 Therapeutic strategies for targeting IL-6 signaling. Current therapeutic regimes designed to clinically suppress IL-6 activities involve the application of the blocking monoclonal antibody MRA (atlizumab, tocilizumab) effective against a range of conditions. This did not distinguish between classical IL-6 signaling and IL-6 trans-signaling. The fusion protein sgp130Fc selectively targets IL-6 trans-signaling, and leaves classical IL-6 signaling intact

considerations have provided a therapeutic rationale for the administration of sgp130 in a series of chronic inflammatory conditions, which are prone to progress to cancer.

References

Aasland D, Oppmann B, Grötzinger J, Rose-John S, Kallen K-J (2002) The upper cytokine binding module and the Ig-like domain of the leukaemia inhibitory factor (LIF) receptor are sufficient for a functional LIFR complex. J Mol Biol 315:637–646

Aasland D, Schuster B, Grötzinger J, Rose-John S, Kallen K-J (2003) Analysis of the leukemia inhibitory factor receptor functional domains by chimeric receptors and cytokines. Biochemistry 42:5244–5252

Abel S, Hundhausen C, Mentlein R, Berkhout TA, Broadway N, Siddall H, Dietrich S, Muetze B, Kallen KJ, Saftig P, Rose-John S, Ludwig A (2004) The transmembrane CXC-chemokine CXCL16 is expressed on vascular cells and shed by the activity of the disintegrin-like metalloproteinase ADAM10. J Immunol 172:6362–6372

Althoff K, Reddy P, Peschon J, Voltz N, Rose-John S, Müllberg J (2000) Contribution of the amino acid sequence at the cleavage site to the cleavage pattern of transmembrane proteins. Eur J Biochem 267:2624–2631

Althoff K, Müllberg J, Aasland D, Voltz N, Kallen K-J, Grötzinger J, Rose-John S (2001) Recognition sequences and structural elements contribute to shedding susceptibility of membrane proteins. Biochem J 353:663–672

Atreya R, Mudter J, Finotto S, Müllberg J, Jostock T, Wirtz S, Schütz M, Bartsch B, Holtmann M, Becker C, Strand D, Czaja J, Schlaak JF, Lehr HA, Autschbach F, Schürmann G, Nishimoto N, Yoshizaki K, Ito H, Kishimoto T, Galle PR, Rose-John S, Neurath MF (2000) Blockade of IL-6 transsignaling abrogates established experimental colitis in mice by suppression of the antiapoptotic resistance of lamina propria T cells. Nat Med 6:583–588

Audet J, Miller CL, Rose-John S, Piret JM, Eaves CJ (2001) Distinct role of gp130 activation in promoting self-renewal divisions by mitogenically stimulated murine hematopoietic cells. Proc Natl Acad Sci U S A 98:1757–1762

Barton BE, Jackson JV (1993) Protective role of interleukin 6 in the lipopolysaccharide-galactosamine septic shock model. Infect Immun 61:1496–1499

Becker C, Fantini MC, Schramm C, Lehr HA, Wirtz S, Nikolaev A, Burg J, Strand S, Kiesslich R, Huber S, Ito H, Nishimoto N, Yoshizaki K, Kishimoto T, Galle PR, Blessing M, Rose-John S, Neurath MF (2004) TGF-beta suppresses tumor progression in colon cancer by inhibition of IL-6 trans-signaling. Immunity 21:491–501

Becker C, Fantini MC, Wirtz S, Nikolaev A, Lehr HA, Galle PR, Rose-John S, Neurath MF (2005) IL-6 signaling promotes tumor growth in colorectal cancer. Cell Cycle 4:217–220

Bleier JI, Pillarisetty VG, Shah AB, DeMatteo RP (2004) Increased and long-term generation of dendritic cells with reduced function from IL-6-deficient bone marrow. J Immunol 172:7408–7416

Campard D, Vasse M, Rose-John S, Poyer F, Lamacz M, Vannier JP (2006) Multilevel regulation of IL-6R by IL-6/sIL-6R fusion protein according to the primitiveness of the peripheral blood-derived CD133+ cells. Stem Cells 24:1302–1314

Chomarat P, Banchereau J, Davoust J, Palucka AKNI (2000) IL-6 switches the differentiation of monocytes from dendritic cells to macrophages. Nat Immunol 1:510–514

Curnow SJ, Scheel-Toellner D, Jenkinson W, Raza K, Durrani OM, Faint JM, Rauz S, Wloka K, Pilling D, Rose-John S, Buckley CD, Murray PI, Salmon M (2004) Inhibition of T cell apoptosis in the aqueous humor of patients with uveitis by IL-6/soluble IL-6 receptor trans-signaling. J Immunol 173:5290–5297

Diao H, Kohanawa M (2005) Endogenous interleukin-6 plays a crucial protective role in streptococcal toxic shock syndrome via suppression of tumor necrosis factor alpha production. Infect Immunol 73:3745–3748

Dillon SR, Sprecher C, Hammond A, Bilsborough J, Rosenfeld-Franklin M, Presnell SR, Haugen HS, Maurer M, Harder B, Johnston J, Bort S, Mudri S, Kuijper JL, Bukowski T, Shea P, Dong DL, Dasovich M, Grant FJ, Lockwood L, Levin SD, LeCiel C, Waggie K, Day H, Topouzis S, Kramer JB, Kuestner R, Chen Z, Foster D, Parrish-Novak J, Gross JA (2004) Interleukin 31, a cytokine produced by activated T cells, induces dermatitis in mice. Nat Immunol 5:752–760

Doganci A, Eigenbrod T, Krug N, De Sanctis GT, Hausding M, Erpenbeck VJ, El-Bdaoui H, Schmitt E, Bopp T, Kallen KJ, Herz U, Schmitt S, Luft C, Hecht O, Hohlfeld M, Ito H, Nishimoto N, Yoshizaki K, Kishimoto T, Rose-John S, Renz H, Neurath MF, Galle PR, Finotto S (2005) The IL-6R alpha chain controls lung CD4+CD4+CD25+T regulatory cell development and function during allergic airway inflammation in vivo. J Clin Invest 115:313–325

Fischer M, Goldschmitt J, Peschel C, Kallen KJ, Brakenhoff JPJ, Wollmer A, Grötzinger J, Rose-John S (1997) A designer cytokine with high activity on human hematopoietic progenitor cells. Nat Biotech 15:142–145

Guillet C, Lelievre E, Plun-Favreau H, Froger J, Chabbert M, Hermann J, Benoit de Coignac A, Bonnefoy JY, Gascan H, Gauchat JF, Elson G (2002) Functionally active fusion protein of the novel composite cytokine CLC/soluble CNTF receptor. Eur J Biochem 269:1932–1941

Hacker C, Kirsch RD, Ju X-S, Hieronymus T, Gust TC, Kuhl C, Jorgas T, Kurz SM, Rose-John S, Yokota Y, Zenke M (2003) Transcriptional profiling identifies Id2 function in dendritic cell development. Nat Immunol 4:380–386

Hegde S, Pahne J, Smola-Hess S (2004) Novel immunosuppressive properties of interleukin-6 in dendritic cells: inhibition of NF-κB binding activity and CCR7 expression. FASEB J 18:1439–1441

Hoebe K, Janssen E, Beutler B (2004) The interface between innate and acquired immunity. Nat Immunol 10:971–974

Humphrey RK, Beattie GM, Lopez AD, Bucay N, King CC, Firpo M, Rose-John S, Hayek A (2004) Maintenance of pluripotency in human embryonic stem cells is Stat3 independent. Stem Cells 22:522–530

Hundhausen C, Misztela D, Berkhout TA, Broadway N, Saftig P, Hartmann D, Fahrenholz F, Postina R, Matthews V, Kallen K-J, Rose-John S, Ludwig A (2003) The disintegrin-like metalloproteinase ADAM 10 is involved in constitutive cleavage of CX3CL1 (fractalkine) and regulates CX3CL1-mediated cell-cell adhesion. Blood 102:1186–1195

Hurst SM, Wilkinson TS, McLoughlin RM, Jones S, Horiuchi S, Yamamoto N, Rose-John S, Fuller GM, Topley N, Jones SA (2001) Control of leukocyte infiltration during inflammation: IL-6 and its soluble receptor orchestrate a temporal switch in the pattern of leukocyte recruitment. Immunity 14:705–714

Jones SA (2005) Directing transition from innate to acquired immunity: Defining a role for IL-6. J Immunol 175:3464–3468

Jones S, Richards PJ, Scheller J, Rose-John S (2005) IL-6 Transsignaling: the in vivo consequences. J Interferon Cytokine Res 25:241–253

Jostock T, Müllberg J, Özbek S, Atreya R, Blinn G, Voltz N, Fischer M, Neurath MF, Rose-John S (2001) Soluble gp130 is the natural inhibitor of soluble IL-6R transsignaling responses. Eur J Biochem 268:160–167

Kallen K-J (2002) The role of transsignalling via the agonistic soluble IL-6 receptor. Biochim Biophys Acta 1592:323–343

Kallen K-J, Grötzinger J, Lelièvre E, Vollmer P, Aasland D, Renné C, Müllberg J, Meyer zum Büschenfelde K-H, Gascan H, Rose-John S (1999) Receptor recognition sites of cytokines are organized as exchangeable modules: transfer of the LIFR binding site from CNTF to IL-6. J Biol Chem 274:11859–11867

Kallen K-J, Grötzinger J, Rose-John S (2000) New perspectives in the design of cytokines and growth factors. Trends Biotechnol 18:455–461

Klouche M, Bhakdi S, Hemmes M, Rose-John S (1999) Novel path of activation of primary human smooth muscle cells: upregulation of gp130 creates an autocrine activation loop by IL-6 and its soluble receptor. J Immunol 163:4583–4589

Lust JA, Donovan KA, Kline MP, Greipp PR, Kyle RA, Maihle NJ (1992) Isolation of an mRNA encoding a soluble form of the human interleukin-6 receptor. Cytokine 4:96–100

Mackiewicz A, Schooltink H, Heinrich PC, Rose-John S (1992) Complex of soluble human IL-6-receptor/IL-6 up-regulates expression of acute-phase proteins. J Immunol 149:2021–2027

März P, Cheng J-C, Gadient RA, Patterson P, Stoyan T, Otten U, Rose-John S (1998) Sympathetic neurons can produce and respond to Interleukin-6. Proc Natl Acad Sci U S A 95:3251–3256

März P, Otten U, Rose-John S (1999) Neuronal activities of IL-6 type cytokines often depend on soluble cytokine receptors. Eur J Neurosci 11:2995–3004

Matthews V, Schuster B, Schütze S, Bußmeyer I, Ludwig A, Hundhausen C, Sadowski T, Saftig P, Hartmann D, Kallen K-J, Rose-John S (2003) Cellular cholesterol depletion triggers shedding of the human interleukin-6 receptor by ADAM10 and ADAM17 (TACE). J Biol Chem 278:38829–38839

McLoughlin RM, Witowski J, Robson RL, Wilkinson TS, Hurst SM, Williams AS, Williams JD, Rose-John S, Jones SA, Topley N (2003) Interplay between IFN-gamma and IL-6 signaling governs neutrophil trafficking and apoptosis during acute inflammation. J Clin Invest 112:598–607

McLoughlin RM, Jenkins BJ, Grail D, Williams AS, Fielding CA, Parker CR, Ernst M, Topley N, Jones SA (2005) IL-6 trans-signaling via STAT3 directs T cell infiltration in acute inflammation. Proc Natl Acad Sci U S A 102:9589–9594

Mitani H, Katayama N, Araki H, Ohishi K, Kobayashi K, Susuki H, Nishii H, Masuya M, Yasukawa K, Minami N, Shiku H (2000) Activity of interleukin-6 in the differentiation of monocytes to macrophages and dendritic cells. Br J Haematol 109:288–295

Mitsuyama K, Tomiyasu N, Suzuki A, Takaki K, Takedatsu H, Masuda J, Yamasaki H, Matsumoto S, Tsuruta O, Toyonaga A, Sata M (2005) A form of circulating interleukin-6 receptor component soluble gp130 as a potential interleukin-6 inhibitor in inflammatory bowel disease. Clin Exp Immunol 143:125–131

Müllberg J, Althoff K, Jostock T, Rose-John S (2000) The importance of shedding of membrane proteins for cytokine biology. Eur Cytokine Netw 11:27–38

Nowell MA, Richards PJ, Horiuchi S, Yamamoto N, Rose-John S, Topley N, Williams AS, Jones SA (2003) Soluble IL-6 receptor governs IL-6 activity in experimental arthritis: blockade of arthritis severity by soluble glycoprotein 130. J Immunol 171:3202–3209

Pasare C, Medzhitov R (2003) Toll pathway-dependent blockade of CD4+CD25+ T cell-mediated suppression by dendritic cells. Science 299:1033–1036

Peters M, Schirmacher P, Goldschmitt J, Odenthal M, Peschel C, Dienes HP, Fattori E, Ciliberto G, Meyer zum Büschenfelde KH, Rose-John S (1997) Extramedullary expansion of hematopoietic progenitor cells in IL-6/sIL-6R double transgenic mice. J Exp Med 185:755–766

Peters M, Müller A, Rose-John S (1998) Interleukin-6 and soluble interleukin-6 receptor: direct stimulation of gp130 and hematopoiesis. Blood 92:3495–3504

Pflanz S, Tacken I, Grötzinger J, Jacques Y, Dahmen H, Heinrich PC, Müller-Newen G (1999) A fusion protein of interleukin-11 and soluble interleukin-11 receptor acts as a superagonist on cells expressing gp130. FEBS Lett 450:117–122

Pflanz S, Hibbert L, Mattson J, Rosales R, Vaisberg E, Bazan JF, Phillips JH, McClanahan TK, de Waal Malefyt R, Kastelein RA (2004) WSX-1 and glycoprotein 130 constitute a signal-transducing receptor for IL-27. J Immunol 172:2225–2231

Richards PJ, Nowell MA, Horiuchi S, McLoughlin RM, Fielding CA, Grau S, Yamamoto N, Ehrmann M, Williams AS, Rose-John S, Topley N, Jones SA (2006) Baculovirus expression and functional characterization of a recombinant human soluble gp130 isoform and its role in the regulation of L-6 trans-signaling. Arthr Rheumat 54:1662–1672

Romano M, Sironi M, Toniatti C, Polentarutti N, Fruscella P, Ghezzi P, Faggioni R, Luini W, van Hinsbergh V, Sozzani S, Bussolino F, Poli V, Ciliberto G, Mantovani A (1997) Role of IL-6 and its soluble receptor in induction of chemokines and leukocyte recruitment. Immunity 6:315–325

Rose-John S (2001) Coordination of interleukin-6 biology by membrane bound and soluble receptors. Adv Exp Med Biol 495:145–151

Rose-John S (2002) GP130 stimulation and the maintenance of stem cells. Trends Biotechnol 20:417–419

Rose-John S, Heinrich PC (1994) Soluble receptors for cytokines and growth factors: generation and biological function. Biochem J 300:281–290

Scheller J, Schuster B, Hölscher C, Yoshimoto T, Rose-John S (2005) No inhibition of IL-27 signaling by soluble gp130. Biochem Biophys Res Commun 326:724–728

Sun Y, März P, Otten U, Ge J, Rose-John S (2002) The effect of gp130 stimulation on glutamate-induced excitotoxicity in primary hippocampal neurons. Biochem Biophys Res Commun 295:532–539

Taga T, Kishimoto T (1997) gp130 and the interleukin-6 family of cytokines. Annu Rev Immunol 15:797–819

Taga T, Hibi M, Hirata Y, Yamasaki K, Yasukawa K, Matsuda T, Hirano T, Kishimoto T (1989) Interleukin-6 triggers the association of its receptor with a possible signal transducer, gp130. Cell 58:573–581

Teague TK, Schaefer BC, Hildeman D, Bender J, Mitchell T, Kappler JW, Marrack P (2000) Activation-induced inhibition of interleukin 6-mediated T cell survival and signal transducer and activator of transcription 1 signaling. J Exp Med 191:915–926

Ulich TR, Yin S, Guo K, Yi ES, Remick D, del Castillo J (1991) Intratracheal injection of endotoxin and cytokines. Interleukin-6 and transforming growth factor beta inhibit acute inflammation. Am J Pathol 138:1097–1102

6 Prevention of Hepatocellular Carcinoma in Chronic Viral Hepatitis Patients with Cirrhosis by Carotenoid Mixture

Hoyoku Nishino

Recent Results in Cancer Research, Vol. 174
© Springer-Verlag Berlin Heidelberg 2007

Abstract

Since the incidence of hepatocellular carcinoma in chronic viral hepatitis patients with cirrhosis is very high, it is valuable to develop effective methods for its prevention. In the present study, the effect of a carotenoid mixture on hepatocellular carcinoma development was examined. Patients were randomly divided into two groups and treated with a carotenoid mixture in addition to conventional antisymptomatic treatment, or antisymptomatic treatment alone. Cumulative incidence of hepatocellular carcinoma development was periodically analyzed using the Kaplan-Meier method. Significantly lower incidence was observed in the carotenoid-treated group compared with the control group in the analysis at year 4.

Introduction

Infection with hepatitis virus is well recognized as one of the important risk factors for liver cancer. In Japan, hepatocellular carcinoma associated with hepatitis C virus infection is continuously increasing, and its prevention is now an urgent social problem. Average incidence of hepatocellular carcinoma in a year has been reported to be about 7% in chronic hepatitis C patients with cirrhosis. In the case of hepatitis B infection, Southeast Asia and Africa are known as severely invaded areas, and in fact, the incidence of liver cancer is very high in these countries. Therefore, we have tried to develop effective methods for prevention against hepatitis virus infection-related liver cancer.

Our previous clinical investigation showed that the serum level of hydrocarbon carotenoids such as beta-carotene, alpha-carotene, and lycopene is lower in liver cancer patients with viral hepatitis than in healthy individuals.

In addition to this clinical observation, we have also found that β-carotene and α-carotene suppressed liver carcinogenesis in animal experiments (Murakoshi et al. 1992). It is particularly interesting that treatment with a mixture of these carotenoids resulted in more effective inhibition than each carotenoid alone. For example, palm fruit carotene mixture, which consisted of β-carotene, α-carotene, and a small portion of other carotenoids such as lycopene showed the highest suppressive effect on liver carcinogenesis in mice compared with β-carotene alone or α-carotene alone at the same dose. Therefore, it may be possible that combined use of various carotenoids improves the efficacy of cancer prevention. It is also possible that a small portion of other carotenoids has potent activity in suppressing liver carcinogenesis. In fact, lycopene was proven to have very high potency in preventing liver cancer in animal experiments (Nishino 1997).

These clinical and experimental observations prompted us to evaluate the effect of a carotenoid mixture on hepatocellular carcinoma development in viral hepatitis patients.

Protocol and Results of the Clinical Trial

The study protocol was approved by the review board for research on human subjects at National Shikoku Cancer Center, Japan. Written informed consent was obtained from each patient.

Patients of viral hepatitis with cirrhosis (more than 90% of these individuals were hepatitis C virus-infected patients) were randomly divided into two groups (Table 1). Patients in group 1 (46 patients) were administered the carotenoid mixture in addition to conventional antisymptomatic treatment. The daily dose of carotenoids was 20 mg in total. The carotenoid mixture contained lycopene 10 mg, β-carotene 6 mg, α-carotene 3 mg, and other small portions of carotenoids such as phytoene and phytofluene, 1 mg. These carotenoids were packed into capsules with α-tocopherol (daily dose, 50 mg). Patients in group 2 (46 patients as the control group) were treated with antisymptomatic treatment alone. Placebo was not used in this study.

These groups were followed up for 2–5 years (3.4 years on average), and hepatocellular carcinoma development was clinically analyzed and recorded. Cumulative incidence of hepatocellular carcinoma development was plotted using the Kaplan-Meier method and compared between the two groups. In this plotting, one patient in group 2 was omitted, since this patient developed liver cancer within 6 months after the entry in the clinical trial.

In the 4th annual analysis, a significant reduction of hepatocellular carcinoma development was observed in group 1 (carotenoid group), as shown in Fig. 1. A greater than 50% reduction of hepatocellular carcinoma incidence was found at 4 years in the group receiving carotenoids, i.e., cumulative incidence of hepatocellular carcinoma in group 1 was 12.3%, while that in group 2 was 34.6% (p<0.02).

Since the effect of the carotenoid mixture treatment was proven to be significant in the annual analysis at year 4, the clinical trial was finalized at this time point, although the duration of the carotenoid administration in the original protocol was scheduled to last an additional 3 years.

Improvement of Cancer Preventive Efficacy by Additional Use of Other Food Factors

Besides hydrocarbon carotenoids, some xanthophylls such as β-cryptoxanthin are also found to be lower in the blood of liver cancer patients with viral hepatitis than in healthy individuals (Jinno et al. 1997). Therefore, additional use of β-cryptoxanthin may improve the efficacy for liver cancer prevention.

We have also found experimentally that myo-inositol may be useful for the prevention of liver carcinogenesis. Since myo-inositol has been known to prevent fatty liver as well as cancer in several organs, such as colon, we evaluated the effect of oral administration of myo-inositol using the experimental model of spontaneous liver carcinogenesis in C3H/He male mice (Nishino et al. 1999). The mean number of liver tumors was significantly decreased by myo-inositol treatment as compared with that in the control group; the control group developed 7.82 tumors/mouse, whereas the 1% myo-inositol-treated group had 0.77 tumors/mouse (p<0.01, Student's t-test).

Based on these clinical and experimental data, we have planned a new clinical trial. Since β-cryptoxanthin is rich in Japanese tangerine oranges, we decided to use them as a form of juice for a clinical trial. The experimental sample contained 3 mg of β-cryptoxanthin and 1 g of myo-inositol in 190 ml canned juice. Hepatitis C virus-infected patients with cirrhosis were ad-

Table 1 Subjects for clinical trial

Group	N	Age	AST (GOT) IU/l	ALT (GPT) IU/l	Platelet(x10⁴/μl)	Observation period (years)
1	46	61.4±9.7	75±44	79±51	10.1±4.1	3.4±1.5
2	46	59.9±8.9	70±37	67±46	10.4±4.9	3.3±1.4
Total	92	60.6±9.3	73±41	73±41	10.3±4.5	3.4±1.5

Mean±SD

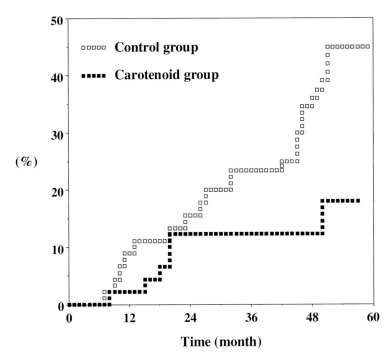

Fig. 1 Effect of carotenoids/ α-tocopherol mixture on hepatocellular carcinoma development in chronic viral hepatitis patients with cirrhosis. Cumulative incidence (%) of hepatocellular carcinoma was plotted using the Kaplan-Meier method and compared between two groups: the carotenoid-treated group and the control group

ministered this preparation (one can per day), in addition to capsules of a carotenoid/ α-tocopherol mixture. In the annual analysis at year 1, none from treated group (n=30) had developed hepatocellular carcinoma. This clinical trial is now on-going.

Analysis of the Mechanism of Action

Carotenoids are well known as natural antioxidants and have potent activity to scavenge free radicals. Since inflammation is accompanied with excess production of free radicals, the scavenging activity of carotenoids against free radicals seems to play an important role in prevention of hepatitis virus infection-related liver carcinogenesis. In addition to the free radical scavenging activity, carotenoid-induced modulation of the expression of various genes also seems to be important. For example, lycopene has been found to increase the promoter activity of anti-oncogenes, such as the RB gene and the Waf1 gene (Table 2).

Discussion

Interferon is well known as an effective treatment for hepatitis patients and has been proven to prevent hepatocellular carcinoma. However, large numbers of patients are nonresponders for interferon treatment. Although repeating administration of interferon is recommended for these cases, it is not always possible to continue. These patients are a high-risk group for future development of hepatocellular carcinoma, and alternative treatments should be tried. In such cases, administration of a carotenoid mixture seems to be valuable.

Table 2 Effect of lycopene on promoter activity of anti-oncogenes

Anti-oncogene	Concentration of lycopene	Induction (fold increased)
RB	2 μM	1.42
	5 μM	3.32
	10 μM	4.04
	20 μM	4.81
Waf1	10 μM	3.49

Lycopene was treated for 24 h.

At present we have selected lycopene, β-carotene, α-carotene, and β-cryptoxanthin as the major components for the carotenoid mixture. In addition to these elements, other natural carotenoids such as zeaxanthin, astaxanthin, and fucoxanthin may also be valuable for clinical use, since these carotenoids showed potent activity in reducing liver carcinogenesis in experimental studies, as shown in Table 3.

In the present study, mixture of carotenoids was packed into capsules with α-tocopherol. α-Tocopherol, a natural antioxidant, was used as a stabilizer for the carotenoid mixture, which is highly sensitive to oxidative stress. In addition, α-tocopherol itself has been proven to have some preventive activity for liver carcinogenesis (Tsuda et al. 1997). Recently, it was also found that tocotrienols, the family of natural vitamin E distributed in various foods with tocopherols, showed potent preventive activity against liver carcinogenesis (Wada et al. 2005). Therefore, combinational use of tocotrienols may be useful for the improvement of efficacy.

Herbal medicine, Sho-saiko-to (TJ-9), has also been reported to prevent hepatocellular carcinoma (Oka et al. 1995). It is of interest that glycyrrhizin, an active component in Sho-saiko-to, was proven experimentally to have preventive activity against liver carcinogenesis (Table 4).

For the mechanism of action analysis, genomics and proteomics seem to be valuable. In fact, comprehensive analysis using DNA array and protein-antibody array has shown the network-like modulation of cellular regulatory systems.

Table 3 Effect of carotenoid on spontaneous liver carcinogenesis in C3H/He male mice

Experiment	n	Percentage of Tumor-bearing mice	Mean number of tumors/mouse	(Inhibition %)
Exp. 1				
Control	14	35.7	1.75	
+Zeaxanthin	12	8.3	0.08	(95.4)
Exp. 2				
Control	15	53.3	0.87	
+Astaxanthin	15	26.7	0.27	(69.0)
Exp. 3				
Control	15	100	5.93	
+Fucoxanthin	15	86.7	3.07	(48.2)

Exp. 1: Zeaxanthin (0.005% in drinking water) was given during the entire experimental period (40 weeks).

Exp. 2: Astaxanthin (0.2 mg suspended in 0.2 ml of corn oil, intragastric gavage, three times per week) was given during the entire experimental period (40 weeks).

Exp. 3: Fucoxanthin (0.001% in drinking water) was given during the entire experimental period (40 weeks).

Table 4 Effect of glycyrrhizin on spontaneous liver carcinogenesis in C3H/He male mice

Exp.	n	Percentage of tumor-bearing mice	Mean number of tumors/mouse	(Inhibition %)
Control	15	80.0	3.07	
+Glycyrrhizin	15	73.3	1.40	(54.4)

Glycyrrhizin (0.005% in drinking water) was given during the entire experimental period (40 weeks).

For example, DNA array analysis for β-cryptoxanthin showed the significant induction of expression in various important genes, such as p16 and p73, and proteome analysis for tocotrienol revealed the increase in pRB2 protein induction (data, not shown). It is of interest that the pattern of modulation for DNA and protein expression has been proven to be unique and specific for each carotenoid. These results support the combined administration of these carotenoids against cancer as a reasonable strategy.

Conclusion

In conclusion, a mixture of various carotenoids seems to be promising for the prevention of liver cancer in hepatitis virus-infected patients with cirrhosis, although a further extended clinical trial is needed to confirm and improve the efficacy of this method.

Acknowledgements

This study was carried out in collaboration with Dr. K. Jinno, Dr. H. Ishikawa and the research groups of Kyoto Prefectural University of Medicine, National Cancer Center Research Institute, National Shikoku Cancer Center, Fruit Tree Research Institute, and Meiji Pharmaceutical University. This work was supported in part by grants from the Program for Promotion of Basic Research Activities for Innovative Biosciences (ProBRAIN), the Ministry of Agriculture, Forestry, and Fisheries, the Ministry of Education, Culture, Sports, Science and Technology, and the Institute of Free Radical Control (IFRC), Japan.

References

Jinno K, Tanimizu M, Ishikawa H, Nishino H, Sakamoto H, Ohshima T (1997) Interventional trial for prevention of hepatocellular carcinoma. J Clin Sci 33:952–963

Murakoshi M, Nishino H, Satomi Y, Takayasu J, Hasegawa T, Tokuda H, Iwashima A, Okuzumi J, Okabe H, Kitano H, Iwasaki R (1992) Potent preventive action of α-carotene against carcinogenesis: Spontaneous liver carcinogenesis and promoting stage of lung and skin carcinogenesis in mice are suppressed more effectively by α-carotene than β-carotene. Cancer Res 52:6583–6587

Nishino H (1997) Cancer prevention by natural carotenoids. J Cell Biochem 27:86–91

Nishino H, Murakoshi M, Masuda M, Tokuda H, Satomi Y, Onozuka M, Yamaguchi S, Bu P, Tsuruta A, Nosaka K, Baba M, Takasuka N (1999) Suppression of lung and liver carcinogenesis in mice by oral administration of myo-inosito. Anticancer Res 19:3663–3664

Oka H, Yamamoto S, Kuroki T, Harihara S, Marumo T, Kim SR, Monna T, Kobayashi K, Tango T (1995) Prospective study of chemoprevention of hepatocellular carcinoma with Sho-saiko-to (TJ-9). Cancer 76:743–749

Tsuda H, Iwahori Y, Hori T, Asamoto M, Baba-Toriyama H, Kim DJ, Kim JM, Uehara N, Iigo M, Takasuka N, Murakoshi M, Nishino H, Kakizoe T (1997) Chemopreventive potential of α-carotene against mouse liver and lung tumor development: Comparison with β-carotene and α-tocopherol. In: Ohigashi H, Osawa T, Terao J, Watanabe S, Yoshikawa T (eds) Food factors for cancer prevention. Springer-Verlag, Tokyo, pp 529–532

Wada S, Satomi Y, Murakoshi M, Noguchi N, Yoshikawa T, Nishino H (2005) Tumor suppressive effects of tocotrienol in vivo and in vitro. Cancer Lett 229:181–191

7 Cox-2 and Cancer Chemoprevention: Picking up the Pieces

Monica M. Bertagnolli

Recent Results in Cancer Research, Vol. 174
© Springer-Verlag Berlin Heidelberg 2007

Abstract

Inhibitors of prostaglandin synthesis show great promise as cancer chemopreventive agents, with efficacy demonstrated in randomized clinical trials. Unfortunately, these agents also cause toxicity in susceptible individuals. The recent reports of cardiovascular adverse events in patients treated with selective Cox-2 inhibitors for colorectal adenoma prevention remind us that all therapies carry risks as well as benefits. This article will discuss the biologic rationale for using selective Cox-2 inhibitors in cancer chemoprevention, and outline new avenues of research necessary to allow their successful use in patients at risk for colorectal cancer.

Introduction

Inducible cyclooxygenase (Cox-2) is a promising target for chemoprevention, with potential for efficacy against a wide range of epithelial tumors. Recent clinical trials of drugs that selectively inhibited Cox-2 showed increased rates of serious cardiovascular disease in patients using these drugs for colorectal cancer chemoprevention for 3 years of continuous drug use. This result led to an examination of the safety and efficacy of all nonsteroidal anti-inflammatory drugs (NSAIDs) and a reassessment of the risks and benefits of selective Cox-2 inhibitors for cancer prevention. This paper will discuss the rationale for directing anti-tumor therapy against Cox-2.

NSAIDs and Colorectal Cancer Chemoprevention

In the early 1980s, a surgeon named William Waddell administered the nonselective NSAID, sulindac, to a patient with familial adenomatous polyposis (FAP). His intention was to treat this patient's desmoid tumor, an FAP-associated neoplasm composed of cells exhibiting the histologic characteristics of a fibrotic or inflammatory process. Sulindac did not alter the natural history of the desmoid tumor, but this drug did induce significant regression of the patient's numerous rectal polyps (Waddell and Loughry 1983). This was the first clinical observation of the chemopreventive potential of NSAIDs.

The primary therapeutic activity of NSAIDs involves inhibition of the cyclooxygenase enzyme, thereby preventing production of active arachidonic acid metabolites from cell membrane phospholipids. Tissue-specific products of cyclooxygenase activity, particularly prostaglandin E_2 (PGE_2), are powerful mediators of inflammation and inhibitors of cellular immune response. At the time of Dr. Waddell's clinical report, the link between epithelial tumors and chronic inflammation was well recognized. In discussing his observation, Dr. Waddell postulated that adenomas were caused by PGE_2-mediated promotion of DNA synthesis and cell proliferation. He theorized that NSAID-associated tumor regression occurred via arrest of tumor cells in the G_1 phase of the cell cycle, an activity observed following prostaglandin inhibition in tumor cell culture studies (Waddell and Loughry 1983). Work over the past 2 decades showed that

PGE_2 mediates a number of additional activities related to tumor formation. PGE_2 binds to specific G-protein-coupled receptors on the epithelial cell surface, initiating signaling cascades that promote cell growth and motility (Coleman et al. 1994). In cell lines, PGE_2 suppresses apoptosis by increasing expression of Bcl-2 and also increases expression of activated MAP kinase, promotes cell migration/invasiveness, and activates epidermal growth factor receptor (EGFR) (Hixon et al. 1994; Pai et al. 2002, 2003; Sheng et al. 1998; Tsujii and DuBois 1995). In addition, PGE_2 induces angiogenesis, thereby providing a mechanism for growth of both primary and metastatic disease (Form and Auerbach 1983; Gately and Kerbel 2003). In animal tumor models, administration of NSAIDs in doses that inhibit tumor formation is associated with reversal of these PGE_2-mediated effects (Buchanan et al. 2003; Jacoby et al. 2000; Leahy et al. 2002).

Colon Cancer Prevention Studies with Nonselective NSAIDs

Throughout the 1990s, data from cancer epidemiology strongly supported a role for NSAIDs in colorectal cancer prevention. Large studies found that frequent NSAID use was associated with an approximately 50% reduction in premalignant adenomas, carcinomas, and even death due to colorectal cancer (Hawk et al. 2004). Animal colon cancer models, both genetic and carcinogen-induced, also showed this relationship. Dr. Waddell's initial observation was confirmed in prospective randomized trials of sulindac for management of patients with FAP (Giardiello et al. 1993; Labayle et al. 1991). These studies documented treatment-associated regression of pre-existing adenomas in FAP patients using sulindac, with this response achieved in approximately 30% of patients over 6 months of treatment. The next goal was to apply this finding to prevention of sporadic disease. Unfortunately, sulindac was poorly tolerated during long-term administration, with many patients experiencing gastrointestinal upset and even episodes of gastric ulceration and bleeding. Because of its better overall tolerance, aspirin was chosen for prevention trials in patients with sporadic colorectal adenomas. Three prospective randomized trials of aspirin have been completed. Overall, these show a roughly 20% reduction in incidence of newly detected colorectal adenomas in patients with a prior history of colorectal adenomas or colorectal cancer (Baron et al. 2002; Benamouzig et al. 2003; Sandler et al. 2003) One study, involving approximately 1,100 patients with sporadic adenomas, showed a significant decrease in recurrent adenomas in a low-dose aspirin arm (81 mg per day; relative risk, 0.81, 95% confidence interval, 0.69;0.96), but not a high-dose aspirin arm (325 mg per day; relative risk, 0.96; 95% confidence interval, 0.81;1.13) (Baron et al. 2002). Nevertheless, the general agreement between these three studies combined with strong epidemiological data led researchers to conclude that aspirin effectively prevented a subset of sporadic colorectal adenomas.

Rationale for Selective Cox-2 Inhibition

In the early 1990s, researchers identified a second cyclooxygenase isoform, termed cyclooxygenase-2 (Cox-2) (O'Banion et al. 1991). Unlike Cox-1, which was constitutively expressed, Cox-2 was induced in response to inflammatory mediators, mitogens, and other cellular stressors. Nonselective NSAIDs, because they inhibit both cyclooxygenase forms, are associated with several serious side effects related to Cox-1 homeostatic activities. These include gastrointestinal ulceration, bleeding susceptibility, and renal toxicity. Selective Cox-2 inhibitors were developed to avoid these complications in patients who required frequent or long-term NSAID use, such as those with severe arthritis or chronic inflammatory conditions. In 1998, these drugs were approved by regulatory agencies for use in patients with severe arthritis.

Studies conducted in the 1980s showed that epithelial tumors contain increased levels of PGE_2 compared to normal tissues (Balch et al. 1982; Bennett et al. 1977). Cox-2 is produced in response to cellular mitogens; therefore it was not surprising that Cox-2 levels were low or absent in normal tissues, and strongly expressed in neoplastic or inflammatory lesions. Preclinical studies showed that Cox-2 mediates tissue-specific prostaglandin and prostacyclin production, and as a result promotes angiogenesis, suppresses apoptosis, and may increase tumor invasiveness by increasing matrix metalloproteinase production. Cox-2 also exhibits peroxidase activity, and as a result may potentiate formation of DNA-damaging agents in susceptible tissues (Fosslein 2000; Seno et al. 2002; Taketo 1998).

Clinical trials of selective Cox-2 inhibitors for prevention of sporadic colorectal adenomas were initiated in 1999. Part of the rationale for these studies was the reduced risk of gastrointestinal, hemorrhagic, or renal toxicity expected for these agents compared to nonselective NSAIDs. Additional data from animal models indicated that selective Cox-2 inhibitors would have greater anti-tumor efficacy than nonselective NSAIDs. In one particularly striking preclinical study, mice with a germline Apc mutation ($Apc\Delta^{716}$) were crossed with animals bearing targeted deletion of the murine Cox-2 gene (Pghs-2–/–). These mice showed a strong gene–dose response to Cox-2 loss(Oshima et al. 1996). The $Apc\Delta^{716}$ Pghs-2+/+ mice developed 652 intestinal tumors on average, in contrast to 224 for $Apc\Delta^{716}$ Pghs-2+/– mice and 93 for $Apc\Delta^{716}$ Pghs-2–/– mice. Tumor reductions of a similar magnitude were observed following treatment of $Apc\Delta^{716}$ mice with a selective Cox-2 inhibitor (Oshima et al. 1996).

Human Trials of Selective Cox-2 Inhibitors

In 1998, celecoxib and rofecoxib were approved by regulatory agencies for treatment of patients with severe arthritis. The first human study of a selective Cox-2 inhibitor for cancer prevention involved 83 patients with familial adenomatous polyposis who had measurable adenomas in the colorectum (Steinbach et al. 2000). This study, reported in 2000, showed that celecoxib use at 400 mg twice daily over a 6-month period produced a 30.7% reduction in polyp burden, where polyp burden was defined as the sum of the diameters of all polyps identified. Three multicenter randomized trials of selective Cox-2 inhibitors for prevention of sporadic colorectal adenomas were initiated in 1999–2000. These studies examined the rates of adenoma detection

by colonoscopy over a 3-year observation period of uninterrupted selective Cox-2 inhibitor use. All patients enrolled in these trials had a prior history of colorectal adenomas. The first trial initiated was a study of rofecoxib in 2,586 patients in the United States. Unfortunately, even before the final efficacy results from this study were known, the investigators reported that long-term rofecoxib use was associated with a significant increase in serious cardiovascular side effects, including myocardial infarction, stroke, and death due to cardiovascular disease (Bresalier et al. 2005). Shortly afterward, this observation was seconded by data from a chemoprevention study involving another selective Cox-2 inhibitor, celecoxib (Solomon et al. 2005). These reports had a profound impact upon the medical and clinical research communities. Selective Cox-2 inhibitors had been widely marketed as safer alternatives to nonselective NSAIDs, and at the time of these reports these drugs were used in many thousands of patients worldwide. These reports of toxicity led clinicians to re-evaluate their use, particularly for chronic treatment of patients with pre-existing cardiovascular disease. At the time of these reports, numerous cancer chemoprevention studies using celecoxib were underway, including trials involving patients with actinic keratoses, superficial bladder tumors, Barrett esophagus, and oral epithelial tumors. Concerns over potential cardiovascular toxicity in these studies led to their suspension in December, 2004. Merck, Inc., the maker of rofecoxib, withdrew this drug from the market. It is interesting to note that, even though nonselective NSAIDs have been in clinical use for many decades, there are no similar long-term cardiovascular risk data for these drugs.

Optimizing Risks and Benefits of Selective Cox-2 Inhibitors for Colorectal Cancer Prevention

At the time of this writing, final data reporting the efficacy of selective Cox-2 inhibitors for colorectal cancer prevention have not yet been published. Fortunately, these studies were all near completion at the time that drug-associated increased cardiovascular risk was identified. As a result, these studies will produce valid efficacy data for the primary prevention endpoint, which involves colonoscopic detection of adenomas after 3 years of planned study drug use. Based upon their demonstrated efficacy in patients with FAP, we can assume that selective Cox-2 inhibitors will be at least as effective or more so than nonselective NSAIDs for colorectal adenoma prevention.

In the short term, the continued use of the selective Cox-2 inhibitors for cancer chemoprevention will depend upon the balance of risks and benefits revealed in these studies. Balancing risks and benefits is a complicated process, and one that must be approached with caution. It is important to remember that the currently available studies were designed to assess prevention of colorectal adenomas, not to determine the cardiovascular effects of selective Cox-2 inhibitors. In considering the anticipated data, it stands to reason that individuals with the highest risk of colorectal neoplasia and the lowest risk of cardiovascular disease will benefit most from selective Cox-2 inhibitors. There are, however, multiple factors involved in risk stratification, and at this time we will be forced to draw conclusions based upon incomplete data.

Some of the variables involved in determining risk and benefit are evident before drug treatment begins. In colorectal tumorigenesis, we know that small tubular adenomas rarely if ever progress to invasive cancer. In addition, it is uncommon for a patient with a single small tubular adenoma to develop recurrent colorectal adenomas. Data from large colonoscopy trials show that patients with multiple adenomas, single adenomas 1 cm or more in diameter, or adenomas with villous or tubulovillous histology are most likely to develop recurrent disease. In evaluating the efficacy of a chemopreventive agent, therefore, it is important to select a study cohort with these characteristics and to evaluate the ability of the drug to inhibit these more advanced lesions. Within the large adenoma prevention trials, it may also be possible to cautiously examine the relationship between pre-existing cardiovascular risk factors, such as diabetes or a history of myocardial infarction, and the risk of cardiovascular complications while using selective Cox-2 inhibitors.

Developing Safer Anti-Cox-2 Treatments

In addition to optimizing patient selection, future work should address ways to reduce the toxicity of selective Cox-2 inhibitors, yet maintain their anti-tumor efficacy. One promising avenue involves altering drug regimens. Carcinogenesis is a decades-long process, and during this time neoplastic lesions progress from initiated but histologically normal cells to increasingly aberrant adenomas to invasive cancer. The available studies of sporadic disease addressed adenoma prevention rather than regression of existing tumors, and the regimens tested consisted of uninterrupted drug use over a 3-year interval. Patients with FAP who were treated with celecoxib demonstrate significant regression of pre-existing adenomas. Therefore, it may not be necessary or even desirable for chemoprevention drugs to be administered in an uninterrupted fashion. For example, a dosing regimen of 6 months on drug with 6 months off drug in patients at high risk for colorectal cancer may permit regression of initiated and/or adenomatous lesions during the treatment phase that do not recur to a significant extent during the rest phase. Intermittent timing of drug use may also reduce toxicity. The time course of development of cardiovascular toxicity in patients treated with selective Cox-2 inhibitors is unknown. These effects, however, were not identified in short-term safety analyses conducted for celecoxib in arthritis patients, and in the chemoprevention trials became evident only after 12–18 months of continuous drug use. Provision of a drug holiday in a chemopreventive regimen may decrease toxicity by reducing cumulative drug exposure, and may even allow recovery of normal homeostatic mechanisms that reduce cardiovascular risk.

It is clear that we must understand the mechanism of activity of cardiovascular toxicity produced by selective Cox-2 inhibitors in order to develop safer anti-Cox-2 regimens. For example, another possibility for reducing cardiovascular risk in Cox-2 chemoprevention may be found in the observation that selective Cox-2 inhibitors promote both hypertension and more advanced cardiovascular disease. If these two conditions are causally linked in users of selective Cox-2 inhibitors, it may be possible to use blood pressure monitoring to identify patients who should discontinue or reduce drug use. The data necessary to draw valid conclusions concerning the cardiovascular risks of selective Cox-2 inhibitors must come from well-designed prospective trials to specifically address cardiovascular endpoints.

Selective Cox-2 inhibitors are not the only compounds that may inhibit the deleterious effects of PGE_2. For example, signaling events downstream of PGE_2 provide additional opportunities for intervention. The targeted inhibitors of related signaling molecules such as EGFR, MAP kinase, and mTOR provide new agents for investigation in chemoprevention trials. An improved understanding of prostaglandin degradation pathways may also be useful. For example, 15-hydroxyprostaglandin dehydrogenase (15-PGDH) is an endogenous Cox-2 antagonist that is downregulated in intestinal tumors (Backlund et al. 2005). 5-PGDH is an NAD+-dependent rate-limiting enzyme mediating the degradation of PGE_2 (Tai et al. 2002), and agents that upregulate 15-PGDH activity include inhibitors of epidermal growth factor receptor activity (Backlund et al. 2005) and the tumor suppressor, TGF-β (Yan et al. 2004). Targeting 15-PGDH or related enzymes may therefore be beneficial in preserving tissue-specific prostaglandin function yet eliminating excess prostaglandin production that is associated with tumorigenesis. Given the deleterious effects associated with chronic suppression of any cell signaling process, new therapies should focus upon restoring the balance of factors found in healthy tissue, rather than chronically suppressing a particular component.

Conclusion

Data from animal models and human trials indicate that Cox-2 is a very important target for cancer prevention. The finding of increased cardiovascular toxicity in patients treated with selective Cox-2 inhibitors for colorectal cancer prevention reminds us of important lessons already learned in breast, lung, and prostate chemoprevention trials, namely that no drug is entirely without risk. In this particular instance, the long-term nature of chemoprevention studies unexpectedly benefited society by identifying serious adverse events associated with a commonly used medication. This should not deter us from the important work of cancer prevention. Despite a newly observed association between long-term selective Cox-2 inhibitor use and cardiovascular disease, Cox-2 remains an important target for cancer prevention.

References

Backlund MG, Mann JR, Holla VR, Buchanan G, Tai HH et al (2005) 12-Hydroxyprostaglandin dehydrogenase is down-regulated in colorectal cancer. J Biol Chem 280:3217–3223

Balch CM, Dougherty PA, Tilden AB (1982) Excessive prostaglandin E_2 production by suppressor monocytes in head and neck cancer patients. Ann Surg 196:645–650

Baron JA, Cole BF, Mott LA (2002) Aspirin chemoprevention of colorectal adenomas. Proceed Am Asso Can Res 43:669

Benamouzig R, Deyra J, Martin A, Girard B, Jullian E et al (2003) Daily soluble aspirin and prevention of colorectal adenoma recurrence: One year results of the APACC trial. Gastroenterology 125:328–336

Bennett A, Tacca MD, Stamford IF, Zebro T (1977) Prostaglandins from tumour of human large bowel. Br J Cancer 6:881–884

Bresalier RS, Sandler RS, Quan H, Bolognese JA, Oxenius B et al (2005) Cardiovascular events associated with rofecoxib in a colorectal adenoma chemoprevention trial. N Engl J Med 352:1092–1102

Buchanan FG, Wang D, Bargiacci F, DuBois RN (2003) Prostaglandin E2 regulates cell migration via the intracellular activation of the epidermal growth factor receptor. J Biol Chem 278:35451–35457

Coleman RA, Smith WL, Narumya S (1994) IUP classification of prostanoid receptors: properties, distribution, and structure of the receptors and their subtypes. Pharm Rev 46:205–229

Form DM, Auerbach R (1983) PGE_2 and angiogenesis. Proc Soc Exp Biol Med 172:214–218

Fosslein E (2000) Biochemistry of cyclooxygenase (COX)-2 inhibitors and molecular pathology of COX-2 in neoplasia. Crit Rev Clin Lab Sci 37:431–502

Gately S, Kerbel R (2003) Therapeutic potential of selective cyclooxygenase-2 inhibitors in the management of tumor angiogenesis. Prog Exp Tumor Res 37:179–192

Giardiello FM, Hamilton SR, Krush AJ, Piantadosi S, Hylind LM et al (1993) Treatment of colonic and rectal adenomas with sulindac in familial adenomatous polyposis. N Engl J Med 328:1313–1316

Hawk ET, Umar A, Viner JL (2004) Colorectal cancer chemoprevention-an overview of the science. Gastroenterology 126:1423–1447

Hixon LJ, Alaberts DX, Krutzsch M, Einsphar J, Brendel K et al (1994) Antiproliferative effect of nonsteroidal anti-inflammatory drugs against human colon cancer cells. Cancer Epidemiol Biomarker Prev 3:433–438

Jacoby RF, Seibert K, Cole CE, Kelloff G, Lubet RA (2000) The cyclooxygenase-2 inhibitor celecoxib is a potent preventive and therapeutic agent in the min mouse model of adenomatous polyposis. Cancer Res 60:5040–5044

Labayle D, Fischer D, Vielh P, Drouhin F, Pariente A et al (1991) Sulindac causess regression of rectal polyps in familial adenomatous polyposis. Gastroenterology 101:635–639

Leahy JM, Ornberg RL, Wang Y, Zweifel BS, Koti AT, Masferrer JL (2002) Cyclooxygenase-2 inhibition by celecoxib reduces proliferation and induces apoptosis in angiogenic endothelial cells in vivo. Cancer Res 62:625–631

O'Banion MK, Sadowski HB, Winn V, Young DA (1991) A serum- and glucocorticoid-regulated 4-kilobase mRNA encodes a cyclooxygenase-related protein. J Biol Chem 266:23261–23267

Oshima M, Dinchuk JE, Kargman SL, Oshima H, Hancock B, Kwong E (1996) Suppression of intestinal polyposis in Apc delta knockout mice by inhibition of cyclooxygenase 2 (COX-2). Cell 87:803–809

Pai R, Sorgehan B, Szabo IL, Pavelka M, Baatar D, Tarnawski AS (2002) Prostaglandin E2 transactivates EGF receptor: a novel mechanism for promoting colon cancer growth and gastrointestinal hypertrophy. Nat Med 8:289–293

Pai R, Nakamura T, Moon WS, Tarnawski AS (2003) Prostaglandins promote colon cancer cell invasion; signaling by cross-talk between two distinct growth factor receptors. FASEB J 17:1640–1647

Sandler RS, Halabi S, Baron JA, Budinger S, Paskett E et al (2003) A randomized trial of aspirin to prevent colorectal adenomas in patients with previous colorectal cancer. N Engl J Med 348:883–890

Seno H, Oshima M, Ishikawa T, Oshima H, Takaku K, Chiba T (2002) Cyclooxygenase-2 and prostaglandin E2 receptor EP2-dependent angiogenesis in Apcdelta 716 mouse intestinal polyps. Cancer Res 62:506–511

Sheng H, Shao J, Morrow JD, Beauchamp RD, DuBois RN (1998) Modulation of apoptosis and Bcl-2 expression by prostaglandin E2 in human colon cancer cells. Cancer Res 58:362–366

Solomon SD, McMurray JJ, Pfeffer MA, Wittes J, Fowler R et al (2005) Cardiovascular risk associated with celecoxib in a clinical trial for colorectal adenoma prevention. N Engl J Med 352:1071–1080

Steinbach G, Lynch PM, Phillips RKS, Wallace MH, Hawk E et al (2000) The effect of celecoxib, a cyclooxygenase-2 inhibitor, in familial adenomatous polyposis. The New England Journal of Medicine 342:1946–1952

Tai HH, Ensor CM, Tong M, Zhou H, Yan F (2002) Prostaglandin metabolizing enzymes. Prostaglandins Other Lipid Mediat 68:483–493

Taketo MM (1998) Cyclooxygenase-2 inhibitors in tumorigenesis (Part II). J Natl Cancer Inst 90:1609–1620

Tsujii M, DuBois RN (1995) Alterations in cellular adhesion and apoptosis in epithelial cells over expressing prostaglanding endoperoxide synthase-2. Cell 83:493–501

Waddell WR, Loughry RW (1983) Sulindac for polyposis of the colon. J Surg Oncol 24:83–87

Yan M, Rerko RM, Platzer P, Dawson D, Willis J et al (2004) 15-Hydroxyprostaglandin dehydrogenase, a COX-2 oncogene antagonist, is a TGF-beta-induced suppressor of human gastrointestinal cancers. Proc Natl Acad Sci U S A 101:17468–17473

Part III Prevention of Female and Male Genital Cancers

8 Human Papillomavirus Vaccine: A New Chance to Prevent Cervical Cancer

Bradley J. Monk, Ali Mahdavi

Recent Results in Cancer Research, Vol. 174
© Springer-Verlag Berlin Heidelberg 2007

Abstract

Human papillomavirus (HPV) is a significant source of morbidity and mortality throughout the world and is the most common sexually transmitted infection in the United States. HPV is the primary etiologic agent of cervical cancer and dysplasia. Thus, cervical cancer and other HPV-associated malignancies might be prevented or treated by HPV vaccines. Recent research on the safety and efficacy of candidate prophylactic vaccines against HPV have shown very promising results, with nearly 100% efficacy in preventing the development of persistent infections and cervical dysplasia. Questions remain, however, concerning the duration of protection, vaccine acceptability, and feasibility of vaccine delivery in the developing world. Screening recommendations might also be modified based on the longer-term follow-up data and cost-effectiveness considerations, but some level of screening is likely to be required for decades following the implementation of vaccine programs.

Introduction

Cervical cancer is a leading cause of cancer mortality among women in developing countries. In the US, even though rates have declined over the past 50 years, there are still more than 9,000 cases of cervical cancer and more than 3,000 deaths from the disease annually (Jemal et al. 2006; Bosch and de Sanjose 2003). Over 99% of cervical cancers are linked to genital infection with HPV, which is the most common viral infection of the reproductive tract worldwide and infects an estimated 660 million people annually. Developed countries have greatly reduced deaths from cervical cancer through screening programs that allow early detection and treatment. However, the difficulties with establishing high-quality cytology-based services in developing countries has hampered the efforts to prevent cervical cancer worldwide. Vaccines against HPV infections have the potential to be a practical and cost-effective way to reduce the incidence of cervical cancer. This article reviews the current status of HPV vaccine development and highlights outstanding research questions. We also review available data on the epidemiology, pathogenesis, and immune responses to HPV infection. Finally, the acceptability and cost-effectiveness of HPV vaccines and the potential to integrate HPV vaccination with the existing immunization programs are discussed.

Human Papillomavirus

More than 40 different HPV types have been identified that infect the anogenital epithelia and other mucosal membranes. Some 13–18 of these types are recognized as high-oncogenic risk HPV types (Fig. 1). It is estimated that HPV-16 accounts for approximately 60% of cervical cancers, with HPV-18 adding another 10%–20%. Other high-risk types include types 31, 33, 35, 39, 45, 51, 52, 56, 58, 59, 68, and 73 (Jansen and Shaw 2004).

In general, HPV infects the basal cells of human epithelial surfaces. Infected basal cells divide; some progeny remain as infected basal cells, while others move away from the basement

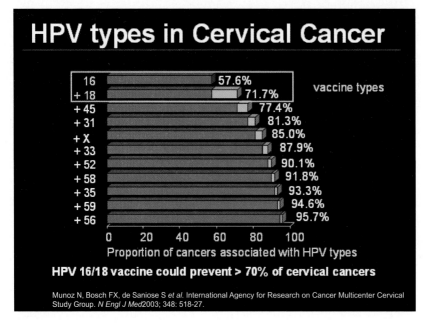

Fig. 1 HPV types in cervical cancer

membrane, differentiate, and become epithelial cells. Virus replication and assembly is tightly linked to the differentiation program of epithelial cells. Infectious virions are produced only in the terminally differentiated cell and are shed as virus-laden squamous cells.

The HPV genome codes for eight proteins (open reading frames). The late L1 and L2 genes code for the viral capsid proteins, the early proteins E1 and E2 are responsible for viral replication and transcription, and E4 seems to aid virus release from infected cells (Spence et al. 2005). The early genes of the high-risk HPV types (E6 and E7) encode the main transforming proteins. These genes are capable of immortalization of epithelial cells and are thought to play a role in the initiation of the oncogenic process. The protein products of these early genes interfere with the normal function of tumor suppressor genes. HPV E6 is able to interact with p53, leading to its dysfunction, thereby impairing its ability to block the cell cycle when DNA errors occur. E6 also keeps the telomerase length above its critical point, protecting the cell from apoptosis. HPV E7 binds to retinoblastoma protein (pRb) and

activates genes that start the cell cycle, leading to tissue proliferation. E5 has also been implicated in cellular transformation.

It is now widely accepted that high-risk HPV infections are a necessary, but not sufficient, cause of virtually all cases of cervical cancer worldwide (Fig. 2) and are a likely cause of a substantial proportion of other anogenital neoplasms and oral squamous cell carcinomas. An estimated 85% of anal cancers; 50% of the cancers of the vulva, vagina, and penis; 20% of oropharyngeal cancers; and 10% of laryngeal and esophageal cancers are attributable to HPV (CDC 2004).

Infection with low oncogenic risk HPV types, such as HPV 6 and 11, can cause benign lesions of the anogenital areas known as condylomata acuminata (genital warts), as well as a large proportion of low-grade squamous intraepithelial lesions of the cervix. Low-risk HPV clinical infections are responsible for substantial morbidity and invoke high costs associated with the treatment of clinically relevant lesions.

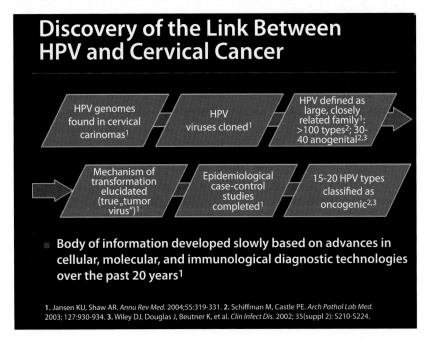

Fig. 2 HPV and cervical cancer

Epidemiology and Pathogenesis

There are an estimated 6.2 million new cases of oncogenic HPV infections occurring in the US each year, and approximately 20 million Americans are infected with HPV at any one time (CDC 2004). High-risk or oncogenic HPV infections can cause precancerous cervical lesions that are detected by routine cytological screening with the Papanicolaou (Pap) test. If these lesions are left undiagnosed they may progress to invasive cervical cancer within a few months to several years (depending on the precancerous lesion grade). Invasive cervical cancer is the second most common cancer in women worldwide. In the US, there are still more than 9,000 cases of cervical cancer and more than 3,000 deaths from the disease annually (Jemal et al. 2006).

Risk determinants for HPV infection that have been identified in various cross-sectional and prospective cohort studies include the number of sexual partners (lifetime and recent), age at first intercourse, smoking, oral contraceptive (OC) use, other sexually transmitted infections (STIs) (e.g., chlamydia and herpes simplex virus), chronic inflammation, immunosuppressive conditions including HIV infection, and parity (Trottier and Franco 2006). Nevertheless, in addition to sexual activity correlates, the most consistent determinant of HPV infection is age, with most studies indicating a sharp decrease in risk after the age of 30. The decrease in risk of HPV infection with increasing age seems to be independent of changes in sexual behavior, suggesting a role for immune response.

The peak in HPV prevalence among women younger than 30 years of age is followed by a decline in prevalence until age 45–50 and then a second peak in the peri- or postmenopausal years (Trottier and Franco 2006). Although the reason for this second, menopausal peak is not clear, it could be attributed to mechanisms, such as reactivation of latent infections acquired earlier in life due to a gradual loss of type-specific immunity or to acquisition of new infections due to sexual contacts with new partners later in life.

For each new case of invasive cancer found by Pap cytology, estimates suggest that there are approximately 50–100 squamous intraepithelial lesions. Women with these precancerous lesions need close monitoring by cytology and, if results persist, by colposcopy and biopsy.

Most infections seem to clear spontaneously; cohort studies have consistently found that only a small proportion of women positive for a given HPV type are found to have the same type in subsequent specimens (Richardson et al. 2003). Whether infections clear completely or the virus remains latent in basal cells at undetectable levels is a matter of debate and cannot be verified empirically. What is clear, however, is the fact that risk of subsequent cervical intraepithelial neoplasia (CIN) is proportional to the number of specimens testing positive for HPV (Ho et al. 1995). This suggests that carcinogenic development results from HPV infections that persist productively (i.e., with sustained viral replication within the squamous epithelium) for prolonged periods of time.

Mao et al. (2006) studied the natural history of high-risk HPVs in the control group of their HPV-16 L1 VLP vaccine clinical trial. They demonstrated that histologic changes become apparent shortly after HPV16 infection. In 11 of the 12 cases, CIN was identified 6–12 months after detection of HPV 16 DNA. Thus, years of persistent infection were not required before significant histologic changes such as CIN2/3 were seen. The median time to clearance of persistent infections (20.7 months) was similar to other previously published reports (Ho et al. 1995).

Immune Responses to HPV

Several studies have demonstrated that virus-neutralizing antibodies mediate protection of animals from experimental papillomavirus infection. For example, passive transfer of sera from virus-like particle (VLP)-vaccinated rabbits to naïve rabbits is sufficient for protection (Breitburd et al. 1995). Similarly, vaccination with L2 peptides protects rabbits from papillomas resulting from viral but not from viral DNA challenge, consistent with the protection mediated by neutralizing antibodies (Embers et al. 2002).

Most of those who develop benign HPV lesions eventually mount an effective cell-mediated immune response that results in lesion regression. Regression of anogenital warts is accompanied histologically by a CD4+ T cell-dominated Th1 response, and data from animal models suggest that the response is modulated by CD4+ T cell-dependent mechanisms. Failure to develop effective cell-mediated immunity to clear or control infection results in persistent infection and, in the case of the high-risk HPVs, an increased probability of progression to high-grade squamous intraepithelial lesions or invasive carcinoma. The increased prevalence of HPV infections and high-grade lesions in immunosuppressed individuals as a consequence of HIV infection demonstrates the importance of CD4+ T cells in the control of HPV infection. The prolonged duration of infection associated with HPV seems to be associated with effective evasion of innate immunity as reflected in the absence of inflammation during virus replication, assembly, and release, and downregulation of interferon secretion and response, thus delaying the activation of adaptive immunity (Stanley 2006b).

The well-characterized foreign (viral) antigens and the well-defined virological, genetic, and pathological progression of HPV have provided a unique opportunity to develop vaccines to prevent HPV infection and the associated pathology.

Vaccine Efficacy

Traditionally, in etiological and cancer prevention studies, the measurable endpoint to determine efficacy of an intervention has been the incidence of cancer itself. But as some cancers take a long time to develop and are not common in a given population, trials with an endpoint of invasive cancer can be prohibitively large and lengthy. In the case of cervical cancer, a disease that can be prevented through proper detection and treatment, a study endpoint of cancer can be ethically impracticable. The US Food and Drug administration Vaccine Advisory Committee has recommended using CIN2/3 as a surrogate marker for cervical cancer in HPV vaccine trials, as this lesion is the intermediate precursor to cervical cancer (Pratt et al. 2001). Since persistent infection with the same high-risk type is considered a predictor for high-grade cervical dysplasia and cancer, it might be a useful surrogate in future vaccine efficacy studies. Indeed, if vaccines prove to be effective against transient or especially persistent HPV infections, it is likely that they will protect women against cervical cancers as well.

Given the mode of transmission of HPV, vaccination of males needs to be considered. Males and females pass this virus back and forth, and logically one would anticipate more effective prevention of transmission if both genders were vaccinated. Because there is little detectable pathology associated with high-risk HPV in males, recommendations for male vaccination may require data from studies of prevention of infection. A vaccine against the nononcogenic HPV types 6 and 11 could be considered in the prophylaxis of genital warts in males to prevent the morbidity associated with this common infection (Shaw 2005).

Prophylactic Vaccine

In general, prophylactic vaccines induce the generation of neutralizing antibody to the pathogen and thus prevent disease on subsequent exposure. Studies exploiting natural papillomavirus infections in the dog, rabbit, and cow, together with HPV1 and HPV11 infections in humans (all situations in which adequate amounts of virus could be obtained), showed clearly that there were serum responses to viral capsid proteins in individuals who were or had been infected (Stanley 1997). In the animal models, seropositive individuals were resistant to subsequent viral challenge. Neutralizing antibody, directed to determinants on the viral capsid L1 protein, was generated in these individuals (Stanley 2006a).

These observations suggested that a vaccine generating such responses must contain L1 protein in the correctly folded, tertiary or native form. Technically, this was very difficult, but a major experimental breakthrough showed that the L1 protein, when expressed by vectors such as recombinant baculovirus or yeast, self-assembled into virus-like particles (VLPs) (Kimbauer et al. 1992). The L1 VLP is a conformationally correct, empty capsid (i.e., it contains no DNA) that appears morphologically identical to, and

contains the major neutralizing epitopes of, the native virion. L1 VLPs closely approximate the antigenic characteristics of wild type virions and have been used extensively in seroepidemiological studies in humans.

Phase I/II clinical trials using HPV L1 VLP delivered intramuscularly have demonstrated the immunogenicity and safety of this vaccine. Koutsky et al. (2002) reported data from a clinical trial of HPV-16 L1 VLPs, indicating for the first time that a vaccine strategy can be implemented in humans to prevent HPV-16 infections and HPV-16-associated premalignant lesions. Young women ($n=2,392$) were assigned to receive placebo or yeast-derived HPV-16 L1 VLPs (40-μg dose) formulated on aluminum adjuvant at month 0, month 2, and month 6 by intramuscular injection. Samples from the genital tract were obtained at enrollment, 1 month after the booster immunization, and every 6 months thereafter. In addition, the women underwent gynecological examinations and were referred for colposcopy according to the protocol. Biopsy tissue was evaluated for intraepithelial neoplasia and analyzed by PCR for the presence of HPV-16 DNA. The assay was validated to have 95% probability to detect 13 copies of HPV-16 DNA per sample. The primary endpoint of the trial was persistent HPV-16 infection, defined by (a) HPV-16 DNA detection in samples obtained at two or more visits at least 4 months apart; (b) a cervical biopsy showing cervical intraepithelial neoplasia or cancer and HPV-16 DNA in the biopsy and in a genital sample collected at the antecedent or subsequent visit; or (c) HPV-16 DNA detected in a sample collected during the last visit before being lost to follow-up.

Women were followed for a median of 17.4 months after completion of the vaccination regimen, at which time 41 cases of persistent HPV-16 infection were accrued. All 41 cases occurred in the placebo group, none in the vaccine group. Of these 41 cases, 31 were persistent HPV-16 infection, five were HPV-16-related CIN1, four were HPV-16-related CIN2, and one occurred in a woman who first tested positive for HPV-16 on the last visit before she was lost to follow-up. These results translate to 100% efficacy (95% confidence interval, 90–100; $p<0.001$). In a follow-up study, Mao et al. (2006) showed that none of the 755 vaccinated women developed CIN2/3 caused by HPV-16 during 48 months of follow-up. After immunization, HPV16 serum antibody titers peaked at month 7, declined through month 18, and remained relatively stable between months 30 and 48. Overall, the observed efficacy for preventing persistent HPV infection was 94%, slightly lower than the 100% reported rate in the interim analysis. Although this study was not designed to evaluate the possible therapeutic effect on women who have evidence of HPV-16 infection before vaccination, the authors found that among the subcohort of women who were HPV-16 DNA-positive at enrollment but anti-HPV-16-seronegative, those who received vaccine were less likely to develop subsequent HPV-16-related CIN2/3 than those who received placebo injections. Despite small numbers, this trend suggests that there may be some benefit to vaccination for women who have recent infections or are early in the natural history of the disease.

In a recent randomized, double-blind, controlled trial, Harper et al. (2004) assessed the efficacy, safety, and immunogenicity of a bivalent HPV-16/18 L1 VLP vaccine (GlaxoSmithKline Biologicals, Rixensart, Belgium) for the prevention of incident and persistent infection with these two virus types, associated cervical cytological abnormalities, and precancerous lesions. They randomized 1,113 women between 15 and 25 years of age to receive three doses of either the vaccine formulated with AS04 adjuvant (aluminum salt and 3-deacylated monophosphoryl lipid A) or placebo on a 0-month, 1-month, and 6-month schedule in North America and Brazil (Table 1). Women were assessed for HPV infection by cervical cytology and self-obtained cervicovaginal samples for up to 27 months, and for vaccine safety and immunogenicity. In the according-to-protocol analyses, vaccine efficacy was 91.6% (95% CI, 64.5–98.0) against incident infection and 100% against persistent infection with HPV-16/18. In the intention-to-treat analyses, vaccine efficacy was 95.1% against persistent cervical infection with HPV-16/18 and 92.9% against cytological abnormalities associated with HPV-16/18 infection. The vaccine was generally safe, well tolerated, and highly immunogenic.

On further analysis of this study, Dubin et al. (2005) observed cross-protection against abnormal cytology (ASCUS or worse) associated with non-HPV-16/18 high-risk types during 12 months of follow-up. This finding challenges the view that cross-protection between HPV types with L1 antigens is unlikely. The identity of the cross-protective epitopes is not yet known; the use of an adjuvant such as AS04 to generate a strong antibody and cellular immune response may contribute to this effect.

Giannini et al. (2005) have recently compared the ability of an HPV-16/18 L1 VLP vaccine formulated with either the AS04 adjuvant system or aluminum salt alone to induce an immune response of high magnitude and persistence. HPV-16/18 L1 VLPs formulated with AS04 adjuvant induced a substantially higher and more persistent response compared with the aluminum-salt-only formulation. The higher antibody responses associated with the AS04 formulation persisted for up to at least 3.5-years after vaccination in human subjects.

Dubin et al. (2005) compared immunogenicity and safety of the HPV-16/18 L1 VLP vaccine formulated with AS04 adjuvant (Cervarix, GlaxoSmithKline Biologicals) in 158 preteen/adolescent (10–14 years) and 458 young women (15–25 years). The vaccine was well tolerated and adverse events were rare in both groups; however, higher antibody titers were observed in preteens/adolescents. They concluded that higher antibody titers in the younger group might result in longer antibody persistence and be particularly advantageous when an HPV vaccine is administered at a young age well before sexual activity.

The results of a randomized, double-blind placebo-controlled multicenter phase II trial of a quadrivalent VLP vaccine were published recently (Villa et al. 2005). The vaccine included four recombinant HPV type-specific VLPs consisting of the L1 major capsid proteins of HPV6, 11, 16, and 18 adsorbed onto amorphous aluminum hydroxyphosphate sulfate adjuvant (GARDASIL, Merck Research Laboratories, Whitehouse Station, NJ, USA). A group of 277 young women (mean age, 20.2 years) were randomly assigned to quadrivalent HPV (20 µg type 6, 40 µg type 11, 40 µg type 16, and 20 µg type 18) L1 virus-like-particle (VLP) vaccine, and 275 young women (mean age, 20.0 years) were assigned to one of two placebo preparations at day 1, month 2, and month 6. In the according-to-protocol cohort, the incidence of persistent HPV 6, 11, 16, or 18 infection or associated disease decreased by 90% (95% CI, 71–97) in women who received the vaccine compared with placebo. The results were similar in an intention-to-treat analysis. All women who received vaccine developed HPV antibody to the four HPV types after the series was completed, and antibody titers were substantially higher than in placebo recipients who had had a previous HPV infection. Mean antibody titers at month 36 remained at or above the titers in women who had a natural HPV infection and cleared the virus. Pain was the most common injection-site adverse event and headache the most common systemic adverse event. There were no vaccine-related serious adverse events (Table 1). A phase III trial of the quadrivalent vaccine, involving 17,800 women aged 16–23 years, has recently been completed. Data from this clinical trial, the Females United to Universally Reduce Endo-ectocervical disease (FUTURE II) study, were presented recently (Skjeldestad et al. 2005). In a subsample of 12,167 women who were ran-

domized to receive quadrivalent HPV 6/11/16/18 recombinant vaccine (GARDASIL, Merck) or placebo and who followed the protocol closely, the vaccine was 100% effective in preventing incident HPV 16/18-related CIN 2/3, adenocarcinoma in situ, and cervical cancer over 2 years of follow-up. The vaccine was well-tolerated and there were no vaccine-related serious adverse events. On June 8, 2006, the FDA announced the approval of GARDASIL, the first vaccine developed to prevent cervical cancer, precancerous genital lesions, and genital warts due to human papillomavirus (HPV) types 6, 11, 16, and 18 (FDA 2006).

From a technical perspective, vaccination with VLPs appears promising. Nevertheless, several practical issues must be addressed before these vaccines can be deployed in clinical practice and public health programs (Table 2).

Studies by the Center for Disease Control and Prevention suggest that some adolescents initiate sexual intercourse very early, in some cases before 13 years of age. Therefore, a vaccination program beginning around 12 years of age might be the ideal. At present, there are two newly licensed vaccines recommended for adolescents;

Table 1 Comparison of quadrivalent and bivalent L1 VLP prophylactic vaccines

Reference	Villa LL et al. 2005	Harper et al. 2004
Design	Randomized double-blind controlled trial	Randomized double-blind controlled trial
Vaccine type	Quadrivalent HPV-6/11/16/18 VLP, L1 capsid component	Bivalent HPV-16/18 VLP, L1 capsid component
Age (years)	16–23	15–25
Trial size	277 Vaccinees 275 placebo	560 Vaccinees 553 placebo
Site	US, Brazil, Europe	US, Canada, Brazil
Antigen	20 µg HPV 6, 40 µg HPV11, 40 µg HPV-16, 20 µg HPV18	20 µg HPV-16, 20 µg HPV-18
Adjuvant	225 µg Aluminum hydroxy phosphate sulfate	500 µg Aluminum hydroxide 50 µg 3-deacylated monophosphoryl lipid (ASO4)
Dose and administration	0.5 ml Intramuscular	0.5 ml Intramuscular
Schedule	0, 2, 6 months	0, 1, 6 months
Follow-up	Up to 35 months	Up to 27 months
Clinical outcome	90% Efficacy preventing HPV-6/11/16/18 infections; 100% efficacy preventing cytological abnormalities	100% Efficacy preventing persistent HPV-16/18 infection; 93% efficacy preventing cytological abnormalities
Major adverse effects	None	None

Table 2 Future HPV immunization programs implementation issues

Potential target populations
9–12 Years of age
Adolescents and young adults
Protection in men
Data on HPV vaccine efficiency in men not yet available
Only vaccinating women might be a good option in some communities
Societal acceptance of vaccines to prevent sexually transmitted infections
Awareness of HPV consequences and ubiquity
Anti-cancer vaccine

Boostrix from GSK for Pertussis, and Menactra from Sanofi-Pasteur for Neisseria meningitidis. An HPV vaccine could be added to a program that administers these to create the foundation of an adolescent check-up. Going forward, a system that routinely provides such a regimen of adolescent vaccinations would help protect a population from cervical cancer and a variety of other diseases. The early years of HPV vaccine availability would necessitate a substantial catch-up effort to vaccinate older individuals who are sexually active (Shaw 2005).

How will HPV vaccines impact recommendations for cervical screening? In the short to medium term, there should be little impact on frequency of screening. Robust field effectiveness for these vaccines has yet to be demonstrated in clinical trials. Since the vaccines may initially cover only types 16 and 18, one must continue to screen for the other 30% of HPV disease caused by the types not in the first versions of these vaccines. It is possible that screening programs may evolve from a cytopathologic basis to a DNA testing base over time. In the longer term, screening recommendations might be modified based on the field data and cost-effectiveness considerations, but some level of screening is likely to be required for decades (Shaw 2005).

Concerns have been raised about the impact of HPV vaccination on both sexual risk behaviors and screening behaviors. Some have expressed concern that adolescents who receive an HPV vaccine may feel less vulnerable to STI and thus practice riskier sexual behaviors; however, there are no published data to support this

concern. Vaccinated women should understand that HPV vaccines will not prevent infection with other sexually transmitted diseases, nor will their introduction eliminate the need for cervical-cancer screening. Screening will continue to be essential to detect cancers and precancerous changes caused by other HPV types, as well as any cancer in women who have not been vaccinated or are already infected with HPV (Kahn 2005).

Vaccination of early adolescents against an STI may pose unique challenges. Adolescents often do not visit their health care provider routinely, and HPV vaccination will require three visits over a 6-month period. Adolescents who may be particularly vulnerable to STI acquisition are less likely to receive preventive health services in general and thus may be more difficult to reach with existing vaccination programs. Parental and adolescent acceptance of vaccination against an STI and provider willingness to recommend such vaccines will also be key determinants of successful vaccine delivery (Zimet et al. 2000). Recent studies demonstrate that although parents generally find STI vaccines acceptable, some do not believe their children are at risk for STIs or express concern that adolescents who are vaccinated may practice riskier sexual behaviors (Zimet et al. 2005).

Finally, questions remain concerning the feasibility of prophylactic HPV vaccines for large-scale immunization programs in less developed countries, where most cervical cancer deaths occur. The vaccines under development require multiple doses and refrigeration, which make administration difficult in developing countries. In addition, it is unclear how to accomplish large-scale vaccination of early adolescents, given that current global vaccination programs are designed to implement vaccination of infants and young children (Lowr and Frazer 2003).

Conclusion and Future Directions

HPV causes the most common viral infection of the reproductive tract worldwide. However, the infection is often transient and self-limited. Several studies have suggested that HPV infection and cervical dysplasia can be prevented by HPV L1 VLP vaccines. The licensure of a vaccine against HPV represents a major public health advance against cervical cancer and other less common cancers including those of the anus, vagina, and vulva. Much still needs to be investigated regarding the local immune responses to the vaccine in the lower genital tract, longevity of immune responses, and alternative delivery routes such as intravaginal, intranasal, and oral administration.

The epidemiology of cervical cancer highlights the need to provide HPV vaccines to persons who may never or rarely be screened, as well as to improve cervical cancer prevention programs so that they will reach the women with the highest risk of disease. However, it will be far easier to recommend routine vaccination than to provide the resources for its routine use, in the United States and throughout the world (Steinbrook 2006).

References

Bosch FX, de Sanjose S (2003) Chapter 1: HPVs and cervical cancer: burden and assessment of casuality. J Natl Cancer Inst Monogr 3–13

Breitburd F, Kimbauer R, Hubbert NL et al (1995) Immunization with virus-like particles from cottontail rabbit papillomavirus (CRPV) can protect against experimental CRPV infection. J Virol 69:3959–3396

Centers for Disease Control and Prevention (2004) Genital HPV infection—CDC Fact Sheet. Centers for Disease Control and Prevention, Atlanta

Dubin G (2005) Enhanced immunogenicity of a candidate HPV 16/18 L1 VLP vaccine with novel ASO4 adjuvant in preteens/adolescents. Poster presentation, 45th ICAAC meeting, Washington, DC, December 2005

Dubin G, Colau B, Zahat T, Quint W, Martin MT, Jenkins D (2005) Cross-protection against persistent HPV infection, abnormal cytology and CIN associated with HPV 16 and 18 related HPN types by a HPV 16/18 L1 VLP vaccine. 22nd International Papilloma Conference, Vancouver, Canada, April–May 2005

Embers ME, Budgeon LR, Pickel M et al (2002) Protective immunity to rabbit oral and cutaneous papillomaviruses by immunization with short peptides of L2, the minor capsid protein. J Virol 76:9798–9805

FDA (2006) FDA licenses new vaccine for prevention of cervical cancer and other diseases in females caused by human papillomavirus. http://www.fda.gov/bbs/topics/NEWS/2006/NEW01385.html. Cited 16 August 2006

Giannini SL, Hanon E, Fourneau MA, Colau B, Suzich J, Losonsky G et al (2005) Superior immune response induced by vaccination with HPV 16/18 L1 VLP formulated with AS04 compared to aluminum salt only formulation. Poster presentation, 4th Annual American Association for Cancer Research (AACR) International Conference on Frontiers in Cancer Prevention Research, Baltimore, MD, September 5, 2005

Harper DM, Franco EL, Wheeler C, Ferris DG, Jenkins D, Schuind A, Zahaf T, Innis B, Naud P, De Carvalho NS, Roteli-Martins CM, Teixeira J, Blatter MM, Korn AP, Quint W, Dubin G(2004) GlaxoSmithKline HPV Vaccine Study Group. Efficacy of a bivalent L1 virus-like particle vaccine in prevention of infection with human papillomavirus types 16 and 18 in young women: a randomized controlled trial. Lancet 364:1757–1765

Ho GY, Burk RD, Klein S, Kadish AS, Chang CJ, Palan P et al (1995) Persistent genital human papillomavirus infection as a risk factor for persistent cervical dysplasia. J Natl Cancer Inst 87:1365–1371

Jansen KU, Shaw AR (2004) Human papillomavirus vaccines and prevention of cervical cancer. Annu Rev Med 55:319–331

Jemal A, Siegal R, Ward E, Murray T, Xu J, Smigal C A et al (2006) Cancer statistics. CA Cancer J Clin 56:106–130

Kahn JA (2005) Vaccination as a prevention strategy for human papillomavirus-related diseases. J Adolesc Health 37:S10–S16

Kirnbauer R, Booy F, Cheng (1992) Papillomavirus L1 major capsid protein self-assembles into virus-like particles that are highly immunogenic. Proc Natl Acad Sci U S A 89:12180–12184

Koutsky LA, Ault KA, Wheeler CM, Brown DR, Barr E, Alvarez FB, Chiacchierini LM, Jansen KU (2002) Proof of Principle Study Investigators. A controlled trial of a human papillomavirus type 16 vaccine. N Engl J Med 347:1645–1651

Lowy DR, Frazer IH (2003) Chapter 16: Prophylactic human papillomavirus vaccines. J Natl Cancer Inst Monogr 111–116

Mao C, Koutsky LA, Ault KA, Wheeler CM, Brown DR, Wiley DJ, Alvarez FB, Bautista OM, Jansen KU, Barr E (2006) Efficacy of human papillomavirus-16 vaccine to prevent cervical intraepithelial neoplasia: a randomized controlled trial. Obstet Gynecol 107:18–27

Pratt D, Goldenthal K, Gerber A (2001) Preventive HPV vaccines. FDA Advisory Committee, Vaccines and Related Biological Products meeting, November 28–29, 2001

Richardson H, Kelsall H, Tellier P, Voyer H, Abrahamowicz M, Ferenczy A et al (2003) The natural history of type-specific human papillomavirus infections in female university students. Cancer Epidemiol Biomarkers Prev 6:485–490

Shaw AR (2005) Human papillomavirus vaccines in development: if they're successful in clinical trials, how will they be implemented? Gynecol Oncol 99:S246–S248

Skjeldestad FE et al (2005) Prophylactic quadrivalent human papillomavirus (HPV) (types 6, 11, 16, 18) L1 virus-like particle (VLP) vaccine (Gardasil™) reduces cervical intraepithelial neoplasia (CIN) 2/3 risk. Infectious Disease Society of America 43rd Annual Meeting, San Francisco, CA, October 7, 2005; Abstract LB-8a

Spence A, Franco E, Ferenczy A (2005) The role of human papillomaviruses in cancer: evidence to date. Am J Cancer 4:49–64

Stanley M (1997) Genital papillomaviruses – prospects for vaccination. Curr Opin Infect Dis 10:55–61

Stanley M (2006a) HPV vaccines. Best Pract Res Clin Obstet Gynaecol 20:279–293

Stanley M (2006b) Immune responses to human papillomavirus. Vaccine 30 [Suppl 1]:S16–S22

Steinbrook R (2006) The potential of human papillomavirus vaccines. N Engl J Med 354:1109–1112

Trottier H, Franco EL (2006) The epidemiology of genital human papillomavirus infection. Vaccine 30 [Suppl 1]:S1–S15

Villa LL, Costa RL, Petta CA, Andrade RP, Ault KA, Giuliano AR, Wheeler CM, Koutsky LA, Malm C, Lehtinen M, Skjeldestad FE, Olsson SE, Steinwall M, Brown DR, Kurman RJ, Ronnett BM, Stoler MH, Ferenczy A, Harper DM, Tamms GM, Yu J, Lupinacci L, Railkar R, Taddeo FJ, Jansen KU, Esser MT, Sings HL, Saah AJ, Barr E (2005) Prophylactic quadrivalent human papillomavirus (types 6, 11, 16, and 18) L1 virus-like particle vaccine in young women: a randomised double-blind placebo-controlled multicentre phase II efficacy trial. Lancet Oncol 6:271–278

Zimet GD, Mays RM, Fortenberry JD (2000) Vaccines against sexually transmitted infections promise and problems of the magic bullets for prevention and control. Sex Transm Dis 27:49–52

Zimet GD, Mays RM, Sturm LA, Ravert AA, Perkins SM, Juliar BE (2005) Parental attitudes about sexually transmitted infection vaccination for their adolescent children. Arch Pediatr Adolesc Med 159:132–137

Prevention and Early Detection of Ovarian Cancer: Mission Impossible?

Robert C. Bast Jr., Molly Brewer, Changping Zou, Mary A. Hernandez,
Mary Daley, Robert Ozols, Karen Lu, Zhen Lu, Donna Badgwell, Gordon B. Mills,
Steven Skates, Zhen Zhang, Dan Chan, Anna Lokshin, Yinhua Yu

Recent Results in Cancer Research, Vol. 174
© Springer-Verlag Berlin Heidelberg 2007

Abstract

Epithelial ovarian cancer is neither a common nor a rare disease. In the United States, the prevalence of ovarian cancer in postmenopausal women (1 in 2,500) significantly affects strategies for prevention and detection. If chemoprevention for ovarian cancer were provided to all women over the age of 50, side effects would have to be minimal in order to achieve an acceptable ratio of benefit to risk. This ratio might be improved by identifying subsets of individuals at increased risk or by bundling prevention of ovarian cancer with treatment for other more prevalent conditions. Approximately 10% of ovarian cancers are familial and relate to mutations of BRCA1, BRCA2, and mismatch repair genes. More subtle genetic factors are being sought in women with apparently sporadic disease. Use of oral contraceptive agents for as long as 5 years decreases the risk of ovarian cancer in later life by 50%. In one study, fenretinide (4-HPR) delayed development of ovarian cancer in women at increased risk of developing breast and ovarian cancer. Accrual to confirmatory studies has been prohibitively slow and prophylactic oophorectomy is recommended for women at increased genetic risk. Vaccines may have a role for prevention of several different cancers. Breast and ovarian cancers express mucins that could serve as targets for vaccines to prevent both cancers. Early detection of ovarian cancer requires a strategy with high sensitivity (>75% for stage I disease) and very high specificity (>99.6%)

to achieve a positive predictive value of 10%. Transvaginal sonography (TVS) has achieved these values in some studies, but is limited by the cost of annual screening in a general population. Two-stage strategies that incorporate both serum markers and TVS promise to be more cost-effective. An algorithm has been developed that calculates risk of ovarian cancer based on serial CA125 values and refers patients at highest risks for TVS. Use of the algorithm is currently being evaluated in a trial with 200,000 women in the United Kingdom that will critically test the ability of a two-stage screening strategy to improve survival in ovarian cancer. Whatever the outcome, additional serum markers will be required to detect all patients in an initial phase of screening. More than 30 serum markers have been evaluated alone and in combination with CA125. Recent candidates include: HE4, mesothelin, M-CSF, osteopontin, kallikrein(s) and soluble EGF receptor. Proteomic approaches have been used to define a distinctive pattern of peaks on mass spectroscopy or to identify a limited number of critical markers that can be assayed by more conventional methods. Several groups are placing known markers on multiplex platforms to permit simultaneous assay of multiple markers with very small volumes of serum. Mathematical techniques are being developed to analyze combinations of marker levels to improve sensitivity and specificity. In the future, serum markers should improve the sensitivity of detecting recurrent disease as well as facilitate earlier detection of ovarian cancer.

Introduction

Although difficult, the development of effective strategies for prevention and particularly for early detection should, in the long run, be achievable goals. The challenge for developing both strategies relates to the fact that ovarian cancer is neither a common nor a rare disease. The lifetime risk of developing ovarian cancer for a woman in the United States is 1 in 70, compared to 1 in 8–9 for breast cancer. Even in postmenopausal women over 50 years of age in whom most epithelial ovarian cancers are diagnosed, the prevalence of the disease is approximately 1 in 2,500. Given the relatively low prevalence of ovarian cancer, any intervention to prevent the disease in the entire population must not only be effective, but must also have very little toxicity. Similarly, an effective screening strategy to detect early-stage disease must not only have high sensitivity, but must also have extremely high specificity to avoid alarming a large number of healthy women and triggering a large volume of inconvenient, morbid, and expensive diagnostic procedures, including exploratory surgery, for women who do not have ovarian cancer.

Despite its relatively low prevalence, ovarian cancer is associated with significant mortality. In 2006, some 20,180 women will develop ovarian cancer in the United States and an estimated 15,310 deaths will occur (Jemel et al. 2006). Five-year survival rates have improved significantly (p<0.05) from 37% in the 1970s to 45% in the 1990s, related in large part to improvements in cytoreductive surgery and combination chemotherapy (Jemel et al. 2006). However, overall survival for women with advanced disease has not improved dramatically over the last three decades and the majority of patients still succumb to the disease. Given the slow pace of progress in the treatment of advanced ovarian cancer, the search for effective strategies for prevention and early detection has become all the more important.

Pathogenesis, Clinical Presentation, and Management

Most ovarian cancers are thought to arise from a single layer of epithelial cells that cover the ovary or line inclusion cysts immediately beneath the ovarian surface. Despite their origin from nondescript epithelial cells, ovarian cancers can differentiate into serous, endometrioid, mucinous, and clear cell histotypes, resembling fallopian tube, endometrium, colonic mucosa, and vaginal rests at the level of morphology and gene expression (Marquez et al. 2005). Ovarian cancer can metastasize through lymphatics and by vascular invasion, but also characteristically spreads over the surface of the peritoneal cavity forming nodules that stud serosal surfaces. Blockade of diaphragmatic lymphatics and leakage of proteinaceous fluid from tumor vessels produce ascites. Recent evidence points to the importance of vascular endothelial growth factor/vascular permeability factor (VEGF/VPF) in stimulating angiogenesis and ascites production (Yoneda et al. 1998).

Some 90% of ovarian cancers are clonal neoplasms that arise from the progeny of single epithelial cells that have undergone multiple genetic and epigenetic alterations (Jacobs et al. 1992). Malignant transformation has been associated with activation of the PI3 kinase (Mills et al. 2001), Ras/MAP/Src (Patton et al. 1998), and STAT3 signaling pathways (Nishimoto et al. 2005), loss of function for p53 (Berchuck et al. 1994) and imprinted tumor suppressor genes (ARHI [Yu et al. 1999], LOT-1 [Abdollahi et al. 1997], PEG3 [Dowdy et al. 2005]), expression of angiogenic factors (VEGF [Yoneda et al. 1998], IL-8 [Yoneda et al. 1998] and bFGF [Yoneda et al. 1998]), and upregulation of mucins (MUC1 [Taylor-Papadimitriou et al. 1999), CA 125 [Bast et al. 1981]). Underlying genetic alterations are thought to result from spontaneous mutations that occur during repair of ovulatory defects or following stimulation with gonadotrophins or androgens.

Although ovarian cancer has been considered a silent killer, the disease is generally symptomatic, even at early stages (Goff et al. 2000). Symptoms, however, are not specific and are generally attributed to benign gastrointestinal, genitourinary, musculoskeletal, or gynecologic conditions. Symptoms such as bloating, gas pains, pelvic discomfort, and urinary frequency have been reported in 89% of patients with disease still limited to the ovaries (stage I) or pelvis (stage II) and in 97% of patients with disease that has spread to the abdomen (stage III) or outside the abdomen (stage IV). Often, ovarian cancer presents at an advanced stage with abdominal distension, ascites, and an adnexal mass that can be palpated on physical examination and imaged by transvaginal ultrasound (TVS) or pelvic computerized tomography. Definitive diagnosis of ovarian cancer generally requires laparoscopy or laparotomy where bilateral salpingo-oophorectomy, total abdominal hysterectomy, omentectomy, and cytoreductive surgery are performed to remove as much of the tumor as possible. Standard postoperative therapy in the United States involves six cycles of intravenous carboplatin and paclitaxel (Berek and Bast 2006) with the possible addition of intraperitoneal chemotherapy (Armstrong et al. 2006).

Epidemiologic Risk Factors

In addition to age over 50 and Caucasian race, an increased number of ovulatory cycles appears to increase risk for ovarian cancer, reflected in an association with early menarche, late menopause, and nulliparity (Berek and Bast 2006). Conversely, factors that decrease the number of ovulatory cycles, including repeated pregnancies, prolonged breast feeding and use of oral contraceptives, decrease the risk of ovarian cancer. A protective effect from tubal ligation suggests that exogenous carcinogens might gain access to the ovary from the uterus through the fallopian tube. However, evidence for viral or strong chemical carcinogens has not been obtained, with the possible exceptions of the use of talc products in all histotypes and of cigarette smoking in mucinous cancers, but not in the more common serous histotype (Berek and Bast 2006). Approximately 10% of ovarian cancers are familial and are associated with mutations in BRCA1, BRCA2 or, less frequently, with the mismatch repair enzymes in the human nonpolyposis colon cancer (HNPCC) syndrome (Berek and Bast 2006).

Prevention of Ovarian Cancer

Familial Ovarian Cancer

In carriers of BRCA1 or BRCA2 mutations, prophylactic bilateral salpingo-oophorectomy will reduce the risk of ovarian cancer by approximately 95%, although primary peritoneal cancers that resemble ovarian cancers histologically can still occur in up to 5% of women even after prophylactic surgery. In specimens obtained at prophylactic oophorectomy, occult cancers have been found in 6% of ovaries from BRCA1 carriers and in 2% of ovaries from BRCA2 carriers (Finch et al. 2006). Small occult cancers have generally been localized to solitary cysts, but have been associated with p53 mutations and reduction of BRCA to homozygosity (Pothuri et al. 2004). As mutation of p53 has been associated with advanced stage disease (Berchuck et al. 1994), these observations suggest that hereditary ovarian cancers may be capable of metastasis while still quite small in volume. A significant number of hereditary cancers may arise in the mucosa of the fallopian tube. Consequently bilateral salpingo-oophorectomy (BSO) is recommended in all BRCA1 and BRCA2 mutation carriers when they have completed child-bearing.

Estimating Risk in Somatic Disease

A strategy for preventing the 90% of ovarian cancers that are sporadic is less clear. Given the incidence and prevalence of ovarian cancer, subpopulations must be identified who are at sufficiently high risk to justify intervention, but not at sufficient risk to warrant prophylactic oophorectomy. More subtle genetic markers such as single nucleotide polymorphisms (SNPs) are being sought to identify women at risk for ovarian cancer (Berchuck et al. 2004). In addition to determining genetic predisposition with greater precision, tests could be developed to detect somatic alterations of the ovarian surface epithelium. Dr. David Fishman has proposed sampling the ovarian surface epithelium at outpatient laparoscopy, providing an ovarian "PAP smear". Cells from the ovarian surface could be examined for alterations in PI3K, RAS/MAP, and

STAT3 signaling, mutation of p53, loss of ARHI expression, upregulation of angiogenic factors, and aberrant expression of CA125 or MUC1. This strategy depends, however, on the assumption that alterations in ovarian surface epithelial cells will reflect the same somatic changes found in cells lining subsurface inclusion cysts where cancers arise more frequently. More than 90% of occult cancers found at prophylactic BSO were found in cysts rather than at the ovarian surface (Pothuri et al. 2004). In addition, Dr. Jeff Boyd and colleagues have found substantial differences in expression array analysis of genes expressed in microdissected surface epithelial cells and in inclusion cysts (Leitao et al. 2003). Another approach that might circumvent this difficulty is optical fluorescence (Brewer et al. 2002) or reflectance spectroscopy of the ovarian surface (Utzinger et al. 2001), which could also be performed at laparoscopy. Analysis of reflected laser light can detect changes in redox potential, vascularity, and cell order, not only at the ovarian surface, but also in subsurface cysts.

Oral Contraceptives

Suppression of ovulation with oral contraceptives for as long as 5 years decreases the incidence of ovarian cancer by 50% (Negri et al. 1991). This may relate in part to suppression of ovulation with a consequent decrease in proliferation of ovarian epithelial cells required to repair ovulatory defects and a reduction in the number of inclusion cysts. Progestins in oral contraceptives also induce apoptosis in ovarian surface epithelial cells (Rodriguez et al. 1998).

Fenretinide and Celecoxib

In one trial of women at increased risk for breast and ovarian cancer conducted in Milan, treatment with fenretinide (4-HPR) delayed development of ovarian cancer for as long as the drug was administered (De Palo et al. 1995, 2002). In cell culture, 4-HPR inhibited growth and induced apoptosis in normal ovarian epithelial (NOE) cells, partially immortalized NOE, and ovarian cancer cells (Brewer, et al. 2005). The strongest

reaction of the p53 pathway in NOE cells was produced by 4-HPR, whereas the drug caused the greatest mitochondrial damage in ovarian cancer cells, suggesting a different mechanism for growth inhibition and/or apoptosis in the normal and malignant cells (Brewer et al. 2005).

A study was initiated some years ago at the Fox Chase Cancer Center in women at high genetic risk for developing ovarian cancer that randomized participants to immediate prophylactic BSO or to treatment with 4-HPR for 6 months prior to surgery to determine whether treatment with 4-HPR would normalize abnormal morphology and biomarkers (Ozols et al. 2003). To date, four patients have been accrued. In an attempt to increase accrual, a similar trial was adopted by the national Gynecologic Oncology Group. Over 30 months, some 20 patients have been registered. Investigators at M.D. Anderson initiated a multicenter randomized double-blind trial comparing effects on ovarian biomarkers of treatment with 4-HPR, oral contraceptives, both agents, or placebos. Women were to be treated for 6 weeks prior to prophylactic BSO. This trial has been closed due to lack of accrual, despite screening several hundred candidates. A group of investigators at the University of Alabama has had greater success in accruing patients to a trial of celecoxib prior to elective TAH and BSO (Barnes et al. 2005). Concern regarding potential cardiovascular toxicity has reduced enthusiasm for long-term trials of uninterrupted COX-2 inhibitors for chemoprevention of cancer (Solomon et al. 2005).

Vaccines

Given the prevalence of epithelial ovarian cancer, a strategy might be considered that links prevention of ovarian cancer to prevention of a more common malignancy, such as breast cancer. Vaccines that stimulate immunity to the MUC-1 mucin core protein that is expressed in most breast cancers have been proposed as preventive agents (Finn 2004). As most ovarian cancers also express the deglycosylated MUC-1 core protein, both forms of cancer might be prevented with a MUC-1 vaccine. A recent epidemiologic study points to an inverse correlation between the number of events that induce anti-MUC1 antibodies and the risk of developing ovarian cancer (Cramer et al. 2005).

Early Detection of Ovarian Cancer

Rationale

When ovarian cancer has not spread beyond the ovaries (stage I), up to 90% of patients can be cured with currently available surgery and chemotherapy. By contrast, disease that has spread from the pelvis (stages III–IV) can be cured in only 30% or less. At present, only 25% of ovarian cancers are diagnosed in stage I. Detection of a larger fraction of patients in stage I might impact favorably on survival.

Given the prevalence of ovarian cancer, there are stringent requirements for an effective screening strategy. As diagnosis of ovarian cancer is generally made at surgery, a positive predictive value of 10% implies ten operations for each case of ovarian cancer diagnosed. To achieve a positive predictive value of 10% with a prevalence of 1 in 2,500 requires a high sensitivity of 75% or greater for early-stage disease and a very high specificity of 99.6%.

Approaches to Screening for Epithelial Ovarian Cancer

Three approaches have been utilized for early detection of ovarian cancer: transvaginal sonography (TVS), serum tumor markers, and a two-phase strategy where an abnormal blood test triggers TVS. Over 70,000 women have been evaluated with TVS alone in three large screening trials in the Japan, the United States, and the United Kingdom (Bourne et al. 1993; Van Nagell et al. 2000; Sato et al. 2001). In prevalence screens, sensitivity for stage I ovarian cancer did not exceed 90% (Bast et al. 2002). Specificity was at the margin of that required to achieve a positive predictive value of 10%, with the most promising results observed in the United States trial (Van Nagell et al. 2000). In the United States, however, the cost of annual screening for all women over the age of 50 would be prohibitive. Annual blood

tests are potentially less expensive, provided that they were sufficiently sensitive and specific. Among the circulating tumor markers for ovarian cancer, CA125 has been evaluated most extensively. CA125 levels have been elevated 10–60 months prior to conventional diagnosis (Bast et al. 2002). In sera from patients with stage I disease found at conventional diagnosis, CA125 is elevated in 50%–60% (Bast et al. 2002). Specificity of a single CA125 determination in apparently healthy women is 99%, but this falls short of the 99.6% specificity required to achieve a positive predictive value of 10%. Specificity of CA125 can, however, be improved by combining CA125 with ultrasound (Jacobs et al. 1999) or by sequential monitoring over time (Skates et al. 1995).

Combination of CA125 and ultrasound

In the United Kingdom, a randomized trial (Jacobs et al. 1995) compared screening with conventional physical examination (10,985 women) to screening with CA125 followed by transabdominal ultrasound (TAU) if CA125 levels were elevated (10,977). When TAU was abnormal, surgery was undertaken. Twenty-nine operations were performed to detect six cancers, yielding a positive predictive value of 21%, or five operations for each case of ovarian cancer detected. Median survival in the screened group (72.9 months) was significantly greater (p=0.0112) than in the control group (41.8 months).

Analysis of Changes in CA 125 Over Time

The trend of CA125 has proven useful in distinguishing malignant from benign disease (Skates et al. 1995). Rising CA125 values are associated with ovarian cancer, presumably related to progressive growth of the source of the antigen. Stable CA125 values, even when elevated, are associated with benign conditions. Steven Skates has developed a computer algorithm that estimates risk of ovarian cancer based on change point analysis. Using changes in CA125 over time to trigger TVS in screening 6,532 women over the age of 50 produced a specificity of 99.8% and a positive predictive value of 19% (Menon et al. 2005). Based on the results of this preliminary study, a large randomized trial (UKCTOCS) was undertaken. A total of 200,000 postmenopausal women have been randomized to three groups: 100,000 controls are followed with conventional pelvic examination annually; 50,000 undergo annual TVS; and 50,000 are monitored with annual CA125 with TVS performed if the risk of ovarian cancer is sufficiently high as judged by the Skates algorithm. Women will be followed for 7 years to determine whether screening improves survival.

Increasing the Sensitivity of Two-Stage Screening Strategies for Ovarian Cancer

Regardless of the outcome of the UKCTOCS trial, CA125 is not likely to provide an optimal initial step in a two-stage screening strategy. At the time of conventional diagnosis, CA125 levels exceed 35 U/ml in 50%–60% of patients with stage I ovarian cancer (Bast et al. 2002). Using change point analysis, the sensitivity of CA125 might be improved by detecting an increase in antigen levels within the normal range. At best, however, the sensitivity of CA125 for early-stage disease is not likely to exceed 80%, as 20% of ovarian cancers express little or no CA125. Greater sensitivity might be achieved with multiple markers, provided that specificity is not compromised. More than 30 markers have been evaluated in combination with CA 125. In these studies, markers have generally been evaluated only two or three at a time, and increased sensitivity has been associated with decreased specificity (Bast et al. 2002).

Novel Markers for Epithelial Ovarian Cancer

Over the last 5 years, several different approaches have been utilized to discover potential markers for ovarian cancer. Mesothelin was recognized by the development of murine monoclonal antibodies against tumor associated antigens (McIntosh et al. 2004). Analysis of growth stimulatory lipids in ovarian cancer ascites detected lysophosphatidic acid (Xu et al. 1998). Biochemical analysis has documented decreased expression of soluble

epidermal growth factor receptor (Baron et al. 2005). Gene expression arrays have detected upregulation of HE4 (Schummer et al. 1999), kallikrein 6 and 10 (Diamandis et al. 2000; Luo et al. 2001), prostasin (Mok et al. 2001), osteopontin (Kim et al. 2002), vascular endothelial growth factor (Lu et al. 2004), and interleukin-8 (Lu et al. 2004). Proteomic analysis has detected peptides that are differentially expressed in serum from ovarian cancer patients and healthy individuals. Investigators have attempted to identify a distinctive pattern of peptide expression in serum or, alternatively, to identify specific peptides and to develop individual assays that can be analyzed in combination with other known markers.

Petricoin et al. generated proteomic spectra using SELDI (surface-enhanced laser desorption and ionization) mass spectroscopy (Petricoin et al. 2002). Sera from 50 healthy women and 50 patients with ovarian cancer were compared using an iterative searching algorithm. A pattern that distinguished ovarian cancer sera was then used to classify serum samples from 66 healthy women and 50 women with ovarian cancer, including 18 with stage I disease. All cancers were correctly classified (93%–100%), as were 95% of 66 healthy individuals (87%–99%). While this is an encouraging preliminary study, few patients with early-stage disease were included. Others investigators have reported difficulty in reproducing the analysis from the primary data (Baggerly et al. 2005).

A second approach has utilized proteomic techniques to identify specific peptides and to develop individual assays that can be analyzed in combination with conventional markers. Zhang et al. utilized sera from five different academic centers to identify upregulation or downregulation of peptides that could be found in all five data sets (Zhang et al. 2004). Three biomarkers were identified: apolipoprotein A1, a truncated form of transthyretin, and a fragment of inter-alpha-1-trypsin inhibitor heavy chain 4 (IATI-H4). Changes in expression of the three markers added 9% sensitivity to CA 125II at a constant specificity of 97%. Interestingly, the IATI-H4 fragment is flanked by potential tissue kallikrein cleavage sites and increased expression of kallikreins has been documented in ovarian cancers (Diamandis et al. 2000; Luo et al. 2001). Thus, the fragment might be generated by proteolytic cleavage by tumor derived kallikreins as normal plasma components percolate through the ovarian cancer stroma, which would provide a strong biologic basis for this marker.

Identification of an optimal combination of biomarkers for early detection of ovarian cancer will require analysis of multiple assays on a common panel of sera from healthy individuals and from ovarian cancer patients at the time of conventional diagnosis. Data of even greater importance must be obtained from prediagnostic samples collected during screening trials from patients destined to develop ovarian cancer. Such serum specimens have generally been preserved in relatively small amounts. Consequently, the simultaneous assay of multiple markers in small volumes of sera will be important for the identification of optimal panels. Luminex technology permits simultaneous multiplexing of several assays in small volumes of serum (Vignali 2000). Sets of beads are marked with different concentrations of a red fluor. Double determinant assays are constructed with primary antibodies reactive with different markers on different sets of beads. Second antibodies reactive with each marker are labeled with a single green fluor. Flow cytometric analysis can permit simultaneous analysis of multiple markers in as little as 50 μL of serum. Promising preliminary data have been obtained by Anna Lokshin at the University of Pittsburgh (Gorelik et al. 2005). Resent unpublished observations from this group indicate that the multimarker approach can achieve a sensitivity of 90%–92% at a specificity of 98%.

To increase sensitivity without losing specificity using multiple markers, sophisticated statistical techniques are required. In two recent studies (Skates et al. 2002, Zhang et al., in revision), CA125II, CA72-4, CA15-3, and M-CSF were measured in a validation set of 60 early-stage ovarian cancer and 98 control sera. At a specificity of 98% that would require TVS in only 2% of patients in a two-stage screening strategy, CA125II exhibited a sensitivity of 48%. At the same level of specificity, artificial neural network analysis with the four markers produced a sensitivity of 72% (Zhang et al., in revision) and a mixture of multivariate normal distributions produced a sensitivity of 75% (Skates et al. 2004). Consequently sensitivity could be increased by 24%–27% without a loss of specificity at the level required for a two-stage screening strategy.

Conclusions

Development of an effective strategy for early detection of ovarian cancer is a work in progress. Two-stage strategies that combine serum markers and TVS promise to be cost-effective. Levels of multiple markers can be combined mathematically to increase sensitivity without sacrificing specificity for an optimal initial stage. Whether the pattern of proteomic expression or the measurement of individual markers will prove most useful remains to be determined. In either case, confirmatory studies will be required before assays become widely available and at present there is no proven screening strategy for ovarian cancer. Given the progress outlined above, however, development of an effective strategy for early detection seems likely within the next decade.

Prophylactic salpingo-oophorectomy remains the most effective strategy for preventing ovarian cancer in carriers of BRCA1, BRCA2, and mismatch repair mutations and is more effective in premenopausal women but renders them menopausal. Genetic and somatic markers for risk are needed to permit effective prevention in subsets of healthy women. Oral contraceptives have decreased risk by 50% in retrospective studies but may increase the risk of breast cancer in BRCA1 women (Narod et al. 2002). Strategies to combine prevention of ovarian cancer with prevention of more prevalent malignancies, such as breast cancer, are particularly attractive, particularly given that the risks profiles are similar.

Acknowledgements

This work was supported in part by the U.T. M.D. Anderson Cancer Center SPORE in Ovarian Cancer 1P50 CA83638-07 and the Fox Chase Cancer Center SPORE in Ovarian Cancer 1P50 CA083638.

References

Abdollahi A, Roberts D, Godwin AK, Schultz DC, Sonoda G, Testa JR, Hamilton TC (1997) Identification of a zinc-finger gene at 6q25: a chromosomal region implicated in development of many solid tumors. Oncogene 14:1973–1979

Armstrong DK, Bundy B, Wenzel L, Huang HQ, Baergen R, Lele S, Copeland LJ, Walker JL, Burger RA; Gynecologic Oncology Group (2006) Intraperitoneal cisplatin and paclitaxel in ovarian cancer. N Engl J Med 5:354:34–43

Baggerly KA, Morris JS, Edmonson SR, Coombes KR (2005) Signal in noise: Evaluating reported reproducibility of proteomic tests for ovarian cancer. J Natl Cancer Inst 97:307–309

Barnes MN, Chhieng DF, Dreher M, Jones JL, Grizzle WE, Jones L, Talley L, Partridge EE (2005) Feasibility of performing chemoprevention trials in women at elevated risk of ovarian carcinoma: initial examination of celecoxib as a chemopreventive agent. Gynecol Oncol 98:376–382

Baron AT, Boardman CH, Lafky JM, Rademaker A, Liu D, Fishman DA, Podratz KC, Maihle NJ (2005) Soluble epidermal growth factor receptor (sEGFR) [corrected] and cancer antigen 125 (CA125) as screening and diagnostic tests for epithelial ovarian cancer. Cancer Epidemiol Biomarkers Prev14:306–318

Bast RC Jr, Feeney M, Lazarus H, Nadler LM, Colvin RB (1981) Knapp RC: Reactivity of a monoclonal antibody with human ovarian carcinoma. J Clin Invest 681:1331–1337

Bast RC Jr, Urban N, Shridhar V, Smith D, Zhang Z, Skates S, Lu K, Liu J, Fishman D, Mills GB (2002) Early detection of ovarian cancer: promise and reality. Cancer Treat Res 107:61–97

Berchuck A, Kohler MF, Marks JR, Wiseman R, Boyd J, Bast RC Jr (1994) The p53 tumor suppressor gene frequently is altered in gynecologic cancers. Am J Obstet Gynecol 170:246–252

Berchuck A, Schildkraut JM, Wenham RM, Claingaert B, Ali S, Henriott A, Halabi S, Rodriguez G, Gertig D, Purdie DM, Keleman L, Spurdle AB, Marks J, Chenevix-Trench G (2004) Progesterone receptor promoter +331A polymorphism is associated with a reduced risk of endometrioid and clear cell ovarian cancers. Cancer Epidemiol Biomarkers Prev 13:2141–2147

Berek JS, Bast RC Jr (2006) Ovarian cancer. In: Kufe DW, Bast RC Jr, Hait W, Hong WK, Pollock RE, Weichselbaum RR, Holland JF, Frei E III (eds) Holland-Frei Cancer Medicine, 7th edn. Decker,Hamilton, Ontario, pp 1543–1568

Bourne TH, Campbell S, Reynolds KM, Whitehead MI, Hampson J, Royston P, Crayford T, Collins WP (1993) Screening for early familial ovarian cancer with transvaginal ultrasonography and colour blood flow imaging. BMJ 306:1025–1029

Brewer M, Utzinger U, Li Y, Atkinson EN, Satterfield W, Auersperg N, Richards-Kortum R, Follen M, Bast R (2002) Fluorescence spectroscopy as a biomarker in a cell culture and in a nonhuman primate model for ovarian cancer chemopreventive agents. J Biomed Opt 1:20–26

Brewer M, Wharton JT, Wang J, McWatters A, Auersperg N, Gershenson D, Bast R, Zou C (2005) In vitro model of normal, immortalized ovarian surface epithelial and ovarian cancer cells for chemoprevention of ovarian cancer. Gynecol Oncol 98:182–192

Cramer DW, Titus-Ernstoff L, McKolanis JR, Welch WR, Vitonis AF, Berkowitz RS, Finn OJ (2005) Conditions associated with antibodies against the tumor-associated antigen MUC1 and their relationship to risk for ovarian cancer. Cancer Epidemiol Biomarkers Prev 14:1125–1131

De Palo G, Mariani L, Camerini T, Marubini E, Formelli F, Pasini B, Decensi A, Veronesi U (2002) Effect of fenretinide on ovarian cancer occurrence. Gynecol Oncol 86:24–27

De Palo G, Veronesi U, Camerini T, Formelli F, Mascotti G, Boni C, Fosser V, Del Vecchio M, Campa T, Costa A (1995) Can fenretinide protect women against ovarian cancer? J Natl Cancer Inst 87:146–147

Diamandis EP, Yousef GM, Soosaipillai AR, Bunting P (2000) Human kallikrein 6 (zyme/protease M/neurosin): a new serum biomarker of ovarian carcinoma. Clin Biochem 33:579–583

Dowdy SC, Gostout BS, Shridhar V, Wu X, Smith DI, Podratz KC, Jiang SW (2005) Biallelic methylation and silencing of paternally expressed gene 3 (PEG3) in gynecologic cancer cell lines. Gynecol Oncol 99:126–134

Finch A, Shaw P, Rosen B, Murphy J, Narod SA, Colgan TJ (2006) Clinical and pathological findings of prophylactic salpingo-oophorectomies in 159 BRCA1 and BRCA2 carriers. Gyn Oncol 100:58–64

Finn O (2004) History of tumour vaccines and novel approaches for preventive cancer vaccines. Dev Biol (Basel) 116:3–12

Goff BA, Mandel L, Muntz HG, Melancon CH (2000) Ovarian carcinoma diagnosis. Cancer 89:2068–2075

Gorelik E, Landsittel DP, Marrangoni AM, Modugno F, Velikokhatnaya L, Winans MT, Bigbee WL, Herberman RB, Lokshin A (2005) Multiplexed immunobead –based cytokine profiling for early detection of ovarian cancer. Cancer Epidemiol Biomarkers Prev 14:981–987

Jacobs IJ, Kohler MF, Wiseman R, Marks J, Whitaker R, Kerns BJM, Humphrey P, Berchuck A, Ponder BAJ, Bast RC Jr (1992) Clonal origin of epithelial ovarian cancer: Analysis by loss of heterozygosity, p53 mutation and X chromosome inactivation. J Natl Cancer Inst 84:1793–1798

Jacobs I, Stabile I, Bridges J, Kemsley P, Reynolds C, Grudzinskas J, Oram D (1999) Multimodal approach to screening for ovarian cancer. Lancet 1:268–271

Jemal A, Siegal R, Ward E, Murray T, Xu J, Smigal C, Thun MJ (2006) Cancer statistics. CA Cancer J Clin 56:106–130

Kim JH, Skates SJ, Uede T, Wong Kk KK, Schorge JO, Feltmate CM, Berkowitz RS, Cramer DW, Mok SC (2002) Osteopontin as a potential diagnostic for ovarian cancer. JAMA 287:1671–1679

Leitao M, Pothuri B, Viale A, Olshen A, Boyd J (2003) Gene expression profiling of ovarian cystic epithelium reveals a quasi-neoplastic phenotype. Gynecol Oncol 88:196

Lu KH, Patterson AP, Wang L, Marquez RT, Atkinson EN, Baggerly KA, Ramoth L, Rosen DG, Liu J, Hellstrom I, Smith D, Hartmann L, Fishman D, Berchuck A, Schmandt R, Whitaker R, Gershenson DM, Mills GB, Bast RC Jr (2004) Selection of potential markers for epithelial ovarian cancer with gene expression arrays and recursive descent partition analysis. Clinical Cancer Res 10:3291–3300

Luo LY, Bunting P, Scorilas A, Diamandis EP (2001) Human kallikrein 10: a novel tumor marker for ovarian carcinoma? Clin Chim Acta 306:111–118

Marquez RT, Baggerly KA, Patterson AP, Liu J, Broaddus R, Frumovitz M, Atkinson EN, Smith D, Hartmann L, Fishman D, Berchuck A, Whitaker R, Gershenson D, Mills GB, Bast RC Jr, Lu K (2005) Patterns of gene expression in different histotypes of epithelial ovarian cancer correlate with those in normal fallopian tube, endometrium and colon. Clin Cancer Res 11:6116–6126

McIntosh MW, Drescher C, Karlan B, Scholler N, Urban N, Hellstrom KE, Hellstrom I (2004) Combining CA 125 and SMR serum markers for diagnosis and early detection of ovarian carcinoma. Gynecol Oncol 95:9–15

Menon U, Skates SJ, Lewis S, Rosenthal A, Rufford B, Sibley K, Macdonald N, Dawney A, Jeyarajah A, Bas RC Jr, Oram D, Jacobs IJ (2005) A prospective study using the risk of ovarian cancer algorithm to screen for ovarian cancer. J Clin Oncol 23:7919–7926

Mills GB, Lu Y, Fang X, Wang H, Eder A, Mao M, Swaby R, Cheng KW, Stokoe D, Siminovitch K, Jaffe R, Gray J (2001) The role of genetic abnormalities of PTEN and the phosphotidylinositol 3-kinase pathway in breast and ovarian tumorigenesis, prognosis and therapy. Semin Oncol 28:125–141

Mok SC, Chao J, Skates S, Wong K, Yiu GK, Muto MG, Berkowitz RS, Cramer DW (2001) Prostasin, a potential serum marker for ovarian cancer: identification through microarray technology. J Natl Cancer Inst 93:1458–1464

Narod SA, Dube MP, Klijn J, Lubinski J, Lynch HT, Ghadirian P, Provencher D, Heimdal K, Moller P, Robson M, Offit K, Isaacs C, Weber B, Friedman E, Gershoni-Baruch R, Rennert G, Pasini B, Wagner T, Daly M, Garber JE, Neuhausen SL, Ainsworth P, Olsson H, Evans G, Osborn M, Couch F, Foulkes WD, Warner E, Kim-Sing C, Olopade O, Tung N, Saal HM, Weitzel J, Merajver S, Gauthier-Villars M, Jernstrom H, Sun P, Brunet JS (2002) Oral contraceptives and the risk of breast cancer in BRCA1 and BRCA2 mutation carriers. J Natl Cancer Inst 23:1773–1779

Negri E, Franceschi S, Tzonou A et al (1991) Pooled analysis of three European case-control studies of epithelial ovarian cancer: Reproductive factors and risk of epithelial ovarian cancer. Int J Cancer 49:50–56

Nishimoto A, Yu Y, Lu Z, Liao W S-L, Bast RC Jr, Luo RZ (2005) ARHI directly inhibits STAT3 translocation and activity in human breast and ovarian cancer cells. Cancer Res 65:6701–6710

Ozols RF, Daly MB, Klein-Szanto A, Hamilton TC, Bast RC, Brewer MA (2003) Chemoprevention of ovarian cancer: The journey begins. Gynecol Oncol 88:S59–S66; discussion S67–S70

Patton SE, Martin ML, Nelson LL, Fang XJ, Mills GB, Bast RC Jr, Ostrowski MC (1998) Activation of the Ras-MAP pathway and phosphorylation of ets-2 at position threonine 72 in human ovarian cancer cell lines. Cancer Res 58:2253–2259

Petricoin EF, Ardekani AM, Hitt BA, Levine PJ, Fusaro VA, Steinberg SM, Mills GB, Simone C, Fishman DA, Kohn EC, Liotta LA (2002) Use of proteomic patterns in serum to identify ovarian cancers. Lancet 359:572–577

Pothuri B, Leitao M, Barakat R, Akram M, Bogomolniy F, Olvera N, Lin O, Soslow R, Robson M, Offit K, Boyd J (2004) Analysis of ovarian carcinoma histogenesis. SGO Abstract #616

Rodriguez GC, Walmer DK, Cline M, Krigman H, Lessey BA, Whitaker RS, Dodge R, Hughes CL (1998) Effect of progestin on the ovarian epithelium of macaques: cancer prevention through apoptosis? J Soc Gynecol Investig 5:271–276

Sato S, Yokoyama Y, Sakamota T, Futagami M, Saito Y (2001) Usefulness of mass screening for ovarian carcinoma using transvaginal ultrasonography. Cancer 89:582–588

Schummer M, Ng WV, Bumgarner RE, Nelson PS, Schummer B, Bednarski DW, Hassell L, Baldwin RL, Karlan BY, Hood L (1999) Comparative hybridization of an array of 21,500 ovarian cDNAs for the discovery of genes overexpressed in ovarian carcinomas. Gene 238:375–385

Skates SJ, Xu F-J, Yu Y-H, Sjövall K, Einhorn N, Chang YC, Bast RC Jr, Knapp RC (1995) Toward an optimal algorithm for ovarian cancer screening with longitudinal tumor markers. Cancer 76:2004–2010

Skates SJ, Horick N, Yu Y, Xu F-J, Berchuck A, Havrilesky L, de Bruijn HW, van der Zee AGJ, Woolas RP, Jacobs IJ, Zhang Z, Bast RC Jr (2004) Pre-operative sensitivity and specificity for early stage ovarian cancer when combining CA 125, CA 15.3, CA 72.4 and M-CSF using mixtures of multivariate normal distributions. J Clin Oncol 22:4059–4066

Solomon SD, McMurray JJ, Pfeffer MA, Wittes J, Fowler R, Finn P, Anderson WF, Zauber A, Hawk E, Bertagnolli M (2005) Adenoma Prevention with Celecoxib (APC) Study investigators. Cardiovascular risk associated with celecoxib in a clinical trial for colorectal adenoma prevention. N Engl J Med 352:1071–1080

Taylor-Papadimitriou J, Burchell J, Miles DW, Dalziel M (1999) MUC1 and cancer. Biochim Biophys Acta. 1455:301–313

Utzinger U, Brewer M, Silva E, Gershenson D, Bast RC Jr, Mitchell MF, Richards-Kortum R (2001) Reflectance spectroscopy for in vivo characterization of ovarian tissue. Lasers Surg Med 28:56–66

Van Nagell JR, Depriest PD, Reedy MB, Gallion HH, Ueland FR, Pavlik EJ, Kryscio RJ (2000) The efficacy of transvaginal sonographic screening in asymptomatic women at risk for ovarian cancer. Gynecol Oncol 77:350–356

Vignali DA (2000) Multiplexed particle-based flow cytometric assays. J Immunol Meth 243:243–255

Xu Y, Shen Z, Wiper DW, Wu M, Morton RE, Elson P, Kennedy AW, Belinson J, Markman M, Casey G (1998) Lysophosphatidic acid as a potential biomarker for ovarian and other gynecologic cancers. JAMA 280:719–723

Yoneda J, Kuniyasu H, Crispens MA, Price JE, Bucana CD, Fidler IJ (1998) Expression of angiogenesis-related genes and progression of human ovarian carcinomas in nude mice. J Natl Cancer Inst 90:447–454

Yu Y, Xu F, Fang X, Zhao S, Li Y, Cuevas B, Kuo W-L, Gray JW, Siciliano M, Mills G, Bast RC Jr (1999) NOEY2 (ARHI), an imprinted putative tumor suppressor gene in ovarian and breast carcinomas. Proc Natl Acad Sci U S A 96:214–219

Zhang Z, Bast RC Jr, Yu Y, Li Jinong, Sokoll LJ, Rai A, Rosenzweig JM, Cameron B, Meng X-Y, Berchuck A, van Haaften-Day C, Hacker NF, de Bruijn HWA, van der Zee A, Jacobs IJ, Fung ET, Chan D (2004) A panel of serum biomarkers identified through proteomic profiling for the detection of early stage ovarian cancer. Cancer Res 64:5882–5890

Zhang Z, Xu F-J, Yu Y, Berchuck A, Havrilesky L, de Bruijn HW, van der Zee A, Woolas RP, Jacobs IJ, Skates S, Bast RC Jr (2006) Detection of Stage I epithelial ovarian cancer using an artificial neural network derived composite index of multiple serum markers. Gynecol Oncol, in revision

Prevention of Prostate Cancer: More Questions than Data

Hans-Peter Schmid, Daniel S. Engeler, Karl Pummer, Bernd J. Schmitz-Dräger

Recent Results in Cancer Research, Vol. 174
© Springer-Verlag Berlin Heidelberg 2007

Abstract

Established risk factors for prostatic adenocarcinoma include increasing age, ethnical origin (race), and familial/hereditary factors. Moreover, the epidemiology of the disease gives some indications that its etiology is probably not only genetic but also environmental. Pathological studies support the fact that geographic differences in incidence and prevalence do not stem from genetic variations as men with the same genetic background raised in different environments present the risk of prostate cancer associated with their country of residency. Prostate cancer is basically an ideal candidate for exogenous preventive measures, such as dietary and pharmacological prevention, due to some specific features: high prevalence, long latency, endocrine dependency, availability of serum markers (prostate-specific antigen) and histological precursor lesions (prostatic intraepithelial neoplasia). Dietary/nutritional factors that may influence disease development include total energy intake (as reflected by body mass index), dietary fat, cooked meat, micronutrients and vitamins (carotenoids, retinoids, vitamins C, D, and E), fruit and vegetable intake, minerals (calcium, selenium), and phytoestrogens (isoflavonoids, flavonoids, lignans). Pharmacological prevention may use drugs that act on intraprostatic testosterone metabolism (finasteride, dutasteride) or induce apoptosis and inhibit tumor growth and metastasis (statins). Since most studies reported to date are case–control analyses, there remain more questions than evidence-based data. However, several large randomized trials are ongoing to clarify the potential for successful prostate cancer prevention. Until we have the results, lifestyle changes could be recommended to men at risk for developing clinical prostate cancer and 5-alpha-reductase inhibitors need to be discussed with men who are concerned about prostate cancer.

Introduction

There are three well-known and indisputable risk factors for prostate cancer, namely increasing age, ethnic origin, and hereditary/familial factors (Aus et al. 2005). International variations in incidence rates for the disease are considerable and it has been suggested that environmental factors may also play a major role. Indeed, data from migration studies clearly demonstrate that the incidence for Asian men increases significantly when moving from their country of origin to the United States (Fig. 1).

Prostatic adenocarcinoma is an ideal candidate for prevention because of several important features including high prevalence of the disease. Endocrine and hormonal dependency makes it susceptible to pharmacological manipulations. Progression is very slow with a long latency period (Schmid et al. 1993). Histological precursor lesions such as prostatic intraepithelial neoplasia (PIN) take about 10 years to develop into early invasive tumor, with clinically significant cancer occurring some 3–4 years later. Prostate-specific antigen (PSA) is a good serum marker for clinical monitoring of disease.

There are, on the other hand, multiple factors potentially influencing the results of trials and making analysis of data more difficult. Among them are validity of studies (case–control, co-

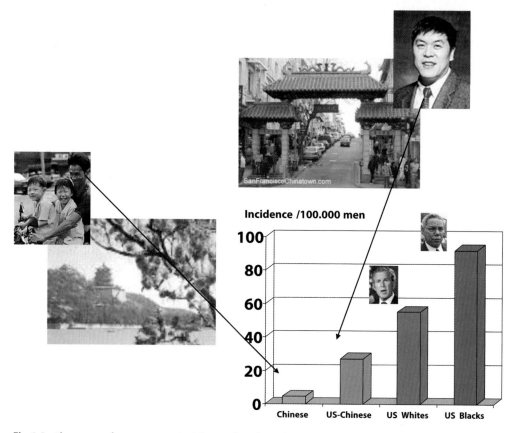

Fig. 1 Incidence rates of prostate cancer in different ethnical populations and the influence of migration

hort, interventional) (Table 1), the follow-up interval in the interventional and most cohort studies, validity of questionnaires, hereditary factors, data from different ethnic backgrounds, correlation between nutrition and lifestyle, and interaction between several nutritional compounds (Schmitz-Dräger et al. 2001).

Dietary/Nutritional Factors

Dietary Fat

High calorie intake has often been associated with an increased risk of prostate cancer. However, the interaction between various compounds (total fat, animal fat, saturated or unsaturated fatty acids, cholesterol, triglycerides, omega-3 fatty acids) is very complex (Wuermli

et al. 2005). Theoretically, high energy intake may stimulate the sympathetic nervous system and basal metabolism and may increase IGF-1 release, thus leading to increased mitosis and cell proliferation (Meyer et al. 1999). The majority of case–control and cohort studies report a positive association between fat consumption and prostate cancer with a relative risk around 2.

Micronutrients

Carotenoids are a group of complex unsaturated hydrocarbons occurring as pigments in plants such as carrots (alpha-, beta-, gamma-carotene) or tomatoes (lycopene). Some carotenoids, but not lycopene, are precursors of vitamin A and they have been shown to act as antioxidants and inhibitors of IGF-1. Giovannucci (1999) reviewed

Table 1 Data on dietary and nutritional factors according to evidence levels

Level Ia	No data
Level Ib	(Selenium)
Level IIa	Lycopene
Level IIb	Dietary fat, vitamin E, rye, soya, and phytoestrogens
Level III	Saturated fat, vitamin E, beta-carotene

Cochrane Collaboration

72 studies concerning intake of tomatoes and tomato-based products and blood lycopene levels in relation to the risk of various cancers. An inverse association was identified in 57 reports and 35 of them were statistically significant. The evidence for a benefit was strongest for tumors of the prostate, lung, and stomach. Conversely, no study indicated that intake of tomatoes or a high serum lycopene level led to an increased risk of cancer of any site.

Vitamins

Numerous studies could demonstrate an inverse correlation between intake of vitamins and incidence of various types of malignant tumors. Of special interest with regard to prostate cancer were vitamins A, C, D, and E.

Vitamin A (retinol) and its precursor (beta-carotene) are found in foods of animal origin (liver, fish oil) or in carrots and green vegetables (spinach, broccoli), respectively. They act as antioxidants by suppressing the carcinogenic potential of free radicals, enhance the immune system, and induce cellular differentiation. Dose-related side effects include hepatotoxicity, central nervous system changes, and mucocutaneous dryness and, therefore, hamper their use in clinical trials (Heinonen et al. 1998).

Vitamin C is a water-soluble antioxidant in fruit and vegetables. The majority of case–control and cohort studies failed to demonstrate any correlation between vitamin C intake or plasma concentrations and occurrence of prostate cancer.

Calcitriol (1,25 dihydroxyvitamin D3) is the active form of vitamin D and responsible for calcium metabolism in kidneys, bone, and gut. A favorable impact of ultraviolet radiation (sun exposure), which is the main source of vitamin D, on the incidence of prostate cancer has been postulated (Hanchette and Schwartz 1992). In primary cultures of prostatic tissues derived from prostate cancer patients, vitamin D3 carried out antiproliferative effects (Peehl et al. 1994). However, the role of vitamin D in prostate cancer promotion and prevention is still controversial.

Vitamin E (alpha-tocopherol) is a fat-soluble potent intracellular antioxidant occurring in lettuce, watercress, and cotton- and hemp-seed oil. In the Finnish alpha-tocopherol beta-carotene (ATBC) trial, 29,133 male smokers aged 50–69 years were randomly assigned to receive alpha-tocopherol (50 mg), beta-carotene (20 mg), both agents, or placebo daily for 5–8 years (Heinonen et al. 1998). However, in this study prostate cancer was only looked at as a secondary end point. A 32% decrease in the incidence and a 41% decrease in mortality from prostate cancer was observed among the subjects receiving alpha-tocopherol compared with those not receiving it. Notably, among men receiving beta-carotene, prostate cancer incidence was 23% higher and mortality was 15% higher compared with those not receiving it. Despite these data, results from other epidemiologic studies do not support a general protective effect of vitamin E.

Minerals

Conversion of vitamin D to the active form 1,25 dihydroxyvitamin D3 is suppressed by high consumption of dietary calcium (milk, cheese) (see also Sect. 2.3). Furthermore, low serum calcium levels stimulate the secretion of parathyroid hormone which promotes the conversion of vitamin D to calcitriol. From a clinical point of view, calcium has been found in excess levels to be associated with an increased rate of prostate cancer progression.

Selenium, a trace element occurring predominantly as selenomethionine in dietary supplements (bread, cereals, fish, chicken, meat), is a key component of a number of functional selenoproteins required for normal health. In a double-blind cancer prevention trial, 974 men with a history of basal cell or squamous cell carcinoma were randomized to either receive 200 µg selenium daily or placebo for a mean of 4.5 years (Clark et al. 1998). Selenium treatment was associated with a 63% reduction in the secondary endpoint of prostate cancer incidence, but the number of cases was rather low. Long-term selenium intake can be determined in toenails. In a nested case–control study within the Health Professionals Follow-Up Study, high levels of selenium in toenails were correlated with a reduced risk for advanced prostate cancer (Yoshizawa et al. 1998). A more recent prospective case–control study did not find a statistically significant difference in toenail selenium levels of patients with newly diagnosed prostate cancer and matched controls (Lipsky et al. 2004). The National Cancer Institute launched a large randomized trial (SELECT study) with four arms to compare selenium (200 µg) plus vitamin E (400 IU) to either agent alone or to placebo. Results will be available presumably after the year 2012 (Table 1).

Phytoestrogens

The major categories of phytoestrogens include isoflavonoids (genistein, daidzein), flavonoids (quercetin), and lignans (enterolactone). The first two groups are found in vegetables such as beans, peas, and especially soy and in fruits; lignans also occur in grains, cereals, and linseeds. The putative biological effects of phytoestrogens are listed in Table 2. In geographic areas with low prostate cancer incidence (Asia, southern Europe) diets are rich in phytoestrogens, which has been confirmed by higher serum levels or urinary concentrations of phytoestrogens compared to Western countries (Adlercreutz et al. 1993). The favorable antitumoral effects of various soy-derived products have been demonstrated in experimental studies; however, clinical data are sparse and assessment of dietary phytoestrogen intake is complex. In an analysis of data from 59 countries, prostate cancer mortality was related to food consumption, tobacco use, socioeconomic factors, reproductive factors, and health indicators (Hebert et al. 1998). Mortality rates were inversely associated with estimated intake of cereals, nuts, oilseed and fish, and soy products were found to be significantly protective.

Pharmacological Prevention

5-Alpha-Reductase Inhibitors

Primary chemoprevention of prostatic carcinoma is an appealing concept with drugs acting on intraprostatic testosterone metabolism. Finasteride and dutasteride are inhibitors of steroid 5-alpha-reductase, the enzyme that converts testosterone to the much more potent androgen dihydrotestosterone.

In the Prostate Cancer Prevention Trial (PCPT), a total of 18,882 men 55 years of age or older were randomly assigned to either receive finasteride (5 mg daily) or placebo for 7 years (Thompson et al. 2003). Digital rectal examination (DRE) was normal in all men and PSA was 3.0 ng/ml or lower. During follow-up, prostatic biopsy was recommended if DRE turned abnor-

Table 2 Potential mechanisms of phytoestrogens on prostatic epithelial cells

Increase of SHBG serum concentration and subsequent decrease of free testosterone through binding to liver estrogen receptors
Decrease of DNA synthesis through inhibition of tyrosine kinase and topoisomerase
Decrease of the effects of free radicals through antioxidant properties
Inhibition of cytochrome P450 activation
Neoangiogenesis inhibition
Inhibition of intraprostatic testosterone metabolism through inhibition of 5-alpha-reductase and aromatase

SHBG Sex hormone binding globulin

Adapted from Schmitz-Dräger et al. 2001

mal or if the annual PSA level, adjusted for the effect of finasteride, increased above 4.0 ng/ml (so-called for cause biopsy). An end-of-study biopsy was planned for all participants. Primary end point was prevalence of prostate cancer during the 7 years of study. Secondary end points included incidence of lower urinary tract symptoms (LUTS) and side effects of finasteride.

Detection rate of prostate cancer was 18.4% in the finasteride group compared to 24.4% in the placebo arm, which translates into a 24.8% reduction in prevalence ($p<0.001$) (Fig. 2). The relative risk reduction was consistent in all subgroups, irrespective of age, ethnical origin, and familial risk. Tumors of Gleason scores 7–10 were more common in the finasteride arm, a fact that sparked much discussion and controversy. In the meantime, this issue could be solved and explained by several arguments. As anticipated, LUTS were more common in the men receiving placebo, whereas sexual side effects were more common in the finasteride group. In conclusion, a careful risk–benefit analysis with the individual patient must be undertaken before finasteride chemoprevention can be recommended.

Statins

3-hydroxy-3-methylglutaryl coenzyme A reductase inhibitors have been shown to induce apoptosis and inhibit tumor growth and metastasis in human cancer cell lines and animal models. In a case–control study, 100 patients with newly diagnosed prostate cancer and 202 controls were checked for any use of statins over a 7-year period through an electronic pharmacy database in the Veterans Administration system (Shannon et al. 2005). Statin use was associated with a significant reduction in prostate cancer risk (odds ratio, 0.38) and the effect was especially pronounced in Gleason scores 7–10. Further studies are needed to determine the role of statins in prostate cancer prevention.

Aspirin

Aspirin and other nonsteroidal anti-inflammatory drugs (NSAID) have been associated with a reduced risk of cancer implicating inflammatory processes in cancer development. Information

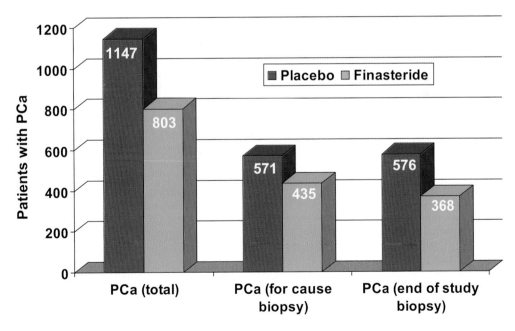

Fig. 2 Prostate Cancer Prevention Trial (PCPT). Patients with prostate cancer (PCa) in the finasteride and placebo group, respectively (absolute numbers)

on NSAID use was obtained from a questionnaire sent to 70,144 men in the American Cancer Society's Cancer Prevention Study II nutrition cohort (Jacobs et al. 2005). Neither current aspirin use nor current use of a NSAID was associated with prostate cancer risk, even at the highest usage level. However, long-duration – 5 or more years – regular use of these agents was associated with reduced risk of prostate cancer (RR, 0.85 for aspirin; RR, 0.82 for NSAID). These results suggest a modest beneficial effect on the incidence of prostate cancer but should be confirmed in further studies.

Physical Activity/Sports

The influence of physical activity on prostate cancer incidence has been looked at in two Scandinavian cohort studies. In a population-based cohort study of 53,242 men aged 19–50 years in Norway, information on physical activity was based on questionnaire responses and a brief clinical examination (Thune and Lund 1994). When occupational and recreational physical activity were combined, a reduced adjusted risk of prostate cancer was observed among men who walked during occupational hours and performed either moderate (RR, 0.61) or regular recreational training (RR, 0.45) relative to sedentary men.

From a Swedish nationwide census, two cohorts of men were identified whose occupational title allowed classification of physical activity levels at work in 1960 and in 1970 (Norman et al. 2002). A third cohort included only men whose jobs required a similar level of activity in both 1960 and 1970. The incidence of prostate cancer was ascertained through record linkage to the Swedish Cancer Register. In all three cohorts, the relative risk for prostate cancer increased with decreasing level of occupational physical activity. Among men with the same physical activity levels in 1960 and 1970, the ratio was 1.11 for men with sedentary jobs as compared with those whose jobs had very high or high activity levels. There was, however, no association between occupational activity and prostate cancer mortality.

Conclusions

There are currently no conclusive study outcomes with respect to prevention of prostate cancer that meet the criteria of evidence-based medicine. Until we have the results of ongoing prospective trials, lifestyle changes could be recommended to men at risk for developing clinical prostate cancer (Aus et al. 2005). These measures may include balanced food intake (Mediterranean style) and physical activity. Chemoprevention at present is not (yet) standard but finasteride must be discussed with the patient.

References

Adlercreutz H, Markkanen H, Watanabe S (1993) Plasma concentrations of phyto-oestrogens in Japanese men. Lancet 342:1209–1210

Aus G, Abbou CC, Bolla M, Heidenreich A, Schmid H-P, van Poppel H, Wolff J, Zattoni F (2005) EAU guidelines on prostate cancer. Eur Urol 48:546–551

Clark LC, Dalkin B, Krongrad A, Combs GF Jr, Turnbull BW, Slate EH, Witherington R, Herlong JH, Janosko E, Carpenter D, Borosso C, Falk S, Rounder J (1998) Decreased incidence of prostate cancer with selenium supplementation: results of a double-blind cancer prevention trial. Br J Urol 81:730–734

Giovannucci E (1999) Tomatoes, tomato-based products, lycopene, and cancer: review of the epidemiologic literature. J Natl Cancer Inst 91:317–331

Hanchette CL, Schwartz GG (1992) Geographic patterns of prostate cancer mortality. Evidence for a protective effect of ultraviolet radiation. Cancer 70:2861–2869

Hebert JR, Hurley TG, Olendzki BC, Teas J, Ma Y, Hampl JS (1998) Nutritional and socioeconomic factors in relation to prostate cancer mortality: a cross-national study. J Natl Cancer Inst 90:1637–1647

Heinonen OP, Albanes D, Virtamo J, Taylor PR, Huttunen JK, Hartman AM, Haapakoski J, Malila N, Rautalahti M, Ripatti S, Maenpaa H, Teerenhovi L, Koss L, Virolainen M, Edwards BK (1998) Prostate cancer and supplementation with alpha-tocopherol and beta-carotene: incidence and mortality in a controlled trial. J Natl Cancer Inst 90:440–446

Jacobs EJ, Rodriguez C, Mondul AM, Connell CJ, Henley SJ, Calle EE, Thun MJ (2005) A large cohort study of aspirin and other nonsteroidal anti-inflammatory drugs and prostate cancer incidence. J Natl Cancer Inst 97:975–980

Lipsky K, Zigeuner R, Zischka M, Schips L, Pummer K, Rehak P, Hubmer G (2004) Selenium levels of patients with newly diagnosed prostate cancer compared with control group. Urology 63:912–916

Meyer F, Bairati I, Shadmani R, Fradet Y, Moore L (1999) Dietary fat and prostate cancer survival. Cancer Causes Control 10:245–251

Norman A, Moradi T, Gridley G, Dosemeci M, Rydh B, Nyren O, Wolk A (2002) Occupational physical activity and risk for prostate cancer in a nationwide cohort study in Sweden. Br J Cancer 86:70–75

Peehl DM, Skowronski RJ, Leung GK, Wong ST, Stamey TA, Feldman D (1994) Antiproliferative effects of 1,25 dihydroxyvitamin D3 on primary cultures of human prostatic cells. Cancer Res 54:805–810

Schmid H-P, McNeal JE, Stamey TA (1993) Observations on the doubling time of prostate cancer: the use of serial prostate-specific antigen in patients with untreated disease as a measure of increasing cancer volume. Cancer 71:2031–2040

Schmitz-Dräger BJ, Eichholzer M, Beiche B, Ebert T (2001) Nutrition and prostate cancer. Urol Int 67:1–11

Shannon J, Tewoderos S, Garzotto M, Beer TM, Derenick R, Palma A, Farris PE (2005) Statins and prostate cancer risk: a case-control study. Am J Epidemiol 162:318–325

Thompson IM, Goodman PJ, Tangen CM, Lucia MS, Miller GJ, Ford LG, Lieber MM, Cespedes RD, Atkins JN, Lippman SM, Carlin SM, Ryan A, Szczepanek CM, Crowley JJ, Coltman Jr CA (2003) The influence of finasteride on the development of prostate cancer. N Engl J Med 349:215–224

Thune I, Lund E (1994) Physical activity and the risk of prostate and testicular cancer: a cohort study of 53,000 Norwegian men. Cancer Causes Control 5:549–556

Wuermli L, Joerger M, Henz S, Schmid H-P, Riesen WF, Thomas G, Krek W, Cerny T, Gillessen S (2005) Hypertriglyceridemia as a possible risk factor for prostate cancer. Prostate Cancer Prostatic Dis 8:316–320

Yoshizawa K, Willett WC, Morris SJ, Stampfer MJ, Spiegelman D, Rimm EB, Giovannucci E (1998) Study of prediagnostic selenium level in toenails and the risk of advanced prostate cancer. J Natl Cancer Inst 90:1219–1224

Part IV Prevention
of Breast Cancer

Primary Prevention of Breast Cancer by Hormone-Induced Differentiation

Irma H. Russo, Jose Russo

Recent Results in Cancer Research, Vol. 174
© Springer-Verlag Berlin Heidelberg 2007

Abstract

Breast cancer is a fatal disease whose incidence is gradually increasing in most industrialized countries and in all ethnic groups. Primary prevention is the ultimate goal for the control of this disease. The knowledge that breast cancer risk is reduced by early full-term pregnancy and that additional pregnancies increase the rate of protection has provided novel tools for designing cancer prevention strategies. The protective effect of pregnancy has been experimentally reproduced in virgin rats by treatment with the placental hormone human chorionic gonadotropin (hCG). HCG prevents the initiation and inhibits the progression of chemically induced mammary carcinomas by inducing differentiation of the mammary gland, inhibiting cell proliferation, and increasing apoptosis. It also induces the synthesis of inhibin, a tumor suppressor factor, downregulates the level of expression of the estrogen receptor alpha (ER-α) by methylation of CpG islands, imprinting a permanent genomic signature that characterizes the refractory condition of the mammary gland to undergo malignant transformation. The genomic signature induced by hCG is identical to that induced by pregnancy and is specific for this hormone. Comparison of the mammary gland's genomic profile of virgin Sprague-Dawley rats treated daily with hCG for 21 days with that of rats receiving 17β-estradiol (E_2) and progesterone (Pg) (E_2+ Pg) revealed that in hCG-treated rats 194 genes were significantly up-modulated (>2.5 log2-folds) ($p<0.01$) and commonly expressed, whereas these genes were not expressed in the E_2+ Pg group. The genomic signature induced by hCG and pregnancy included activators or repressors of transcription genes, apoptosis, growth factors, cell division control, DNA repair, tumor suppressor, and cell-surface antigen genes. Our data indicate that hCG, like pregnancy, induces permanent genomic changes that are not reproduced by steroid hormones and in addition regulates gene expression through epigenetic mechanisms that are differentiation-dependent processes, leading us to conclude that hormonally induced differentiation offers enormous promise for the primary prevention of breast cancer.

Introduction

Breast cancer, the fatal disease most frequently diagnosed in American women, is increasing in incidence at a rate of approximately 6% per year in women from all ethnic groups (Greenlee et al. 2001; Jemal et al. 2002). Similar trends are observed worldwide, even in countries characterized by their low breast cancer incidence (De Waard and Thijssen 2005; Forbes 1997; Howe et al. 2001). Improved detection methods, the identification of women at higher risk by family history or detection of germline mutations in the BRCA1 and BRCA2 genes (Warmuth et al. 1997), and diagnosis at an early stage have resulted in a decline in breast cancer mortality in the United States (Greenlee et al. 2001; Jemal et al. 2002; Forbes 1997). Although genetic predisposition accounts for fewer than one in ten cases of breast cancer, women that are carriers of BRCA1/BRCA2 germline mutations are at an

85% lifetime risk of developing breast cancer, with a significantly earlier age of onset of the disease (Chang and Elledge 2001). Current strategies to prevent breast cancer in women at high risk are prophylactic mastectomy, oophorectomy, or antiestrogen therapy (Armstron et al. 2005), whereas for the general population, trials of dietary changes with reduced fat intake designed to mimic the diets of countries with low breast cancer incidence are advocated. Opponents of this approach argue that only a lifetime dietary change can decrease the risk of breast cancer, and therefore major dietary changes undertaken now may not alter breast cancer incidence for another generation (Tymchuk et al. 2000). Another strategy capitalizes in a unique feature of breast cancer, its estrogen dependence, which can be manipulated to control growth or prevent tumor development utilizing either selective estrogen receptor modulators (SERMs), such as tamoxifen (King et al. 2001; Narod et al. 2000; Baum 2002; Mouridsen et al. 2001; Robertson et al. 2001), or aromatase inhibitors (AIs), such as Arimidex, Letrozole, and Exemestane (Janov et al. 2001; Tymchuk et al. 2000). However, the inability to predict precisely who will develop breast cancer has required the implementation of broad, population-based strategies utilizing preventative measures that have significant side effects and require a protracted treatment. These drawbacks have made these strategies not widely acceptable to a majority of treated women who would not have developed breast cancer even if untreated (Gail et al. 1989).

In light of the fact that more than 50% of breast cancer cases remain unexplained by personal characteristics and other traditionally accepted risk factors, that once the disease becomes metastatic it becomes incurable (Mirza et al. 2002), and the observed worldwide increased incidence of the disease, effective interventions for its primary prevention are urgently required (De Waard and Thijssen 2005; Dunn et al. 2000; Hoffmann et al. 2001; Matsumoto and Yamane 2000; Mirza et al. 2002).

Up to now the possibilities of successfully preventing breast cancer have been hindered by the lack of identification of a definitive causal agent or a mechanism responsible of its initiation. Currently, only inheritance of cancer-predisposing genes (Mirza et al. 2002; King et al. 2001; Lynch and Casey 2001; Narod et al. 2000; Khurana et al. 2000; Narod 2001; Riggs 2001; Stoutjesdijk and Barentsz 2001; Hartmann et al. 2001), and radiation exposure at a young age (McGregor et al. 1977; Boice et al. 1991; Clemons et al. 2000; Cutuli et al. 2001; Janov et al. 2001) have been identified as a mechanism or causal agent associated with cancer initiation. Multidisciplinary studies based on epidemiological, endocrinological, experimental, and statistical findings have found a direct association of breast cancer risk with nulliparity, confirming conclusions reached by the Italian physician Bernardino Ramazzini, who, almost 300 years ago, considered breast cancer an occupational disease because of its association with celibacy and nulliparity in nuns (Ramazzini 1961). A large body of evidence has confirmed that nulliparity increases breast cancer risk by 30% when compared with parous women (Blair et al. 1999; Ewertz et al. 1990; Fraumeni et al. 1969). A reduction in lifetime breast cancer risk has been found to be conferred by an early first full-term pregnancy (Trapido 1983; MacMahon et al. 1970; Chie et al. 2000; Holmberg et al.2001; Vessey et al. 1985; Kelsey and Horn-Ross 1993; Lambe et al. 1996). In addition, a greater number of full-term pregnancies increases the protection. Each additional birth after the first reduces the breast cancer risk by 7% in the absence of breastfeeding (Collaborative Group on Hormonal Factors in Breast Cancer 2002). Breastfeeding confers an additional protection of 4.3% reduction in risk for each year a woman breastfeeds (Collaborative Group on Hormonal Factors in Breast Cancer 2002), even if they are carriers of BRCA1 germline mutations (Jernstrom et al. 2004).

Physiological Basis of Breast Cancer Prevention

The above-described epidemiological observations indicating that pregnancy significantly reduces the lifetime risk of developing breast cancer provide a window of opportunity for learning how and why this physiological condition exerts such a protective effect. Due to the complexity of the carcinogenic process, this event does not explain all the aspects of this complex disease; nevertheless, data obtained in experimental models have served as a blue print for developing a new paradigm in breast cancer prevention (I.H. Russo and J. Russo 1993, 1994, 1996; I.H. Russo et al. 1990a, b; J. Russo et al. 1977; Srivastava et al. 1998; Mgbonyebi et al. 1996; Tahin et al. 1996; J. Russo and I.H. Russo 2000; Alvarado et al. 1993, 1994). Our studies have unraveled the biological principle underlying the protection conferred by an early first full-term pregnancy, demonstrating experimentally that it induces in the breast the expression of a specific signature in response to the differentiation of this organ driven by the reproductive process. This signature serves, in turn, as a biomarker associated with lifetime decreased breast cancer risk. More importantly, we have harnessed this biological principle by demonstrating in an experimental model that a short treatment with human chorionic gonadotropin (hCG), a placental hormone secreted during pregnancy, induces the same genomic signature as pregnancy, inhibiting not only the initiation but also the progression of mammary carcinomas, stopping the development of early lesions, such as intraductal proliferations, and carcinomas in situ (CIS) (Srivastava et al. 1998). These observations indicate that hCG administered for a very short period of time has significant potential as a chemopreventive agent, exerting a long-lasting inhibition of the transforming potential of the normal cell without altering the organ's physiology. This new biological concept implies that when the genomic signature of protection or refractoriness to carcinogenesis is acquired, the hormonal treatment with hCG is no longer required, contrasting with the need of continuous administration of currently used chemopreventive agents for suppressing a metabolic pathway or abrogating the function of an organ (King et al. 2001; Narod et al. 2000).

Epidemiological and Clinical Basis for the New Paradigm

Epidemiological and clinical evidence indicates that endocrinological and reproductive influences play major roles in breast cancer. It has long been known that the incidence of breast cancer is greater in nulliparous than in parous women (Nix 1964; Kelsey and Horn-Ross 1993; Lambe et al. 1996; J. Russo et al. 1982). Changes in lifestyle, that in turn influence the endocrinology of women, have been observed during the last decades in American women, namely a progressive decrease in the age of menarche (Tanner 1973; Kelsey and Horn-Ross 1993) and a progressive increase in the age at which a woman bears her first child (Lambe et al. 1996). The significance of these changes is highlighted by the reduction in breast cancer risk associated with late menarche and the completion of a full-term pregnancy before age 24, with further reduction in the lifetime breast cancer risk as the number of pregnancies increases (Kelsey and Horn-Ross 1993; Lambe et al. 1996; J. Russo et al. 1982). Women who undergo their first full-term pregnancy after age 30, on the other hand, appear to be at higher risk of breast cancer development than nulliparous women, suggesting that parity-induced protection against breast cancer is related to the timing of a first full-term pregnancy. Pregnancy is also associated with a transient increase relative to nulliparous women, lasting 10–15 years, followed thereafter by a decreased risk; the protection conferred lasts a lifetime (Lambe et al. 1996). Of interest is the fact that women from different countries and ethnic groups exhibit a similar degree of parity-induced protection from breast cancer, regardless of the endogenous incidence of this malignancy (Rao et al. 1994; Coe 1998). This observation suggests that the reduction in breast cancer risk associated with early first full-term pregnancy does not result from factors specific to a particular environmental, genetic, or socioeconomic setting, but rather from an intrinsic effect of parity on the biology of the breast (Apter 1996; Coe 1998; Gaudette et al. 1996; Kelsey and Horn-Ross 1993; Lambe et al. 1996; Rao et al. 1994; J. Russo et al. 1982; Shivvers and Miller 1997). Environmental, genetic, and socioeconomic factors, among others, affect the endocrine milieu, indirectly influencing the breast's susceptibility to developing cancer. These observations indicate that an early first full-term pregnancy modifies, through mechanisms still poorly understood, specific biological characteristics of the breast that result in a lifetime decreased risk of cancer development

Experimental Animal Studies: Role of Pregnancy and Chorionic Gonadotropin in Mammary Gland Differentiation and Cancer Initiation

Experimental studies have contributed to clarifying the mechanisms of this protection by demonstrating the role played by pregnancy-induced terminal differentiation of the mammary gland on the susceptibility of the mammary epithelium to carcinogenesis (Nandi et al. 1995; Rao et al. 1994; J. Russo et al. 1979, 1982, 1992; J. Russo and I.H. Russo 1980a, b; 1993, 1994). These observations indicate that the terminally differentiated state of lactation should be reached for attaining protection, although other mechanisms have been proposed for the protective effect of early first full-term pregnancy, including the occurrence of sustained changes in the level or regulation of hormones that affect the breast (I.H. Russo et al. 1991; Sinha et al. 1983). Regardless the intervening mechanism, the end result of the first pregnancy is a dramatic modification of the architecture of the breast (Nandi et al. 1995; I.H. Russo et al. 1991; I.H. Russo and J. Russo 1998; J. Russo et al. 1979, 1982, 1992; Sinha et al. 1983).

The induction of mammary cancer in rodents with a polycyclic aromatic hydrocarbon (PAH) such as 7,12-dimethylbenz(a)anthracene (DMBA) requires that the carcinogen be administered to young nulliparous females (J. Russo et al. 1977). In Sprague-Dawley rats, if the females have completed a full-term pregnancy with or without lactation, prior to carcinogen exposure, carcinoma incidence is dramatically decreased (J. Russo et al. 1979, 1982; J. Russo and I.H. Russo 1980a, b, 1994). The inhibitory effect of pregnancy on mammary cancer initiation can be mimicked in virgin rats by treatment with the glycoprotein placental hormone chorionic gonadotropin (hCG). Administration of hCG as a daily intraperitoneal injection for 21 days, followed by a 21-day resting period prior to carcinogen administration results in a dose-related reduction in tumor incidence and number of tumors per animal (I.H. Russo and J. Russo 1993, 1994; I.H. Russo et al. 1990a, b; J. Russo et al. 1977). This phenomenon is in great part mediated by the induction of mammary gland differentiation, the inhibition of cell proliferation, an increase in the DNA repair capabilities of the mammary epithelium, decreased binding of the carcinogen to the DNA, and activation of genes controlling programmed cell death (PCD) and of tumor suppressor genes (Alvarado et al. 1993, 1994; Mgbonyebi et al. 1996; I.H. Russo and J. Russo 1994, 1996; J. Russo et al. 1982; J. Russo and I.H. Russo 2000; Srivastava et al. 1998; Tahin et al. 1996). Our results indicate that hCG activates physiological and phylogenetically conserved forms of active cell death, such as PCD or apoptosis, which are associated with specific phases of development that control cell proliferation and differentiation (J. Russo and I.H. Russo 2000). Among the tumor suppressor genes activated by hCG is inhibin, a gene product primarily found in testes and ovary (Alvarado et al. 1993). Inhibin-deficient mice homozygous for the null allele identifies α-inhibin as an important negative regulator of cell proliferation. Our results indicate that inhibin mediates the differentiating action of both pregnancy and hCG on the mammary gland, in which it might act as an autocrine and/or paracrine growth regulator (I.H. Russo and J. Russo 1994).

Role of hCG in Breast Cancer Progression

Our studies of the protective effect of hCG-induced differentiation on experimental mammary carcinogenesis led us to postulate the possibility that hCG might be useful in preventing the development of breast cancer in women. The fact that the time of initiation of breast cancer in the female population is not known represented a major drawback for accomplishing the goal of instituting a truly preventative hormonal treatment. Thus, it had to be assumed that all women are at risk of being the carriers of initiated lesions. This assumption requires that before the hormonal treatment is initiated it has to be proven that it either inhibits the progression of putatively initiated cells, or at least does not cause tumor progression. Based upon our previous observations that the chemical carcinogen DMBA induces neoplastic transformation in the mammary gland by acting on the highly proliferating TEBs of the virgin animal (I.H. Russo and J. Russo 1996; J. Russo et al. 1979, 1982), and that once initiated these structures progress to intraductal proliferations (IDPs) within

3 weeks of exposure to the carcinogen (Srivastava et al. 1998; J. Russo et al. 1982), we tested the effect of hCG on tumor progression by administering 8 mg DMBA/100 g body weight to 45-day-old virgin Sprague-Dawley rats. Twenty days later, when IDPs were already evident, the animals were treated with 100 IU/hCG per day for 40 days (DMBA+hCG group). Age-matched untreated, hCG–, and DMBA+ saline-treated rats were used as controls. Tissues were collected at the time of DMBA administration and at 5, 10, 20, and 40 days of hCG injection, and 20 days after cessation of treatment (I.H. Russo and J. Russo 1996; J. Russo and I.H. Russo 2000).

Mammary Gland Development
Under the Influence of hCG

The development of the mammary gland in the rat requires the evaluation of changes in the parenchyma of the gland, since, unlike women, no significant external changes occur in this organ after puberty (I.H. Russo and J. Russo 1996). The

six pairs of the mammary gland of the young virgin rat is composed of ducts ending in club-shaped terminal end buds (TEBs), which are multilayered structures measuring 100–140 μm in diameter. They are lined by a 3- to 10-layer thick cuboidal epithelium that rests on a discontinuous layer of myoepithelial cells (J. Russo et al. 1977; I.H. Russo and J. Russo 1996; J. Russo and I.H. Russo 1980). After the beginning of ovarian function, the mammary ducts undergo further longitudinal lengthening and branching with sprouting of a few alveolar buds (ABs) that progressively evolve to lobular structures (Fig. 1). The lobules found in the rat mammary gland can be classified according to their degree of development as lobule type 1 (Lob 1), which consists of clusters of approximately 10 ± 4 ductules per unit. Individual ductules are lined by a single layer of cuboidal epithelial cells and few myoepithelial cells. With further growth, Lob 1 evolve to lobules type 2 (Lob 2), which are larger and composed of approximately 40 ± 7 ductules; these progress to lobules type 3 (Lob 3), that contain approximately 60 ± 12 ductules or alveoli

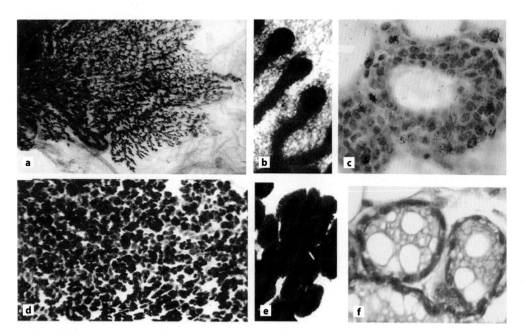

Fig. 1 a Whole mount of a virgin rat mammary gland, 55 days of age (toluidine blue, ×2). **b** Terminal end buds (TEBs) (toluidine blue, ×10). **c** TEB is a multilayer structure measuring 100–140 μm in diameter. The TEB is lined by a three- to ten-layer-thick cuboidal epithelium that rests on a discontinuous layers of myoepithelial cells. **d** Whole mount of a pregnant rat mammary gland, 75 days of age (toluidine blue, ×2). **e** Lobule type 3 (toluidine blue, ×10). **f** Histological section of the ductules of a lobule type 3 containing secretory material (H&E, ×40)

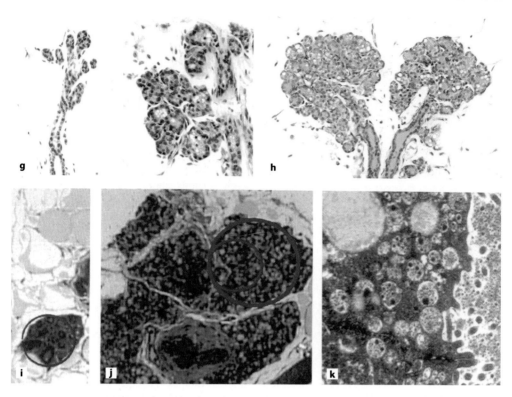

Fig. 1 *(continued)* **g–i** The lobules found in the rat mammary gland can be classified according to their degree of development as Lob 1, which consists of clusters of approximately 10±4 ductules per unit (**g**). Individual ductules are lined by a single layers of cuboidal epithelial cells (ECs) and few myo-ECs. With further growth, Lob 1 evolves to Lob 2, which is larger, and composed of approximately 40±7 ductules (**h**). Lob 3 contains approximately 60±12 ductules or alveoli per lobule (**i**); **j–l** Under the effect of hCG, the mammary gland forms lobules type 4 (**j**) that are formed by more than 80 ductules per lobular unit containing material in their lumen (**k**). Electron microscopy section in **l**, shows the proteinaceous and lipid composition of the milk secretion. (Uranyl acetate and lead citrate, ×4,000)

per lobule (I.H. Russo et al. 1990a). The administration of 100 IU/hCG per day for 40 days to young virgin rats deeply affects the development of the mammary gland, profoundly modifying the relative proportions of Lob 1, Lob 2, and Lob 3. While the concentration of Lob 1 in the mammary gland of untreated or saline-injected control virgin rats decreases slightly as a consequence of aging, in hCG-treated animals the number of Lob 1 decreases slightly by the 10th day of hormonal treatment, and even further between the 20th and 40th days. After cessation of treatment, their number increases sharply, reaching the same values found in control animals. Lob 2 are practically nonexistent in the 45-day-old animals; they first became evident when the animals

reach the age of 75 days, and their percentage increases even further in the next 10 days, reaching its peak in the 85-day-old animals, remaining unchanged thereafter. With hCG treatment, the lobules type 2 develop in a biphasic pattern. Their concentration increases progressively from 70 to 85 days of age, decrease significantly by the time the animals reach the age of 105 days, and increase again after cessation of treatment. Lob 3 formation, on the other hand, starts at the 10th day of treatment, it increases progressively between the 20th and 40th days, decreasing only after cessation of the hormonal treatment due to their regression to Lob 2. The resulting recovery of this type of lobule is absent in control animals.

Effect of hCG on Terminal End Buds, Intraductal Proliferations, and Ductal Carcinomas in Situ

The mammary gland of 45-day-old virgin rats contains the highest number of terminal end buds (TEBs). In animals of the saline control group, the number of TEBs decreased slightly as a function of age, as has been previously described, whereas in the DMBA group their number remained constant. In both hCG-treated groups, a reduction in the relative percentage of TEBs was observed as early as 5 days after the initiation of treatment, and more sharply between the 10th and the 20th days, to reach a plateau thereafter. The percentage of TEBs in these two groups of animals was significantly lower than the values found in the saline control and DMBA groups ($p<0.01$). A more noticeable effect of the hormonal treatment occurred at the level of intraductal proliferations (IDPs) and ductal carcinoma in situ (DCIS). In DMBA-treated animals, there were 5.80 IDPs per gland when they reached the age of 105 days, that is, 25-fold higher than the values observed in the hCG-treated animals, in which there were 0.23 IDP/gland. These differences were still significant in the 125-day-old animals. The number of DCISs was also higher in the DMBA-treated group, and their number was decreased by 13-fold by hCG treatment. The number of DCISs increased slightly when the animals reached the age of 125 days, averaging 1.76 DCISs/gland; however, it was still significantly lower than that observed in the DMBA group of animals that contained 23 DCISs/gland. Occasional lactating adenomas were observed in both hCG- and DMBA+hCG-treated animals (J. Russo and I.H. Russo 2000).

Effect of hCG Treatment on DMBA-Induced Tumor Progression

While mammary tumors were palpated as early as 25 and 30 days after carcinogen administration in the DMBA+hCG and DMBA groups, respectively, none of the animals in the saline control or the hCG-treated groups developed tumors. In the group of animals treated with DMBA, the number of palpable tumors contin-

ued increasing until the end of the experiment. In the DMBA+hCG group, the number of palpable tumors reached a plateau when the animals were 105 days old, and no additional tumors were detected in the 125-day-old animals. The highest total number of tumors and number of tumors per animal were observed in the DMBA group, while the DMBA+hCG group showed a reduction in the total number of palpable tumors and number of tumors per animal at all the time points studied. The histopathological analysis of both palpable tumors and microscopic lesions revealed that most of them were adenocarcinomas with papillary, cribriform, or comedo features. Only three fibroadenomas developed in the DMBA group and two in the DMBA+hCG group. The hormonal treatment reduced the incidence of adenocarcinomas more noticeably, from 8.3 in the DMBA to 1.8 adenocarcinomas per animal in the DMBA+hCG group (Table 1) (J. Russo and I.H. Russo 2000).

In summary, hCG treatment inhibited the progression of mammary carcinomas by stopping the development of early lesions, i.e., IDPs and carcinomas in situ (CISs). These findings indicated that hCG has a significant potential as a chemopreventive agent not only before the cell is initiated, but also after the carcinogenic process has been initiated and is vigorously progressing. Ours was the first report to indicate that a hormone preventive agent such as hCG is able to stop the initiated cells by inhibiting the formation of the intermediate step represented by the CIS, what ultimately results in a lower incidence of invasive tumors (J. Russo and I.H. Russo 2000).

Direct Effects of hCG on Mammary Epithelial Cells

Inhibitory Effect of DMBA-Induced Mammary Carcinogenesis in Ovariectomized Animals

In order to determine if hCG has a direct effect in the mammary gland, the experimental protocol depicted in Table 2 was utilized. Ovariectomy was performed after DMBA administration (group 3) and compared with intact animals in group 1. As expected, the tumor incidence and the number of tumors per animals were signifi-

Table 1 Effect of hCG treatment on the progression of DMBA-induced mammary tumors

Group/treatment	Age/days of treatment[a]	Tumor incidence			
		No. animals with tumors/total No. of animals[c]	%	No. tumors per animal/total no. tumors[d]	No. AdCa per animal/ total no. Od AdCa[h]
DMBA + saline	70/5	0/11	0.00	0.00/0	0.00/0
DMBA + saline	75/10	4/11	36.36	0.36/4	0.36/4
DMBA + saline	85/20	7/11	63.63	1.45/16	1.45/16
DMBA + saline	105/40	11/11	100.0	7.45/82	7.45/82
DMBA + saline	125/20[b]	11/11	100.0	8.54/94[e]	8.27/91
DMBA + hCG	70/5	1/16	6.25	0.06/1	0.06/1
DMBA + hCC	75/10	3/16	18.75	0.18/3	0.18/3
DMBA + hCG	85/20	8/16	50.00	0.87/14	0.87/14
DMBA + hCG	105/40	13/16	81.25	2.00/32[f]	1.93/31
DMBA + hCG	125/20[b]	13/16	81.25	1.57/30[g]	1.81/29

[a]Age of the animals (in days) at the time of sacrifice/days of treatment with 100 IU hCG/day

[b]Twenty days post-termination of the 40 day-hCG treatment

[c]Number of animals with tumors/total number of animals per group/treatment and age group

[d]Number of tumors per animal/total number of tumors from each specific group/treatment and animal age group

[e]Three out of 94 tumors were fibroadenomas

[f]One out of 32 tumors was a fibroadenoma

[g]One out of 30 tumors was a fibroadenoma

[h]Number of invasive adenocarcinomas (Ad-Ca) per animal/total number of adenocarcinomas per group/treatment and animal age group

DMBA 7,12-dimethylbenz(a)anthracene, hCG human chorionic gonadotropin

Table 2 Effect of ovariectomy and hCG treatment in DMBA-induced mammary carcinogenesis

Group	Number of animals	Number of animals with tumor/ number of animals	%	Number of tumors	Tumors/ animal
1. DMBA + saline	18	18/18	100	60	3.30
2. DMBA + hCG	20	9/20	45	20	1.00
3. OV+ DMBA	18	1/18	6	4	0.22
4. OV + DMBA + hCG	20	0/20	0	0	0.00
5. OV + DMBA + EP	18	6/18	33	8	0.44
6. OV+ DMBA + EP+ hCG	20	2/20	10	2	0.10

DMBA 7,12-dimethylbenz(a)anthracene, hCG human chorionic gonadotropin, OV ovariectomy, EP estrogen + progesterone

cantly reduced by ovarian ablation as well as by hCG (groups 2 and 4). Estrogen supplementation in the ovariectomized animals reestablished the tumor incidence and number of tumors per animal (group 5); however, hCG significantly reduced, in those supplemented animals, the number of tumors per animal as well as the incidence (group 6). These data clearly indicate that hCG has a direct effect on the mammary gland independently of ovarian function. This also suggests that hCG could be a tumoristatic agent in postmenopausal women, even in presence of hormone replacement therapy.

Effect on Human Breast Epithelial Cells in Vitro

Treatment of human breast epithelial cells with hCG inhibits the proliferative activity of the cells and induces activation of apoptotic genes. Inhibition of cell growth was observed only in HBEC, whereas the urothelial cells T24 were not affected by this treatment (Fig. 2). MCF-10F cells exhibited activation of the apoptotic genes TRPM2, ICE, TGF-β, p53, bax, and p21WAFI/CIP[1] (Fig. 3). BPl-E cells, derived from BP-transformed MCF-10F cells were also growth-inhibited; however, the pattern of gene activation differed from that exhibited by the parent cells (Fig. 4). BP1-E cells exhibited activation of only ICE, bax, and p21WAFI/CIP[1] and significantly downregulated bcl2, but did not modify TGF-β,p53, or c-myc expression. The urothelial cells did not show activation of any of the apoptotic genes. The lack of activation of the genes that control programmed cell death in these latter cells coincides with the selectivity of hCG in the inhibition of in vitro cell proliferation, which was observed only in HBEC, but not in T24 cells (Tahin et al. 1996). This specificity of action might be attributed to a receptor-mediated effect of hCG on human breast epithelial cells, whose presence has recently been reported in rat mammary epithelial cells.

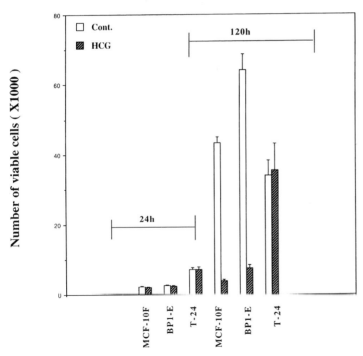

Fig. 2 Effect of hCG treatment on cell growth. MCF-10F, BPI-E, and T24 cells were treated daily with 100 IU/ml hCG and harvested at 24 and 120 h for cell growth determination by WST-colorimetric assay. Control cells were treated with vehicle only. Values represent the mean number of viable cells (×1000) ±SD of three wells from two experiments. (Reprinted with permission from: Srivastava et al. 1998)

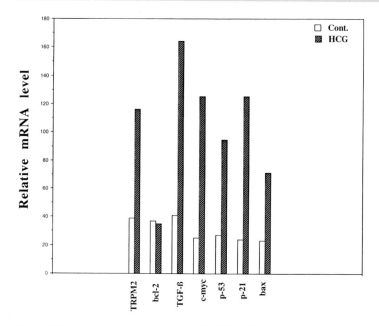

Fig. 3 Histogram showing the expression of TRPM2, ICE, bcl-2, TGFβ, c-myc, p53, p21, and bax mRNA relative to their respective controls in MCF-10F cells treated with hCG for 24 h. Relative MRNA content was determined by scanning laser densitometry of autoradiographs, and equalized by detection of β-actin. (Reprinted with permission from Srivastava et al. 1998)

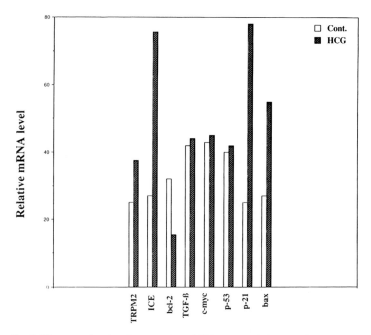

Fig. 4 Histogram showing the expression of TRPM2, ICE, bcl-2, TGFβ, c-myc, p53, p21, and bax MRNA relative to their respective controls in BPI-E cells treated with hCG for 24 h. Relative MRNA content was determined by scanning laser densitometry of autoradiographs, and equalized by detection of β-actin. (Reprinted with permission from Srivastava et al. 1998)

Increased expression of TRPM2 and TGF-β genes have been shown during chemotherapeutic regression of a mouse bladder tumor (Buttyan et al. 1989), regressing human breast cancer cells, and in prostatic tumors after hormone withdrawal (Armstrong et al. 1992; Kyprianou et al. 1991). In our experimental model, activation of these genes occurred only in MCF-10F but not in the chemically transformed and T24 cell lines. This observation supports the concept that activation of these two genes might be dependent on specific cell characteristics. The association between the induction of cell growth inhibition and TRPM2 activation has also been reported to be stimulated in MCF-7 cells by 1,25dihydroxyvitamin D3 (Simboli-Campbell et al. 1996). ICE gene expression was increased by hCG treatment in MCF-10F and BPI-E cells by the hormonal treatment. This gene, which belongs to a protease family has been shown to be relevant in the in-

duction of apoptosis (Fig. 5) (Tewari et al. 1995; Fernandes-Ainemri et al. 1995a, b; Harvey et al. 1998). Increases in the levels of ICE (caspase-1) mRNA have been associated with apoptosis in mammary epithelial cells by loss of attachment to extracellular matrix proteins and treatment of some tumor cell lines with chemotherapeutic drugs (Boudrau et al. 1995). Several lines of evidence indicate that the induction of apoptosis can be mediated by both p53 and c-myc, which are the major players in the context of growth arrest and apoptosis (Evan and Littlewood 1993). We have found that hCG treatment significantly induced the expression of p53 and p21WAF1/CIP1 in MCF-10F cells, an observation that suggested that the cell growth arrest was mediated by the tumor suppressor p53 through its downstream target gene p21WAF1/CIP1 (Evan and Littlewood 1993; El-Deiry et al. 1993). Nevertheless, BPI-E cells exhibited an inhibition in their

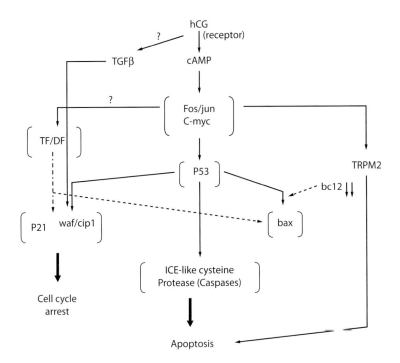

Fig. 5 Postulated model of hCG-induced cell cycle arrest and apoptosis in human breast epithelial cells. In the presence of hCG for 24 h breast epithelial cells bind the hormone to a putative membrane receptor. This triggers a cascade of programmed cell death gene activation through the CAMP-PKA pathway, as well as through activation of TGF-β. HCG treatment activates (upregulates) TRPM2, ICE, TGF-β, p53, and p21 in MCF-10F cells; in BP1-E cells it activates TRPM2, ICE, p21, and bax, but does not activate TGF-β, c-myc, or p53, leading us to postulate that p21 and bax activation in these cells proceeds through an alternative pathway, i.e., TF/DF (bent arrow). (Reprinted with permission from Srivastava et al. 1998)

in vitro growth and induced p21WAFI/CIPI mRNA, but the expression of c-myc and p53 genes was not modified by the hormonal treatment. These observations might indicate that cell growth and activation of the apoptotic genes have been independently modulated by other genes and/or other external factors. Recent evidence has shown both p53-dependent and p53-independent apoptosis pathways (Sakamuro et al. 1995; Ronen et al. 1996). Thus, our observation that p53 was significantly activated by hCG treatment in MCF-10F but not in BP1-E cells led us to postulate that the activation of apoptotic genes might have occurred through those two different pathways for the inhibition of in vitro cell proliferation (Fig. 5). Our observations suggested that in MCF-10F cells hCG arrested the progression of the cell cycle by inducing (probably through its receptor) the CAMP-PKA and p53, as well as the TGF-β pathways to act on their target gene p21WAF1/CIP1, proceeding then toward cell cycle arrest and apoptosis (Fig. 6). In the case of the chemically transformed cell line, TGF-β, p53, and c-myc did not express any changes in their level of expression, although there was a profound induction of p21WAF1/CIP1 mRNA, thus

suggesting that this gene was induced by hCG independently of p53, probably via transcription factor (TF), differentiation factor (DF) (Fig. 5), as has been shown in other systems (Johnson et al. 1994).

ICE class proteases (caspases) have been shown to play an important role in p53-mediated apoptosis (Harris 1996), though the molecular details are not fully understood. This mechanism is supported by our findings that hCG treatment induces an increase in the expression of both p53 and ICE in MCF-10F cells. Another possible involvement of p53 in apoptosis is the regulation by members of the bcl2 multiprotein family (Stroebel et al. 1996; Merlo et al. 1997). Some of the members of the bcl2 family such as bcl2 and bcl-XL, are blockers of cell death, while others, e.g., Bax and bcl-XS, are promoters of apoptosis (Stroebel et al. 1996; Merlo et al. 1997). Recent studies have indicated that bax can be activated by both p53-dependent and -independent pathways in different systems (Stroebel et al. 1996). In the present study, hCG treatment induced bax expression in both MCF-10F and BP1-E cells, but it markedly reduced bcl2 expression in BP1-E cells only. The fact that p53, bax, and bcl2 expres-

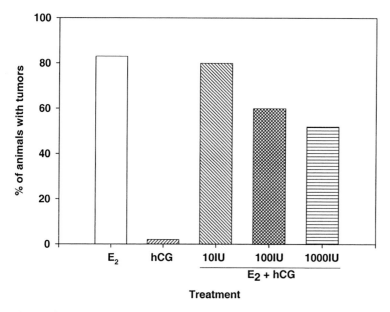

Fig. 6 Effect of hCG treatment on the growth of tumors formed by MCF-7 cells inoculated in nude mice. E_2, animals treated with 17-β-estradiol; hCG, animals treated with hCG alone; E_2+hCG, animals implanted with one pellet of 17-β-estradiol and treated with 10, 100, or 1,000 IU of hCG/day for 50 days. (Reprinted with permission from J. Russo and I.H. Russo 2004)

sion are differently modulated by the hormonal treatment is a strong indication that alternative pathways might be operational in the activation of apoptotic genes by hCG. In these studies, we observed that control cells exhibited an elevation in the level of expression of apoptotic genes. After 120 h in culture, the level of expression of TRPM2, ICE, TGF-B, bax, and p21WAF1/CIP1 genes was increased in MCF-10F. In BP1-E cells, TRPM2, ICE, and p21WAF1/CIP1 were higher at 120 h in culture than at 24 h. The similarities in the activation of gene expression between levels in 24-h-treated and 120-h controls indicate that hCG accelerates the process of gene activation, a phenomenon that has been reported to be associated with confluence (Merlo et al. 1997).

In conclusion, our results demonstrate that the 24-h hCG treatment of immortalized and chemically transformed human breast epithelial cells activates apoptotic genes even before the arrest of cell growth becomes evident. Of relevance is the fact that hCG, which is an inhibitor of in vitro cell proliferation and in vivo acts as a preventive and tumoristatic agent (I.H. Russo et al. 1990b; Alvarado et al. 1994), may utilize different pathways for activating apoptotic genes, depending upon the degree of expression of neoplastic phenotypes (J. Russo et al. 2001; Calaf and Russo 1993; Mgbonyebi et al. 1997; Albini et al. 1997). Taken together, the results of the present study demonstrate that the growth inhibitory effect of hCG is associated with its ability to activate the expression of apoptotic genes. The importance of our present findings lies in the potential use of hCG as a chemopreventive and chemotherapeutic agent in breast cancer.

Tumoristatic Effect of hCG on Malignant Human Breast Epithelial Cells Transplanted into a Heterologous Host

The observation that hCG had an inhibitory effect on chemically induced rat mammary carcinomas led us to test whether this hormone had an effect on the in vivo growth of malignant human breast epithelial cells. For this purpose, MCF-7 cells, a cell line derived from a metastatic breast carcinoma, were injected to Balb/c nude mice (nu/nu). The animals were divided into five groups: the animals of four groups had implanted a silastic tube containing 5 mg 17-β-estradiol in the interscapular region 5 days after castration, and one group was castrated but did not receive the estrogen supplementation. The cells were injected in the mammary fat pad of mice in all the groups at a concentration of 1×10^6 cells. HCG was administered to the group of animals that did not receive the estrogen at a dose of 1,000 IU/day, and to the three estrogen-supplemented groups at the doses of 10, 100, or 1,000 IU/day. The animals that received estradiol pellets alone had an incidence of 85% tumor formation. The group of animals injected with hCG alone did not develop tumors. Animals that received estradiol pellets and also hCG exhibited a reduction in both tumor incidence and tumor size that were dose-dependent. These studies led us to conclude that the treatment with hCG abrogates the effect of the estrogen growth dependency of MCF-7 cells in a heterologous hosts (Fig. 6).

Genomic Signature Induced by hCG and Pregnancy

RNA was obtained from mammary glands of rats in their 15th and 21st day of pregnancy or hCG treatment, and 21 and 42 days postpartum or post-treatment, respectively. RNAs were analyzed utilizing two membranes for each animal and compared with mRNA of age-matched virgin control rats. RNAs were hybridized to cDNA array membranes that contained 5,800 rat genes (Research Genetics, Huntsville, AL). Cluster analysis was performed using the Jaidexp (Java Analysis information & Data Exploration) specific program, version 1:0 and statistically analyzed. Four clusters of genes were identified (Fig. 7): cluster A shows genes that were overexpressed (threefold) at 15 and 21 days of pregnancy/hCG treatment, but decreased to control values after 21 and 42 days postpartum or post-treatment, respectively. These genes, which included beta casein and alpha lactalbumin, are related to the secretory properties of the mammary epithelium (Mailo et al. 2002). Similar genes were identified using the DD technique, as explained above. Cluster B was composed of genes that were increased threefold at 21 days of pregnancy/treatment and continued rising, reaching the highest peak at 21 days, decreas-

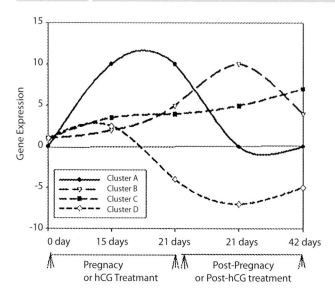

Fig. 7 Cluster analysis of rat mammary gland gene expression during and after pregnancy and hCG. (Reprinted with permission from J. Russo and I.H. Russo 2004)

ing by 42 days postpartum/post-hCG treatment. Among these genes were the fatty acid binding protein, the EST Rn.37635 with high homology to BCL7B gene, cathecol-O-methyltransferase, and the EST genes Rn. 5953, Rn.22912, and Rn.4339 (Mailo et al. 2002). The upregulation of cathecol-O-methyltransferase is significant because it can be involved in the conjugation of estradiol and cathecol estrogens, reducing the carcinogenic effect of these hormones. Genes related to the apoptotic pathways, such as testosterone repressed prostate message 2 (TRPM2), interleukin 1β-converting enzyme (ICE), bcl2, bcl-XL, bcl-XS, p53, p21, and c-myc were also upregulated from three to fivefold (Mailo et al. 2002) (Fig. 7). We have shown that the activation of programmed cell death genes occurred through a p53-dependent process, modulated by c-myc and with partial dependence on the bcl2-family related genes (Srivastava et al. 1998, 1999; J. Russo and I.H. Russo 2000). In this cluster were also included inhibins A and B, heterodimeric nonsteroidal secreted glycoproteins with tumor suppressor activity (Sun 1984; Vermeulen et al. 1976). We have found that inhibins are not present in the normal resting mammary gland, but are induced by pregnancy or hCG treatment (Alvarado et al. 1993, 1994). We have also shown that hCG has an autocrine or paracrine effect on mammary epithelial cells (J. Russo and I.H.

Russo 2000). HCG also activates the cluster B of genes in DMBA-induced mammary tumors, indicating that this hormone acts through the same pathways for exerting its preventative and therapeutic effects (Fig. 7). Cluster C (Fig. 7) represents genes whose level of expression progressively increased with time of pregnancy or hCG treatment, reaching their highest levels between 21 and 42 days postpartum or after the end of treatment. Among these were known genes such as those coding for a fragment of glycogen phosphorylase, AMP-activated kinase, bone morphogenetic protein 4, and vesicle-associated protein 1 (149). G/T mismatch-specific thymine DNA glycosylase gene, which was observed to be upregulated in the Lob 3 of the human breast, was also increased by fivefold in this model. These data indicate that the activation of genes involved in the DNA repair process is part of the signature induced in the mammary gland by either pregnancy or hCG treatment of virgin animals. These observations confirm our previous findings that in vivo the ability of the cells to repair carcinogen-induced damage by unscheduled DNA synthesis and adduct removal is more efficient in the parous and in the hCG-treated virgin than in the untreated virgin animal mammary gland (J. Russo et al. 1982; Tay and Russo et al. 1981a, b, 1983). Therefore, a principal mechanism mediating the protection from mammary carcinogen-

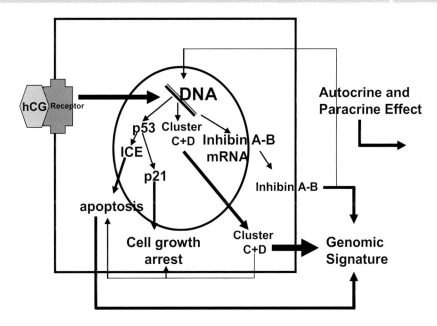

Fig. 8 Postulated mechanism of action of hCG. The hormone binds to a specific membrane receptor, activating genes identified to be specific for pregnancy or hCG-induced differentiation and that have been found to be correlated with the lobular development of the mammary tissue. Thus, a pathway of activation of p53 and ICE may lead to apoptosis or through p21 to cell growth arrest. Activation of inhibin A and B may lead to differentiation through autocrine or paracrine mechanisms. The activation of genes (clusters c and d) are responsible for the refractoriness of the gland to carcinogenesis. (Reprinted with permission from J. Russo and I.H. Russo 2004)

esis conferred by either full-term pregnancy or hCG treatment is the enhancement of the ability of the cells to repair DNA damage, which is in turn the determinant of the lower susceptibility to carcinogenesis. Cluster D consists of genes coding for pro-alpha collagen III, pro collagen II alpha 1, BTG1, and thymosin beta 4, which were upregulated more than threefold at the 15th day of pregnancy or hCG treatment, downregulated at the 21st day in both pregnant and hCG-treated animals, and remained downregulated up to 42 days (Mailo et al. 2002) (Fig. 7). Cluster D, in combination with Cluster C, is a component of the signature induced by hCG in the mammary gland (Fig. 8).

These data demonstrate that the genomic signature of the mammary gland induced in virgin animals by exogenous administration of hCG is similar to that induced by pregnancy, and that specific genomic profiles are still manifested by 42 days after termination of treatment. The importance of these specific signatures is highlighted by the fact that administration of car-

cinogen to hCG-treated or control virgin rats whose mammary glands appear morphologically similar will induce a markedly different tumorigenic response, supporting the concept that the differentiation induced by hCG is expressed at genomic level, and results in a shift of the susceptible cells to refractory cells. The permanence of these changes, in turn, makes them ideal surrogate markers for the evaluation of hCG effect as a breast cancer preventive agent.

Unifying Concepts

Based in our knowledge of the pathogenesis of mammary cancer we have tested the effect of hCG hormone on the early phases of tumor progression, namely from TEBs damaged by DMBA to IDPs, in situ carcinomas, and invasive carcinomas, and demonstrate that this hormone inhibits the progression of 7,12-dimethylbenz(a)anthracene (DMBA)-induced mammary tumors. Treatment of young virgin rats with hCG induced a profuse lobular development of the mammary gland, practically eliminating the highly proliferating TEBs, with overall reduction in the proliferative activity of the mammary epithelium and induction of the synthesis of inhibin, a secreted protein with tumor-suppressor activity. The hormonal treatment induced differentiation of the mammary gland, which was manifested at morphological, cell kinetic, and functional levels. The morphological changes consisted of progressive branching of the mammary parenchyma and lobule formation. They were accompanied by reduction in the rate of cell proliferation. The functional changes comprised increased synthesis of inhibin, β-casein, and other milk-related bioactive peptides. In addition, hCG increased the expression of the programmed cell death TRPM2, ICE, p53, c-myc, and bcl-XS, also inducing apoptosis and downregulation of cyclins. Programmed cell death genes were activated through a p53-dependent process, modulated by c-myc, with partial dependence on the bcl-2 family-related genes. Of relevance was the observation that lobular development, which reached its maximal expression after the 15th day of hCG treatment, regressing after hormone withdrawal, was preceded by activation of genes associated with the expression of programmed cell death, and furthermore, that the expression of these genes was still elevated 20 days after cessation of treatment. Data generated with the new tools provided by the cDNA microarray techniques have demonstrated that while lobular development regressed after the cessation of hormone administration, programmed cell death genes remained activated, but more importantly a new set of genes (cluster C) reached maximum expression, whereas others (cluster D) are downregulated. The genes in clusters C and D are those providing the genomic signature that is specific for hCG and pregnancy. The genomic signature is specific for pregnancy and hCG and significantly different from that induced by other hormones such as estrogen and progesterone.

Altogether these mechanisms play a role in the protection exerted by hCG from chemically induced carcinogenesis, and might even be involved in the life-time reduction in breast cancer risk induced in women by full term and multiple pregnancies. The implications of these observations are twofold: on one hand, they indicate that hCG, like pregnancy, may induce early genomic changes that control the progression of the differentiation pathway; and on the other hand that these changes are permanently imprinted in the genome, regulating the long-lasting refractoriness to carcinogenesis). The permanence of these changes, in turn, makes them ideal surrogate markers of the hCG effect in the evaluation of this hormone as a breast cancer preventive agent.

References

Albini A, Pagliefi L, Orengo G, Carlene S, Aluigi M, De Maachi R, Matteucci C, Mantovani A, Carozzi S, Benelli R (1997) The B-core fragment of human chorionic gonadotropin inhibits growth of Kaposi's sarcoma derived cells and a new immortalized Kaposi's sarcoma cell line. AIDS 11:713–721

Alvarado ME, Alvarado NE, Russo J, Russo IH (1994) Human chorionic gonadotropin inhibits proliferation and induces expression of inhibin in human breast epithelial cells in vitro. In Vitro 30:4–8

Alvarado MV, Russo J, Russo IH (1993) Immunolocalization of inhibin in the mammary gland of rats treated with hCG J Histochem Cytochem 41:29–34

Apter D (1996) Hormonal events during female puberty in relation to breast cancer risk. Eur J Cancer Prev 5:476–482

Armstrong DK, Issacs JT, Ottaviano YL and Davidson NE (1992) Programmed cell death in an estrogen-independent human breast cancer cell line MDA-MB-468. Cancer Res 52:3418–3424

Baum M (2002) The ATAC (Arimidex Tamoxifen Alone or in Combination) adjuvant breast cancer trial in post-menopausal patients: factors influencing the success of patient recruitment. Eur J Cancer 38:1984–1986

Blair A, Zahm SH, Silverman DT (1999) Occupational cancer among women: Research status and methodologic considerations. Am J Ind Med 36:6–17

Boice JD Jr, Preston D, Davis FG, Monson RR (1991) Frequent chest X-ray fluoroscopy and breast cancer incidence among tuberculosis patients in Massachusetts. Radiat Res 125:214–222

Boudrau N, Sympson CJ, Werb Z, Bissell MJ (1995) Suppression of ICE and apoptosis in mammary epithelial cells by extracellular matrix. Science 267:891–893

Buttyan R, Olsson CA, Pintar J, Chang C, Bandyk Ng P, Sawczuk IS (1989) Induction of the TRPM2 gene in cells undergoing programmed cell death. Mol Cell Biol 9:3473–3481

Calaf G, Russo J (1993) Transformation of human breast epithelial cells by chemical carcinogens. Carcinogenesis 14:483–492

Chang J, Elledge RM (2001) Clinical management of women with genomic BRCA1 and BRCA2 mutations. Breast Cancer Res Treat 69:101–113

Chie WC, Hsieh C, Newcomb PA, Longnecker MP, Mittendorf R, Greenberg ER, Clapp RW, Burke KP, Titus-Ernstoff L, Trentham-Dietz A, MacMahon B (2000) Age at any full-term pregnancy and breast cancer risk. Am J Epidemiol 151:715–722

Clemons M, Loijens L (2000) Goss P Breast cancer risk following irradiation for Hodgkin's disease. Cancer Treat Rev 26:291–302

Coe K (1998) Breast cancer in Hispanic women. Women and Cancer 1:38–43

Collaborative Group on Hormonal Factors in Breast Cancer (2002) Breast cancer and breastfeeding: Collaborative reanalysis of individual data from 47 epidemiological studies in 30 countries including 50302 women with breast cancer and 96973 women without disease. Lancet 360:187–195

Cutuli B, Borel C, Dhermain F, Magrini SM, WassermanTH, Bogart JA, Provencio M, de Lafontan B, de la Rochefordiere A, Cellai E, Graic Y, Kerbrat P, Alzieu C, Teissier E, Dilhuydy J, Mignotte H, Velten (2001) M Breast cancer occurred after treatment for Hodgkin's disease: analysis of 133 cases. Radiother Oncol 59:247–255

De Waard F, Thijssen JH (2005) Hormonal aspects in the causation of human breast cancer: epidemiological hypotheses reviewed with special reference to nutritional status and first pregnancy. J Steroid Biochem Mol Biol 97:451–458

Dunn BK, McCaskill-Stevens W, Kramer B, Ford LG (2000) Chemoprevention of breast cancer: The NSABP's breast cancer prevention trial. J Women's Cancer 2:177–191

El-Deiry W, Tokino T, Velculescu VE, Levy DB, Parsons R, Trent JM, Lin D, Mercer WE, Kinzler KW, Vogelstein (1993) B WAF1, a potential mediator of p53 tumor suppression. Cell 75:817–825

Evan GI, Littlewood TD (1993) The role of c-myc in cell growth. Curr Opin Genet Dev 3:44–49

Ewertz M, Duffy SW, Adami HO, Kvale G, Lund E, Meirik O, Mellemgaard A, Soini I, Tulinius H (1990) Age at first birth parity and risk of breast cancer: a meta-analysis of 8 studies from the Nordic countries. Int J Cancer 46:597–603

Fernandes-Alnemri T, Litwack G, Alnemri ES (1995a) Mch2, a new member of the apoptotic ced-3/ice cysteine protease gene family. Cancer Res 55:2737–2742

Fernandes-Ainemri T, Takashi A, Armstrong R, Krebs J, Fritz L, Tommaselli KJ, Wang L, Yu Z, Croce C M, Saiveson G, Earnshaw W C, Litwack G, Alnemri ES (1995b) Mch3, a novel human apoptotic cysteine protease highly related to CPP32. Cancer Res 5:6045–6052

Forbes JF (1997) The incidence of breast cancer: the global burden public health considerations. Semin Oncol 4 1 [Suppl 1]:S1-20–S1-35

Fraumeni JF Jr, Lloyd JW, Smith EM, Wagoner JK (1969) Cancer mortality among nuns: Role of marital status in etiology of neoplastic disease in women. J Natl Cancer Inst 2:455–468

Gail MH, Brinton LA, Byar DP, Corle DK, Breen SB, Schairer C, Mulvihill JJ (1989) Projecting individualized probabilities of developing breast cancer for white females who are being examined annually. J Natl Cancer Inst 81:1879–1886

Gaudette LA, Silberberger C, Altmayer CA, Gao RN (1996) Trends in breast cancer incidence and mortality. Health Reports 8:29–37

Greenlee RT, Hill-Harmon MB, Murray T, Thun M (2001) Cancer Statistics 2001. CA Cancer J Clin 1:15–36

Harris CC (1996) Structure and function of the p53 tumor suppressor gene: clues for rational cancer therapeutic strategies. J Natl Cancer Inst 88:1442–1455

Hartmann LC, Sellers TA, Schaid DJ, Frank TS, Soderberg CL, Sitta DL, Frost MH, Grant CS, Donohue JH, Woods JE, McDonnell SK, Vockley CW, Deffenbaugh A, Couch FJ, Jenkins RB (2001) Efficacy of bilateral prophylactic mastectomy in BRCA1 and BRCA2 gene mutation carriers. J Natl Cancer Inst 93:1633–1637

Harvey KJ, Blomquist JFI, Ucker DS (1998) Commitment and effector phases of the physiological cell death pathway elucidated with respect to Bcl-2 caspase and cyclin-dependent kinase activities. Mol Cell Biol 18:2912–2922

Hoffmann D, Hoffmann I, El-Bayoumy K (2001) The less harmful cigarette: a controversial issue, a tribute to Ernst L Wynder. Chem Res Toxicol 14:767–790

Holmberg E, Holm LE, Lundell M, Mattsson A, Wallgren A, Karlsson P (2001) Excess breast cancer risk and the role of parity age at first childbirth and exposure to radiation in infancy. Br J Cancer 85:362–366

Howe HL, Wingo PA, Thun MJ, Ries LA, Rosenberg HM, Feigal EG, Edwards BK (2001) Annual report to the nation on the status of cancer (1973 through 1998), featuring cancers with recent increasing trends. J Natl Cancer Inst 93:824–842

Janov AJ, Tulecke M, O'Neill A, Lester S, Mauch PM, Harris J, Schnitt SJ, Shapiro (2001) CL Clinical and Pathologic Features of Breast Cancers in Women Treated for Hodgkin's Disease: A Case-Control Study. Breast J 7:46–52

Jemal A, Thomas A, Murray T, Thun M (2002) Cancer Statistics 2002. CA Cancer J Clin 52:23–47

Jernstrom H, Lubinski J, Lynch HT, Ghadirian P, Neuhausen S, Isaacs C, Weber BL, Horsman D, Rosen B, Foulkes WD, Friedman E, Gershoni-Baruch R, Ainsworth P, Daly M, Garber J, Olsson H, Sun P, Narod SA (2004) Breast-feeding and the risk of breast cancer in BRCA1 and BRCA2 mutation carriers. J Natl Cancer Inst 96:1094–1098

Johnson M, Dimitrov D, Vojta .PJ, Barrett JC, Noda A, Pereira-Smith OM, Smith JR (1994) Evidence for a p53-independent pathway for upregulation of SDI/CIPI/WAFI/p21 RNA in human cells. Mol Carcinog 1:59–64

Kelsey JL, Horn-Ross PL (1993) Breast Cancer: Magnitude of the problem and descriptive epidemiology . Epidemiol Rev 15:7–16

Khurana KK, Loosmann A, Numann PJ, Khan SA (2000) Prophylactic mastectomy – pathologic findings in high-risk patients. Arch Pathol Lab Med 124:378–381

King MC, Wieand S, Hale K, Lee M, Walsh T, Owens K, Tait J, Ford L, Dunn BK, Costantino J, Wickerham L, Wolmark N, Fisher B (2001) Tamoxifen and breast cancer incidence among women with inherited mutations in BRCA1 and BRCA2: National Surgical Adjuvant Breast and Bowel Project (NSABP-P1) Breast Cancer Prevention Trial. JAMA 286:2251–2256

Kyprianou N, English HF, Davidson NE, Issacs JT (1991) Programmed cell death during regression of MCF-7 human breast cancer following estrogen ablation. Cancer Res 51:162–166

Lambe M, Hsieh CC, Chan HW, Ekbom A, Trichopoulos D and Adami H O (1996) Parity age at first and last birth and risk of breast cancer: A population-based study in Sweden. Breast Cancer Res Treat 38:305–311

Lynch HT, Casey MJ (2001) Current status of prophylactic surgery for hereditary breast and gynecologic cancers. Curr Opin Obstet Gynecol 13:25–30

MacMahon B, Cole P, Lin TM et al (1970) Age at first birth and breast cancer risk. Bull World Health Organ 43:209–221

Mailo D, Russo J, Sheriff F, Hu YF, Tahin Q, Mihaila D, Balogh G, Russo IH (2002) Genomic signature induced by differentiation in the rat mammary gland. Proc Am Assoc Cancer Res 43:5368a

Matsumoto H, Yamane T (2000) Green tea and cancer prevention. J Womens Cancer 2:153–158

McGregor DH, Land CE, Choi K, Tokuoka S, Liu PI, Wakabayashi I, Beebe GW (1977) Breast cancer incidence among atomic bomb survivors Hiroshima and Nagasaki 1950–1989. J Natl Cancer Inst 59:799–811

Merlo GR, Cella N, Hynes N (1997) Apoptosis is accompanied by changes in Bcl-2 and Bax expression induced by loss of attachment and inhibited by specific extracellular matrix proteins in mammary epithelial cells. Cell Growth Differ 8:251–260

Mgbonyebi O P, Tahin Q, Russo J, Russo IH (1996) Serum levels of chorionic gonadotropin in treated female rats during the progression of DMBA-induced tumorigenesis. Proc Am Assoc Cancer Res 37:1564a

Mgbonyebi OP, Russo J, Russo IH (1997) Induction of reversible growth arrest of immortal and neoplastic human breast epithelial cells by human chorionic gonadotropin (hCG). Proc Am Assoc Cancer Res 38:294–295

Mirza AN, Mirza NQ, Vlastos G, Singletary SE (2002) Prognostic factors in node-negative breast cancer: a review of studies with sample size more than 200 and follow-up more than 5 years. Ann Surg 235:10–26

Mouridsen H, Gershanovich M, Sun Y, Perez-Carrion R, Boni C, Monnier A, Apffelstaedt J, Smith R, Sleeboom HP, Janicke F, Pluzanska A, Dank M, Becquart D, Bapsy PP, Salminen E, Snyder R, Lassus M, Verbeek JA, Staffler B, Chaudri-Ross HA, Dugan M (2001) Superior efficacy of letrozole versus tamoxifen as first-line therapy for postmenopausal women with advanced breast cancer: results of a phase III study of the International Letrozole Breast Cancer Group. J Clin Oncol 19:2596–2606

Nandi S, Guzman RC, Yang J (1995) Hormones and mammary carcinogenesis in mice rats and humans: a unifying hypothesis. Proc Natl Acad Sci U S A 92:3650–3657

Narod S (2001) Prophylactic mastectomy in carriers of BRCA mutations. N Engl J Med 345:1498; author reply 1499–1500

Narod SA, Brunet JS, Ghadirian P, Robson M, Heimdal K, Neuhausen SL, Stoppa-Lyonnet D, Lerman C, Pasini B, de los Rios P, Weber B, Lynch H (2000) Tamoxifen and risk of contralateral breast cancer in BRCA1 and BRCA2 mutation carriers: a case-control study. Hereditary Breast Cancer Clinical Study Group. Lancet 356:1876–1881

Nix JT (1964) Study of the relationship of environmental factors to the type and frequency of cancer causing death in nuns 1963. Hosp Prog 45:71–74

Ramazzini B (1965) De virginum vestalium valetudine tuenda dissertatio (a dissertation on the care of the health of nuns). J Occup Med 7:516–520

Rao DN, Ganesh B, Desai PB (1994) Role of reproductive factors in breast cancer in a low-risk area: a case-control study. Br J Cancer 70:129–152

Riggs T (2001)Prophylactic mastectomy in carriers of BRCA mutations. N Engl J Med 345:1499–500

Robertson JF, Nicholson RI, Bundred NJ, Anderson E, Rayter Z, Dowsett M, Fox JN, Gee JM, Webster A, Wakeling AE, Morris C, Dixon M (2001) Comparison of the short-term biological effects of 7alpha-[9-(4,4,5,5,5-pentafluoropentylsulfinyl)-nonyl]estra-1,3,5, (10)-triene-3,17beta-diol (Faslodex) versus tamoxifen in postmenopausal women with primary breast cancer. Cancer Res 61:6739–6746

Ronen D, Schwartz D, Teitz Y, Goldfinger N, Rotter V (1996) Induction of HL-60 cells to undergo apoptosis is determined by high levels of wild type p-53 protein whereas differentiation of the cells is mediated by lower p53 levels. Cell Growth Differ 7:21–30

Russo IH, Russo J (1993) Chorionic gonadotropin: a tumoristatic and preventive agent in breast cancer in drug resistance in oncology In: Teicher BA (ed), Marcel Dekker, pp 537–560

Russo IH, Russo J (1994) Role of hCG and inhibin in breast cancer (review). Int J Oncol 4:297–306

Russo IH, Russo J (1996) Mammary gland neoplasia in long-term rodent studies. Environ Health Perspect 104.938–967

Russo IH, Russo J (1998) Role of pregnancy and chorionic gonadotropin in breast cancer prevention. In: Birkhauser MH, Rozenbaum H (eds) Proc IV European Congress on Menopause. ESKA, Paris, pp 133–142

Russo IH, Koszalka M, Russo J (1990a) Effect of human chorionic gonadotropin on mammary gland differentiation and carcinogenesis. Carcinogenesis 11:1849–1855

Russo IH, Koszalka M, Russo J (1990b) Human chorionic gonadotropin and rat mammary cancer prevention. J Natl Cancer Inst 82:1286–1289

Russo IH, Koszalka M, Russo J (1991) Comparative study of the influence of pregnancy and hormonal treatment on mammary carcinogenesis. Br J Cancer 64:481–484

Russo J, Russo IH (1980a) Influence of differentiation and cell kinetics on the susceptibility of the mammary gland to carcinogenesis. Cancer Res 40:2677–2687

Russo J, Russo IH (1980b) Susceptibility of the mammary gland to carcinogenesis. II Pregnancy interruption as a risk factor in tumor incidence. Am J Pathol 100:497–512

Russo J, Russo IH (1993) Developmental pattern of the human breast and susceptibility to carcinogenesis. Eur J Cancer Prevent 2:85–100

Russo J, Russo IH (1994) Toward a physiological approach to breast cancer prevention. Cancer Epidemiol Biomarkers Prev 3:353–364

Russo J, Russo IH (2000) Human chorionic gonadotropin in breast cancer prevention In: Ethier SP (ed) Endocrine oncology. Humana Press, Totowa, NJ, pp 121–136

Russo J, Janssens J, Russo IH (2000) Recombinant human chorionic gonadotropin (r-hCG) significantly reduces primary tumor cell proliferation in patients with breast cancer. Breast Cancer Res Treat 64:161a

Russo J, Saby J, Isenberg W, Russo IH (1977) Pathogenesis of mammary carcinoma induced in rats by 7,12-dimethylbenz(a)anthracene. J Natl Cancer Inst 59:435–445

Russo J, Wilgus G, Russo IH (1979) Susceptibility of the mammary gland to carcinogenesis. I Differentiation of the mammary gland as determinant of tumor incidence and type of lesion. Am J Pathol 96:721–734

Russo J, Tay LK, Russo IH (1982) Differentiation of the mammary gland and susceptibility to carcinogenesis. Breast Cancer Res Treat 2:5–73

Russo J, Rivera R, Russo IH (1992) Influence of age and parity on the development of the human breast Breast Cancer Res Treat 23:211–218

Sakamuro D, Eviner V, Elliott KJ, Showe L, White E, Prendergast GC (1995) C-myc induces apoptosis in epithelial cells by both p-53 dependent and p53 independent mechanisms. Oncogene 11:2411–2418

Shivvers SA, Miller DS (1997) Preinvasive and invasive breast and cervical cancer prior to or during pregnancy. Clin Perinatol 24:369–389

Simboli-Campbell M, Narvaez CJ, Tenniswood M, Welsh (1996) JE 1,25- Dihydroxyvitamin D3 induces morphological and biochemical markers of apoptosis in MCF-7 breast cancer cells. J Steroid Biochem Mol Biol 58:367–376

Sinha DK, Patzik JE, Dao TL (1983) Progression of rat mammary development with age and its relationship to carcinogenesis by a chemical carcinogen. Int J Cancer 31:321–327

Srivastava P, Russo J, Russo IH (1998) Chorionic gonadotropin inhibits rat mammary carcinogenesis through activation of programmed cell death. Carcinogenesis 18:1799–1808

Srivastava P, Russo J, Russo IH (1999) Inhibition of rat mammary tumorigenesis by human chorionic gonadotropin is associated with increased expression of inhibin. Mol Carcinog 26:10–19

Stoutjesdijk MJ, Barentsz JO (2001) Prophylactic mastectomy in carriers of BRCA mutations. N Engl J Med 345:1499, author reply 1499–1500

Strobel T, Swanson L, Korsmeyer S, Cannistra SA (1996) Bax enhances pacitaxel-induced apoptosis through a p53-independent pathway. Proc Natl Acad Sci U S A 93:14094–14099

Sun M (1984) Panel says Depo-Provera not proved safe. Science 226:950

Tahin Q, Mgbonyebi OP, Russo J, Russo IH (1996) Influence of hormonal changes induced by the placental hormone chorionic gonadotropin on the progression of mammary tumorigenesis. Proc Am Assoc Cancer Res 37:1622a

Tanner JM (1973) Trend towards earlier menarche in London, Oslo, Copenhagen, the Netherlands and Hungary. Nature 243:95–96

Tay LK, Russo J (1981a) 7,12-dimethylbenz [a] anthracene-induced DNA binding and repair synthesis in susceptible and non-susceptible mammary epithelial cells in culture. J Natl Cancer Inst 7:155–161

Tay LK, Russo J (1981b) Formation and removal of 7,12-dimethylbenz [a] anthracene-nucleic acid adducts in rat mammary epithelial cells with different susceptibility to carcinogenesis. Carcinogenesis 2:1327–1333

Tay LK, Russo J (1983) Metabolism of 7,12-dimethylbenz(a)anthracene by rat mammary epithelial cells in culture. Carcinogenesis 4:733–738

Tewari M, Quan LT, O'Rourke A, Desnoyers S, Zeng Z, Beidler DR, Poirier GG, Salvesen GS, Dixit VM (1995) Yama/CPP32, a mammalian homolog of CED-3, is a Crm A-inhibitable protease that cleaves the death substrate poly(ADP-Ribose) polymerase. Cell 81:801–809

Trapido EJ (1983) Age at first birth parity and breast cancer risk. Cancer 51:946–948

Tymchuk CN, Tessler SB, Barnard RJ (2000) Changes in sex hormone-binding globulin insulin and serum lipids in postmenopausal women on a low-fat high-fiber diet combined with exercise. Nutr Cancer 38:158–162

Vermeulen A, Dhnodt M, Their YK, Van Der Kerckhove D (1976) Plasma sex steroid and gonadotropin levels in control and silastic vaginal medroxyprogesterone acetate-impregnated ring cycles. Fertil Steril 27:773–779

Vessey MD, McPherson K, Roberts MM, Neil A, Jones L (1985) Fertility and the risk of breast cancer. Br J Cancer 52:625–628

Warmuth MA, Sutton LM, Winer EP (1997) A review of hereditary breast cancer: From screening to risk factor modification. Am J Med 102:407–415

12

The Genomic Signature of Breast Cancer Prevention

Jose Russo, Gabriela Balogh, Daniel Mailo, Patricia A. Russo, Rebecca Heulings, Irma H. Russo

Recent Results in Cancer Research, Vol. 174
© Springer-Verlag Berlin Heidelberg 2007

Abstract

Early pregnancy imprints in the breast permanent genomic changes or a *signature* that reduces the susceptibility of this organ to cancer. The breast attains its maximum development during pregnancy and lactation. After menopause, the breast regresses in both nulliparous and parous women containing lobular structures designated Lob.1. The Lob 1 found in the breast of nulliparous women and of parous women with breast cancer never went through the process of differentiation, retaining a high concentration of epithelial cells that are targets for carcinogens and therefore susceptible to undergoing neoplastic transformation, these cell are called Stem cells 1, whereas Lob 1 structures found in the breast of early parous postmenopausal women free of mammary pathology, on the other hand, are composed of an epithelial cell population that is refractory to transformation called Stem cells 2. The degree of differentiation acquired through early pregnancy has changed the genomic signature that differentiates the Lob 1 from the early parous women from that of the nulliparous women by shifting the Stem cell 1 to a Stem cell 2, making this the postulated mechanism of protection conferred by early full-term pregnancy. The identification of a putative breast stem cell (Stem cell 1) has reached in the last decade a significant impulse and several markers also reported for other tissues have been found in the mammary epithelial cells of both rodents and humans. The data obtained thus far is supporting the concept that the lifetime protective effect of an early pregnancy against breast cancer is due to the complete differentiation of the mammary gland, which results in the replacement of the *Stem cell 1* that is a component of the nulliparous breast epithelium with a new stem cell, called *Stem cell 2*, which is characterized by a specific genomic signature. The pattern of gene expression of the stem cell 2 could potentially be used as useful intermediate end points for evaluating the degree of mammary gland differentiation and for evaluating preventive agents such as human chorionic gonadotropin.

The Structure of the Human Breast

The breast tissue of normally cycling nonpregnant adult women contains three identifiable types of lobules, the lobules type 1 (Lob 1) and the more developed lobules type 2 (Lob 2) and type 3 (Lob 3) (Fig. 1) (J. Russo et al. 1988, 1992, 1994; J. Russo and I.H. Russo 1987a, b, 2004). The lobular composition of the breast of sexually mature women is determined by numerous endogenous and exogenous factors. Principal among them are age, and hence, number and regularity of menstrual cycles, endocrine imbalances, use of exogenous hormones, environmental exposures that could act as endocrine disruptors, and the physiological status of pregnancy. The breast attains its maximum development during pregnancy; it occurs in two distinctly dominant phases: an early stage, characterized by ductal lengthening and profuse branching, sustained by active cell proliferation at the distal end of the ductal tree; the rapid increase in number of newly formed ductules results in the progression of Lob 2 to Lob 3 (I.H. Russo et al. 1989; I.H. Russo and J. Russo 1994; J. Russo and I.H. Russo 1987a, b, 2004). The beginning of secretory activity is indicative of the progression from ductules to secretory acini, which are characteristics of the fully differentiated Lob 4 (Fig. 1) (I.H. Russo et al. 1989; I.H. Russo and J. Russo 1994; J. Russo and I.H. Russo 1987, 2004; Vorherr 1974).

In nulliparous women, the breast contains a great number of undifferentiated structures such as terminal ducts and Lob 1 that remains almost constant throughout their lifespan. The Lob 2 are present in moderate numbers during the early reproductive years and Lob 3 are almost totally absent, suggesting that a certain percentage of Lob 1 might have progressed to Lob 2, but very few Lob 2 have progressed to Lob 3 (J. Russo et al. 1992; J. Russo and I.H. Russo 2004). In parous women, on the other hand, a history of one or more full-term pregnancies between the ages of 14 and 20 years correlates with a significant increase in the number of Lob 3. This type of lob-

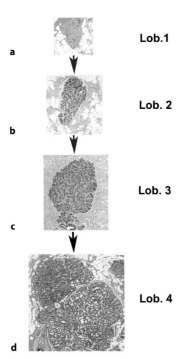

Fig. 1 a Histological sections of lobule type 1, **b** lobule type 2, **c** lobule type 3, and **d** lobule type 4. All the histological sections have been stained with H & E and photographed at ×2.5 magnification

ules remains present as the predominant structure until a woman reaches the age of 40. Their percentage decreases after the fourth decade of life, due to their involution to Lob 1 (I.H. Russo et al. 1989; I.H. Russo and J. Russo 1994; J. Russo and I.H. Russo 1987, 2004; Vorherr 1974).

Genetic influences are responsible of at least 5% of the breast cancer cases; they also seem to influence the pattern of breast development and differentiation, as evidenced by the study of prophylactic mastectomy specimens obtained from women with familial breast and breast/ovarian cancer, or proven to be carriers of the *BRCA1* gene, as determined by linkage analysis (J. Russo et al. 2001a; J. Russo and I.H. Russo 2004). Morphological and architectural analysis of prophylactic mastectomy specimens revealed that these characteristics were similar in breasts obtained from either nulliparous or parous women. In both groups of women, the breast tissues were predominately composed of Lob 1 and only a few specimens contained Lob 2 and Lob 3, in frank contrast with the predominance of Lob 3 found in parous women without familial history of breast cancer (J. Russo et al. 2001a, b; J. Russo and I.H. Russo 2004). The developmental pattern of the breast of parous women of the familial breast cancer group was similar to that of nulliparous women and less developed than the breast of parous women without a history of familial breast cancer. The breast of women belonging to the familial breast cancer group also presented differences in the branching pattern of the ductal tree, observations that suggested that the genes that control lobular development might have been affected in women carrying breast cancer predisposing genes (J. Russo et al. 1994, 2001a, b; J. Russo and I.H. Russo 2004).

The Role of Breast Architecture and the Pathogenesis of Breast Cancer

An important concept that emerged from the study of breast development is that the terminal ductal lobular unit (TDLU), which had been identified as the site of origin of the most common breast malignancy, the ductal carcinoma (J. Russo et al. 1990; J. Russo and I.H. Russo 2004; Wellings et al. 1975), corresponds to a specific stage of development of the mammary parenchyma, the Lob 1. This observation is supported by comparative studies of normal and cancer-bearing breasts obtained at autopsy. It was found that the nontumoral parenchyma in cancer-associated breasts contained a significantly higher number of hyperplastic terminal ducts, atypical Lob 1 and ductal carcinomas in situ originated in Lob 1 than those breasts of women free of breast cancer. These observations indicate that the Lob 1 is affected by preoplastic as well as by neoplastic processes (J. Russo and I.H. Russo 1998; J. Russo et al. 1994, 2000; J. Russo and I.H. Russo 1994, 2004; Vorherr 1974). The finding that the Lob 1, which are undifferentiated structures, cause the most aggressive neoplasm, acquires relevance in light of the fact that these structures are more numerous in the breast of nulliparous women, who are in turn at a higher risk of developing breast cancer. The Lob 1 found in the breast of nulliparous women never went through the process of differentiation; these contain what we have called Stem cell 1 (Figure 2), whereas the same structures, when found in the breast of postmenopausal parous women contained Stem cell 2 (Fig. 2) (J. Russo and I.H. Russo 1997, 2004). More differentiated lobular structures have been found to be affected by neoplastic lesions as well, although they trigger tumors whose malignancy is inversely related to the degree of differentiation of the parent structure, i.e., Lob 2 bring about lobular carcinomas in situ, whereas Lob 3 give rise to more benign breast lesions, such as hyperplastic lobules, cysts, fibroadenomas, and adenomas, and Lob 4 to lactating adenomas (J. Russo et al. 1990). Each specific compartment of the breast gives rise to a specific type of lesion and also provides the basis for a new biological

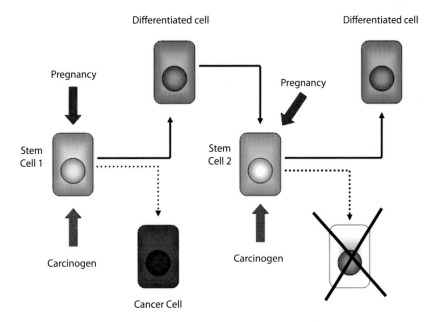

Fig. 2 Breast cancer originates in undifferentiated terminal structures of the mammary gland, the Lob 1, which contain the Stem cell 1 that is the target of the neoplastic event. Early parity induces differentiation of the mammary gland, thus creating the stem cell 2. Even though differentiation significantly reduces cell proliferation in the mammary gland, the mammary epithelium remains capable of responding with proliferation to given stimuli, such as a new pregnancy. Under these circumstances, however, the cells that are stimulated to proliferate are from structures that have already been primed by the first cycle of differentiation, that are able to metabolize the carcinogen and repair the induced DNA damage more efficiently than the cells of the nulliparous gland, and are less susceptible to carcinogenesis. However, if the shifting of Stem cell 1 to Stem cell 2 has not been completed, a carcinogenic stimulus powerful enough may overburden the system, thereby successfully initiating a neoplastic process (Reprinted with permission from J. Russo et al. 2005)

concept that the differentiation of the breast determines the susceptibility to neoplastic transformation (J. Russo et al. 1975).

The finding that the most undifferentiated structures bring about the most aggressive neoplasms support our hypothesis that the presence of Lob 1 explains the higher breast cancer risk of nulliparous women, since they represent the population with the highest concentration of undifferentiated structures in the breast (J. Russo et al. 1994; J. Russo and I.H. Russo 1987, 1998, 1999). Nontumoral breast tissues from cancer-bearing lumpectomy or mastectomy specimens removed from nulliparous women have an architecture dominated by Lob 1; their overall architecture is similar to that of nulliparous females free of mammary pathology (J. Russo et al. 1994). Although the breast tissues of parous women from the general population contain predominantly Lob 3 and a very low percentage of Lob 1, in those parous women that have developed breast cancer their breast tissues have also the Lob 1 as the predominant structure, appearing in this sense similar to those of nulliparous women (J. Russo et al. 1992, 1994; J. Russo and I.H. Russo 2004). It is of interest to note that all the parous breast cancer patients we have studied had a history of late first full-term pregnancy or familial history of breast cancer. The analysis of these samples allowed us to conclude that the architecture of the breast of parous women with breast cancer differs from that of parous women without cancer. The similarities found between the architecture of the breast of nulliparous women and that of parous women with cancer support the hypothesis that the degree of breast development is of importance in the susceptibility to carcinogenesis, and, furthermore, that parous women who develop breast cancer might exhibit a defective response to the differentiating influence of the hormones of pregnancy (J. Russo et al. 1992, 1994) and therefore they are hosting numerous Stem cells 1 that are susceptible to carcinogenesis (Fig. 2). Since ductal breast cancer originates in Lob 1 or TDLU (J. Russo et al. 1990; Wellings et al. 1975), and the epidemiological observation that nulliparous women exhibit a higher incidence of breast cancer than parous women (Henderson et al. 1974, 1993; Kelsey et al.1993; Lambe et al. 1996; MacMahon et al.

1970; Trapido 1983; Vessey et al. 1985) indicates that Lob 1 in these two groups of women might be biologically different or exhibit different susceptibility to carcinogenesis (J. Russo et al. 1989, 1992, 1993, 1994, 2000). Even though the Lob 1 is the hallmark of the postmenopausal breast, we postulate that the degree of differentiation acquired through early pregnancy has caused a genomic signature that differentiates the Lob 1 from the early parous women from that of the nulliparous women by shifting the Stem cell 1 to a Stem cell 2 that is refractory to carcinogenesis (Fig. 2). This is supported by recent data obtained in the rat model (J. Russo and I.H. Russo 1997) in which a cluster of genes remain activated in the involuted gland after pregnancy, conferring a special genomic signature to the gland that is responsible for its refractoriness to chemical carcinogenesis. Thus the refractoriness is produced by the shifting of the compartments of Stem cells 1 to other stem cells called Stem cells 2 (Fig. 2) (J Russo et al. 2001; J. Russo and I.H. Russo 1997). The advances of the human genome project and the availability of new tools for genomic analysis, such as cDNA array, tissue array, laser capture micro dissection (LCM), and bioinformatics techniques have permitted the identification of clusters of genes that are differentially expressed in populations that differ in their breast cancer risk (Balogh et al. 2006). Furthermore, those clusters of genes whose expression may be affected by early pregnancy and that can be proven functionally relevant in protecting the breast from cancer development could serve as markers for evaluating cancer risk in large populations.

Genomic Changes Induced by Pregnancy in Breast Epithelial Cells

The collections of normal breast tissue that adhere to well-established parameters of normality are extremely difficult to obtain (J. Russo et al. 1988), mainly because the normal human breast tissue must be obtained from women with different reproductive histories. One group must represent the low-risk group composed of postmenopausal women without breast cancer who completed their first full-term pregnancy (FFTP) before age 24. The second group for comparison is postmenopausal women without breast cancer who are nulliparous. The selection of postmenopausal women must be those who are at least 1 year after their last menses if menopause occurred naturally or basal serum follicle stimulating hormone (FSH) greater than 40 ng/ml if menopause was surgical and the participant is less than 60 years old. The age at menarche, day of last menstruation, number of miscarriages, year of first full-term pregnancy, number of pregnancies, and no replacement therapy or previous surgical procedures for benign or malignant diseases of the breast are important conditions for the selection of the samples to be analyzed and as a consequence limit the number of samples available for a large study.

The breast epithelial cells and the stroma of the lobules type 1 found in the breast tissue of postmenopausal parous women has a genomic signature different from similar structures derived from postmenopausal nulliparous women (J. Russo and I.H. Russo 1997). Those genes that are significantly different are grouped in major categories based on their putative functional significance. Among them are those gene transcripts related to a) immune-surveillance, b) DNA repair and programmed cell death, and c) transcription, chromatin structure/activators/co activator (Balogh et al. 2006) (Table 1).

Role of Immune Surveillance-Related Genes in the Parous Breast

In breast epithelial cells of parous women, four gene transcripts were significantly upregulated (Table 1). The cytoplasmic Toll/interleukin-1 receptor (TIR) (Sanghavi et al. 2004) signaling domain is known to be instrumental in inducing a signaling cascade upon recognition of specific ligand, triggering innate immune responses (Yamamoto and Akira 2004). The T cell receptor Vβ 1 (TCRβ) in breast tumors recognize specific cytotoxic T lymphocytes in a major histocompatibility complex (MHC) unrestricted fashion (Ito et al. 1997; Kirii et al. 1998). The breast epithelial cells of the parous breast also have upregulated the MHC class I HLA-A24. HLA-A24-binding peptides have the capacity to elicit anti-tumor cytotoxic T lymphocytes (CTL) in vitro (Nukaya

et al. 1999). It has been shown that HLA class I antigen downregulation is associated with worse clinical course of ovarian carcinoma, which may reflect the escape of tumor cells from immune recognition and destruction (Vitale et al. 2005). The epithelial cells of the parous breast also upregulated the expression of interleukin 22 receptor (Table 1). Interleukin-22 (IL-22) is a member of interferon/IL-10 family, which plays an important role in immune response through activation of the STAT 3 signal transduction pathway (Wei et al. 2003; Donnelly et al. 2004; Wolk et al. 2004). The enhanced immune-surveillance mechanism that has been imprinted because of the differentiation cycle induced by pregnancy could be one of the protective factors induced by the cells against neoplastic initiation or progression. Contrary to the postmenopausal parous breast epithelial cells, those cells derived from the lobules type 1 of the postmenopausal nulliparous women presented an upregulation of the gene transcript for the dendritic cell protein (GA17). The potential role of this dendritic cell protein in the epithelial cells of the nulliparous breast could be explained by the recent publication of Thomachot et al. (2004), who have found that primary breast carcinomas are frequently infiltrated by dendritic cells. The breast carcinoma cells produce soluble factors, which may attract dendritic cells and their precursors in vivo and promote the differentiation of the latter into Langerhans cells and immature dendritic cells with altered functional capacities. The infiltration of breast cancer by these altered dendritic cells may contribute to the impaired immune response against the tumor (Thomachot et al. 2004). This mechanism was partly driven by a TGFβ-dependent mechanism since a pan-TGFβ polyclonal antibody completely blocks breast cancer cell-induced Langerhans cell differentiation and partly reduces immature dendritic cell development (Thomachot et al. 2004). These data indicate that if this mechanism takes place in the nulliparous breast the dendritic cells normally present in the breast tissue under the action of initiated breast epithelia will be unable to initiate the immune surveillance mechanism of protection. This is supported by the data that TGFβ is not overexpressed in the nulliparous mammary gland (D'Cruz et al. 2002).

Table 1 Genes differentially expressed in the postmenopausal breast of parous and nulliparous women

Gene name	Parous	Nulliparous	P-value	Function
Sterile alpha and TIR motif containing 1	1.96 ± 0.09	1.00 ± 0.36	0.011	Gene transcripts with immune-surveillance function
T cell receptor V-beta 1 (TCRB)	1.69 ± 0.09	0.98 ± 0.19	0.0044	
Interleukin 22 receptor, alpha 2	2.49 ± 0.41	0.79 ± 0.31	0.0797	
MHC class I HLA-A24 glycoprotein mRNA, 3' end	1.59 ± 0.04	0.41 ± 0.03	0.0001	
Dendritic cell protein	0.92 ± 0.35	1.63 ± 0.29	0.055	
Excision repair cross-complementing rodent repair deficiency, complementation group 2 (xeroderma pigmentosum D)	1.62 ± 0.13	0.94 ± 0.32	0.027	Gene transcripts with DNA repair and programmed cell death functions
RAD51-like 1 (S. cerevisiae)	2.01 ± 0.06	0.79 ± 0.38	0.1917	
Excision repair cross-complementing rodent repair deficiency, complementation group 6	1.67 ± 0.41	0.6 ± 0.49	0.044	
TP53-activated protein 1	0.87 ± 0.24	1.77 ± 0.1	0.0001	
Homo sapiens, similar to NBR2, clone MGC:5031, mRNA, complete cds	1.60 ± 0.43	0.83 ± 0.18	0.046	
Ribosomal protein S3	1.74 ± 0.11	0.77 ± 0.31	0.1458	
Likely ortholog of mouse putative IKK regulator SIMPL	1.67 ± 0.15	0.98 ± 0.31	0.027	
BCL2-associated X protein	1.91 ± 0.15	0.95 ± 0.13	0.0011	
Transcription elongation regulator 1-like	2.10 ± 0.34	0.98 ± 0.38	0.019	Gene transcripts with, translation, transcription function
LIM domain-binding 2	1.82 ± 0.11	0.92 ± 0.27	0.0059	
Heart and neural crest derivatives expressed 2	0.87 ± 0.36	1.52 ± 0.02	0.0003	
Bromodomain adjacent to zinc finger domain, 2A	1.69 ± 0.38	0.90 ± 0.16	0.03	
Processing of precursor 5, ribonuclease P/MRP subunit (S. cerevisiae)	1.50 ± 0.08	0.88 ± 0.26	0.016	
Zinc finger CCCH type domain containing 5	1.56 ± 0.08	0.83 ± 0.16	0.0023	
Zinc finger protein and BTB domain containing 11	1.64 ± 0.22	0.66 ± 0.22	0.0052	
HMT1 (hnRNP methyltransferase, S. cerevisiae)-like 1	1.62 ± 0.11	0.65 ± 0.18	0.0013	
BarH-like homeobox 1	1.57 ± 0.26	0.62 ± 0.3	0.015	
SOX2 overlapping transcript (noncoding RNA)	1.54 ± 0.07	0.60 ± 0.26	0.0036	
SRY (sex determining region Y)-box 30	1.51 ± 0.23	0.54 ± 0.16	0.0037	
Eukaryotic translation initiation factor 3, subunit 5 epsilon, 47 kDa	1.59 ± 0.34	0.5 ± 0.02	0.0052	

Table 1 *(continued)* Genes differentially expressed in the postmenopausal breast of parous and nulliparous women

Gene name	Parous	Nulliparous	P-value	Function
BTB and CNC homology 1, basic leucine zipper transcription factor 2	0.93 ± 0.19	1.83 ± 0.28	0.01	Gene transcripts with, translation, transcription function
Ring finger protein 146	1.67 ± 0.12	0.73 ± 0.09	0.1309	
Integral membrane protein 2B (AT rich interactive domain 5B (MRF1-like)	0.96 ± 0.33	2.09 ± 0.47	0.027	

The Role of DNA Repair and Programmed Cell Death Genes in the Parous Breast

DNA repair is central to the integrity of the human genome and reduced DNA repair capacity has been linked to genetic susceptibility to cancer. A reduced DNA repair is associated with risk of breast cancer in women. The epithelial cells of the breast from parous women present four DNA repair-related genes that are upregulated significantly when compared with the same gene expression in the epithelial cells of the nulliparous breast (Table 1). The Excision Repair Cross-Complementing Rodent Repair Group 2 (ERCC2), a major DNA repair protein, is involved in nucleotide excision repair and basal transcription (Caggana et al. 2001; Sancar and Tang 1993; Troelstra et al. 1992; Zhou et al. 2002). ERCC6 corrects the repair defect of Cockayne's syndrome complementation group B (Troelstra et al. 1992). The *ERCC6* gene in humans directs the excision nuclease to RNA polymerase stalled at a lesion in the transcribed strand and thus ensures preferential repair of this strand compared to the nontranscribed strand (Sancar and Tang 1993). The ribosomal protein S3 (RPS3) is also upregulated in the breast of postmenopausal parous women. Ribosomal protein S3 (RPS3) is a multifunctional ribosomal protein that is a structural and functional component of the ribosome, and also a DNA repair enzyme involved in the DNA base excision repair pathway (Lim et al. 2002; Lyamouri et al. 2002). RPS3 functions not only as a DNA repair endonuclease and ribosomal protein S3, but has also been related to apoptosis. Deletion analysis reveals that the two functions of rpS3, DNA repair and apoptosis, use independent functional domains (Jang et al. 2004). The RAD51-like 1 that is involved

in the homologous recombination repair is an essential process for the maintenance and variability of the genome. In eukaryotes, the Rad epistasis group proteins serve the main role for meiotic recombination and/or homologous recombination repair (Osakabe et al. 2002). In humans, interaction of RAD51 with proteins such as BRCA1 and BRCA2 has provided insight into the mechanism of how these molecules function as tumor suppressors (Ashley and Plug 1998; Essers et al. 1997; Ghabrial et al. 1998; Leasure et al. 2001; Tsuzuki et al. 1996). These data indicate that the activation of genes involved in the DNA repair process is part of the signature induced in the mammary gland by pregnancy. These observations confirm previous findings that in vivo the ability of the cells to repair carcinogen-induced damage by unscheduled DNA synthesis and adduct removal is more efficient in the mammary gland of parous rats (Tay and Russo 1981a, b). For these reasons, they have been included as a property of the Stem cells 2.

In the parous breast, two gene transcripts are significantly upregulated with a functional role in program cell death (Table 1). Tumor necrosis factor alpha (TNF-alpha) is a cytokine that acts as an important mediator of the apoptotic process, also demonstrating selective cytotoxicity against malignant breast tumor cells. Activation of this cytokine requires the interaction with mouse pelle-like kinase (SIMPL) (Kwon et al. 2004). An ortholog of the mouse putative IKK regulator SIMPL is upregulated significantly in the breast tissue of postmenopausal parous women. Overexpression of SIMPL leads to the activation of NF-κB-dependent promoters and inactivation of SIMPL inhibits IRAK/mPLK as well as tumor necrosis factor receptor type I-induced NF-κB activity (Vig et al. 2001). The BCL2-associated X protein is also upregulated in the breast epithelial cells of parous women. Bax is a pro-apoptotic gene whose transcription is stimulated by active p53, including the pro-apoptotic gene p21, a cell cycle regulator (Falke et al. 2004; Qin et al. 2004). As indicated above, the ribosomal protein S3 (RPS3), which is also upregulated in the parous breast tissue, activates caspase-8/caspase-3 and sensitizes cytokine-induced apoptosis (Jang et al. 2004). These two transcripts, BCL2-associated X protein and RPS3, are part of the genomic signature of the Stem cell 2. Supporting evidence for this finding comes from the rat experimental model in which postpregnancy involuted mammary gland exhibits a genomic signature characterized by an elevated expression of genes involved in programmed cell death pathways, such as testosterone-repressed prostate message 2 (TRPM2), interleukin 1β-converting enzyme (ICE), bcl-XL, bcl-XS, p53, p21, and c-myc, which can be from three- to fivefold upregulated (J. Russo and I.H. Russo 2004; Srivastava et al. 1997, 1999).

Role of the Transcription, Translation Factor Regulators, and Chromatin Structure-Related Genes in the Parous Breast

The larger groups of gene transcripts, which are significantly different in the breasts of the parous compared with the nulliparous woman, belong to the transcription and translation factor regulators (Table 1). Among the transcription factors are the LIM domain-binding 2 and SOX 2, which are significantly upregulated in the epithelial cells of the parous breast. LIM domain-containing proteins contribute to cell fate determination, the regulation of cell proliferation, and differentiation by activating transcription of cell-type-specific genes, but this activation requires cooperation with other nuclear factors (Cassata et al. 2000; Dawid et al. 1995; Goyal et al. 1999; Harris et al. 2002; Johnson et al. 1997). For example, it has been found that the nuclear domain 10 protein (NDP52), which is also upregulated in the parous breast epithelial cells, interact with the Lim domain (Korioth et al. 1995). SOX1/2/3 interact with various partner transcription factors and participate in defining distinct cell states that depend on the partner factors; thus the regulation of SOX2 and its partner factors, exemplified by Pax6, determines the spatiotemporal order of the occurrence of cell differentiation (Kondoh et al. 2004). Therefore it is possible to postulate that SOX2 could play an important role in the differentiated breast epithelial cells of the parous breast. Interestingly, SOX-2 is a transcription factor that is expressed by self-renewing and multipotent stem cells of the embryonic neuroepithelium (Komitova and Eriksson 2004; Miyagi et al. 2004; Stevanovic 2003). SOCK 2 is also considered a stem cell marker (Ginis et al. 2004). Therefore, although we do not know its role in the breast epithelial cell, it could well represent the marker of the differentiated Stem cell 2 previously postulated (J. Russo and I.H. Russo 1997). Furthermore, genes of the Sox family encode evolutionarily conserved HMG box-containing transcription factors, which play key roles in various events of cell determination/differentiation during development (Bullejos et al. 2000; Cremazy et al. 2001; De Martino et al. 1999; Koopman et al. 2004). The SOX 30 or sex determination region Y (SRY) is also significantly upregulated in the parous breast epithelial cells. Sox 30 family proteins are characterized by a unique DNA-binding domain, a HMG box, which shows at least 50% sequence similarity with mouse Sry, the sex-determining factor. Osaki et al. have shown specific expression of Sox30 in normal testes, but not in maturing germ cell-deficient testes. This suggests that the expression of this gene in the breast could be a marker of differentiation and part of the signature induced by pregnancy in the breast epithelial cells. In this category can also be included the BarH-like homeobox 1 gene, which was significantly upregulated in the parous breast epithelial cells (Table 1). The BarH1 and BarH2 (Bar) *Drosophila* genes are homeobox-containing genes, which are required for the fate determination of external sensory organs in the fly. They have also been identified in mouse and human (Bulfone et al. 2000). Although the function of this gene in the mammary gland is not clearly understood, it is known that it plays an important role during mouse neurogenesis in the migration and survival of cerebellar granule cells and precerebellar neurons and that it functionally links Barhl1 to the NT-3 signaling pathway during cerebellar development (Bermingham et al. 2001; Bulfone et al. 2000; Li et al. 2004). BarH1 could be considered another marker of the differentiated Stem cell 2 in the breast epithelia of the parous woman.

The transcription factors associated with chromatin remodeling complexes such as the zinc finger and BTB domain containing 11 and the bromodomain adjacent to zinc finger domain 2A (BAZ2A) (Table 1), are significantly upregulated in the parous breast epithelial cells. The zinc finger and BTB domain containing 11 is highly conserved in a large family of eukaryotic proteins and is crucial for the latter's diverse roles in mediating interactions among proteins that are involved in transcription regulation and chromatin structures (Chen et al. 2004; Hoatlin et al. 1999). The bromodomain adjacent to zinc finger domain 2A (BAZ2A) is a structural motif characteristic of proteins involved in chromatin-dependent regulation of transcription. Bromodomain proteins have been identified as integral components of chromatin remodeling complexes and frequently possess histone acetyltransferase activity. The novel gene, termed BAZ2A, is localized to chromosomes 12q24.3-qter. Their encoding genes have been identified at translocation breakpoints, and at least one, CBP, is a tumor suppressor gene (Jones et al. 2000). This special function in chromatin structure makes them candidates markers of the differentiated Stem cell 2.

Another group of genes associated with their function as co activator and in chromatin remodeling seems to play an important role in the signature induced by pregnancy in the breast epithelial cells (Table 1). One of them is the p300/CBP-associated factor (PCAF), which is significantly upregulated in the epithelial cells of the parous breast tissue. p300/CBP-associated factor (PCAF) is a co-activator of the tumor suppressor, p53. PCAF participates in p53's transactivation of target genes through acetylation of both bound p53 and histones within p53 target promoters (Watts et al. 2004). Interestingly enough, various kinds of cofactors, such as steroid receptor co-activator-1 (SRC-1), transcription intermediary factor 2 (TIF2), and amplified in breast cancer 1 (AIB1), have also been reported to interact with nuclear receptors in a ligand-dependent man-

ner and enhance transcriptional activation by the receptor via histone acetylation/methylation and recruitment of additional co-activator, such as CREB-binding protein (CBP)/p300 (Iwase 2003). The role of p300/CBP-associated factor in the differentiated breast epithelial cells of parous women could be similar to the effect of transretinoic acid (ATRA) treatment of metastatic breast cancer cells, which, by increasing the protein levels of the histone acetyl transferases p300 and CBP, suppresses the level of histone deacetylase and increases the level of acetylated histone H4. ATRA has also been shown to decrease Bcl-2, increase Bax, and decrease VEGF (Hayashi et al. 2003). Bax is upregulated in the postmenopausal parous breast epithelial cells.

The suppressor of hairy wing homolog 4 is significantly upregulated in the epithelial cells of the parous breast (Table 1). This gene transcript has been shown in *Drosophila* (Chen and Corces 2001), can bind chromatin insulators, and is thought to regulate gene expression by establishing higher-order domains of chromatin organization. Chromatin insulators, or boundary elements, affect promoter–enhancer interactions and buffer transgenes from position effects (Byrd and Corces 2003; Chen and Corces 2001; Pai et al. 2004; Parnell et al. 2003). Although we do not know how the suppressor of hairy-wing can regulate the chromatin organization of the breast epithelial cell, it is possible that mechanism of this nature works in silencing or repressing certain genes that control proliferation or at the same time may increase repair of damage and specific response to hormones. A similar function in chromatin remodeling could be played by the suppressor of Ty homolog 3, which has been found to be significantly upregulated in the parous breast epithelial cells (Table 1). Suppressors of Ty (SPT) genes were originally identified through a genetic screen for mutations in the yeast *Saccharomyces cerevisiae* that restore gene expression disrupted by the insertion of the transposon Ty. Classic members of the SPT gene family, SPT11, SPT12, and SPT15, encode for the histones H2A and H2B and for TATA-binding protein (TBP), respectively. In addition, accumulating evidence suggests that SPT gene products play more diverse roles, including roles in DNA replication as well as DNA recombination and developmental regulation (Yamaguchi et al. 2001). For example, it has been reported that the function of H2A and H2B in one repression assay was found to be dependent on three SPT (suppressor of Ty) genes whose products are important for chromatin-mediated repression. These results suggest that repressive chromatin structure may be established through the interactions of the Spt proteins with these histones (Recht et al. 1996). Of interest is that SPT gene, which is upregulated because of the differentiation cycle induced by pregnancy, is a suppressor of mutations induced by the retrotransposon Ty in *Saccharomyces cerevisiae*. All SPT genes isolated to date suppress Ty-induced mutations by altering transcription. Suppressor of hairy-wing and the suppressor of Ty homolog 3 are considered part of the unique signature to the Stem cells 2 of the parous breast and be functionally involved in the protection conferred by an early pregnancy against cancer in this organ.

Genomic Profile of the Nulliparous Breast

The genes defining the genomic signature of the nulliparous breast or Stem cells 1 separate this epithelia from the more differentiated Stem cells 2, resulting from the pregnancy (Table 1). An interesting gene that is downregulated in the parous breast and significantly upregulated in the nulliparous breast tissue is the cryptic gene (Table 1). This gene was found using a differential display screening approach to identify mesoderm-specific genes, relying upon the differentiation of embryonic stem cells in vitro. The cryptic gene encodes a secreted molecule containing a variant epidermal growth factor-like (EGF) motif. The name "cryptic" was based on its predicted protein sequence similarity with Crypto, which encodes an EGF-related growth factor. Based on their strong sequence similarities, it was proposed that Cryptic, Crypto, and the Xenopus FRL-1 gene define a new family of growth factor-like molecules, which was named the CFC (Crypto, Frl-1, and Cryptic) family (Shen et al. 1997). In the mouse, Cryptic is not expressed in adult tissues, whereas Cr-1 is expressed at a low level in several different tissues, including the mammary gland. In the mammary gland, expres-

sion of Cr-1 in the ductal epithelial cells increases during pregnancy and lactation and immunoreactive and biologically active Cr-1 protein can be detected in human milk. Overexpression of Cr-1 in mouse mammary epithelial cells can facilitate their in vitro transformation and in vivo these Cr-1-transduced cells produce ductal hyperplasias in the mammary gland. Recombinant mouse or human Crypto can enhance cell motility and branching morphogenesis in mammary epithelial cells and in some human tumor cells. These effects are accompanied by an epithelial-mesenchymal transition associated with a decrease in beta-catenin function and an increase in vimentin expression. Expression of Crypto is increased several-fold in human colon, gastric, pancreatic, and lung carcinomas and in a variety of different types of mouse and human breast carcinomas. More importantly, this increase can first be detected in premalignant lesions in some of these tissues. In mammary epithelial cells, part of these responses may depend on the ability of CR-1 to transactivate erb B-4 and/or fibroblast growth factor receptor 1 through an src-like tyrosine kinase (Salomon et al. 2000). Altogether, the upregulation of this gene in the nulliparous breast is very important because it confirms the ability of these cells to proliferate and even to respond readily to growth factors, which if acting in a damaged cell will impulse it to cell transformation. We consider that this gene is part of the signature of the Stem cells 1.

The Odz (odd Oz)/ten homolog 3 is upregulated significantly in the nulliparous breast epithelial cells (Table 1). The product of the *Drosophila melanogaster* odd Oz (odz)/Tenascin-major (ten-m) pair-rule gene consists of eight epidermal growth factor (EGF)-like repeats followed by a novel 1,800 amino acid polypeptide stretch unique to proteins of the Odz/Ten-m family (Dgany and Wides 2002). Odz is a type I transmembrane protein with the vast C-terminal portion in the intracellular space and with the EGF repeats deployed extracellularly (Dgany and Wides 2002). Expression of the Odz2 gene is restricted to the nervous system. The expression patterns suggest that each of the genes has its own distinct developmental role. Comparisons of *Drosophila* and vertebrate Odz expression patterns suggest evolutionarily conserved functions (Ben-Zur et al. 2000; Levine et al. 1994). Its discovery in the breast epithelial cells of the nulliparous breast is new and opens the door for a growth regulatory function and is considered part of the signature of the Stem cells 1.

In the nulliparous breast cells, we have identified the bric-a-brac (BTB) and cap-n-collar(CNC) homology 1(BACH1), and the HAND2 gene (heart and neural crest derivatives expression 2) (Table 1). The gene, termed *BACH1*, encodes a 736-amino-acid polypeptide with 80.3% identity to the murine Bach1 protein and contains a Cap'n'collar (CNC)-type basic leucine zipper (bZip) domain and a protein interaction motif, the BTB domain (Ohira et al. 1998). Its role in the breast epithelial cells may be more related to regulation of transcription (Aiyer et al. 2005; Dai and Cserjesi 2002; Dai et al. 2004; Murakami et al. 2004; Russell et al. 1998). *HAND2* is required for vasculature development (Morikawa and Cserjesi 2004), regulates cell type-specific expression of norepinephrine in concert with Phox2a homeodomain (Xu et al. 2003), and mediates dorsoventral (DV) patterning in the anterior pharyngeal arches (Miller et al. 2003). Considering all this evidence, it is possible to speculate that HAND2 could play an important role in the development of the mammary gland and be part of the genomic signature of the Stem cells 1 (Table 1). Overexpression of this gene could maintain a low branching pattern of the gland that can be overcome by the hormonal stimulation of pregnancy.

Genomic Differences in the Stroma of the Breast of Nulliparous and Parous Women

The laser-captured microdissection of the stroma of the lobules type 1 of the parous and nulliparous breast present significantly up- and downregulated genes. Among them is neuropilin 2 (Table 2). Neuropilins and group A plexins are components of receptor complexes for class 3 semaphorins, gradients of which help to guide migration of neural progenitor cells and axonal growth cones during development and guide regenerating axons (Ara et al. 2005; Watanabe et al. 2004). Npn2 facilitates VEGF-induced retinal neovascularization (Fukahi et al. 2004; Shen et al. 2004), small lymphatic vessels and capillaries (Yuan et al. 2002). The upregulation of the neuropilin 2 in the stroma of the parous lobules 1 could play a role in the orientation and branching organization of the ductal structures and could act by inhibiting cell proliferation of the adjacent epithelial cells, as has been shown that the proliferative activity of the ductular structures of the parous breast is significantly lower than the Lob.1 of the nulliparous breast (J. Russo et al. 1999). The reverse effect to increase cell proliferation by VEGF in the breast carcinoma and trophoblast cells indicates that the biological actions of VEGF and/or neuropilin 2 on certain cell types may differ from the effects of this molecule on vascular endothelial cells (Endo et al. 2004).

Thy 1 cell surface antigen is upregulated in the stroma cells of the parous breast tissue (Table 2). Sca-1 and Thy-1 are considered markers on hematopoietic progenitor cells (Boyum et al. 2204). Thy 1 is also considered a marker of stem cells in hepatoblastoma (Fiegel et al. 2004). Thy-1 expression is induced by transformation of keratocytes to corneal fibroblasts and myofibroblasts, suggesting a potential functional role for Thy-1 in stromal wound healing and providing a surface marker to distinguish the normal keratocyte from its repair phenotypes (Pei et al. 2004). Thy-1 (CD90) is a small GPI-anchored protein that is particularly abundant on the surface of mouse thymocytes and peripheral T cells. Thy-1 could be involved in the maintenance of T cell homeostasis in the absence of TCR triggering, as well as potentiating Ag-induced T cell responses (Haeryfar and Hoskin 2004). We do not know in which specific cells of the stroma the Thy1 is expressed, but its function in the interlobular stroma is either by increasing the fibroblast differentiation or by acting as immune modulators in conjunction with the other gene transcripts also upregulated in the epithelium of the Lob.1 of the parous woman (Table 1). Distinct subpopulations of fibroblasts contribute, based on the expression of the Thy-1, in affecting proliferation and myofibroblast differentiation (Zhou et al. 2004). These data are of interest in that the changes observed in the interlobular stroma may also be a reflection of the genomic changes in the breast epithelial cells or vice versa.

Table 2 Known genes differentially expressed in the stroma of the Lobules type 1 of the breast of nulliparous and parous women

Gene name	Parous	Nulliparous	P-value
PFTAIRE protein kinase 1	0.98 ± 0.31	1.79 ± 0.13	0.0161
Human epididymis-specific 3 beta	0.96 ± 0.50	2.00 ± 0.17	0.0320
Ligand of neuronal nitric oxide synthase with carboxyl-terminal PDZ domain	0.92 ± 0.34	2.20 ± 0.45	0.0025
Homolog of mouse C2PA	0.69 ± 0.47	1.92 ± 0.09	0.0304
Sorting nexin 17	0.27 ± 0.39	1.60 ± 0.41	0.0011
Chloride channel 3	0.17 ± 0.52	1.53 ± 0.25	0.0129
Neuropilin 2	2.46 ± 0.59	0.98 ± 0.15	0.0282
DnaJ (Hsp40) homolog, subfamily C, member 8	2.26 ± 0.58	0.98 ± 0.41	0.0058
Chaperonin-containing TCP1, subunit 6B (zeta 2)	2.31 ± 0.58	0.95 ± 0.17	0.0290
Hypothetical protein FLJ13660 similar to CDK5 activator-binding protein C53	2.56 ± 0.51	0.94 ± 0.49	0.0001
Keratin, hair, basic, 5	1.73 ± 0.41	0.91 ± 0.16	0.0296
Adaptor-related protein complex 1, mu 2 subunit	2.01 ± 0.49	0.88 ± 0.39	0.0026
Kallikrein 11	1.81 ± 0.58	0.85 ± 0.27	0.0330
Protein phosphatase 1G (formerly 2C), magnesium-dependent, gamma isoform	1.90 ± 0.48	0.85 ± 0.27	0.0131
Amyloid beta (A4) precursor protein-binding, family B, member 2 (Fe65-like)	2.16 ± 0.47	0.84 ± 0.33	0.0037
Human DNA sequence from clone 71L16 on chromosome Xp11. Contains a probable zinc finger protein (pseudo)gene, an unknown putative gene, a pseudogene with high similarity to part of antigen KI-67, a putative chondroitin 6-sulfotransferase-like gene an	2.22 ± 0.44	0.81 ± 0.20	0.0095
Sialyltransferase 6 (N-acetyllacosaminide alpha 2,3-sialyltransferase	1.96 ± 0.52	0.76 ± 0.42	0.0023
Nuclear factor I/X (CCAAT-binding transcription factor)	1.97 ± 0.46	0.70 ± 0.40	0.0007
Uridine monophosphate synthetase (orotate phosphoribosyl transferase and orotidine-5'-decarboxylase	1.66 ± 0.57	0.70 ± 0.18	0.0509
M-phase phosphoprotein homolog	1.85 ± 0.43	0.68 ± 0.04	0.0351
Integrin, alpha M (complement component receptor 3, alpha; also known as CD11b (p170), macrophage antigen alpha polypeptide)	1.98 ± 0.56	0.65 ± 0.19	0.0248
Thy-1 cell surface antigen	1.58 ± 0.48	0.57 ± 0.37	0.0039
Jun B proto-oncogene	1.55 ± 0.38	0.56 ± 0.37	0.0000

JunB (Table 2) is a component of the Jun family genes of the activating protein-1 transcription factors that are important in the control of cell growth and differentiation and neoplastic transformation. Recently, it was demonstrated that transgenic mice specifically lacking JunB expression in the myeloid lineage developed a myeloproliferative disease, eventually progressing to blast crisis that resembled human chronic myeloid leukemia (Passegue et al. 2004; Yang et al. 2003). JunB is upregulated in the interlobular stroma of the parous women (Table 2) and it is of great interest that junB regulates the numbers of hematopoietic stem cells (Passegue et al. 2004) and therefore it may control the stem cells present in the epithelial cell compartment. This is supported by the increasing number of examples on the importance of mesenchymal–epithelial interactions in physiological (e.g., embryonic development) and pathological (tumorigenesis) processes. In the breast, there is a well-controlled balance of cell proliferation and differentiation, which forms the basis for a proper histoarchitecture of the lobular structure. In the skin, it has been shown that the specific function of c-Jun and JunB in the mesenchymal–epithelial interaction is regulating the expression of interleukin-1 (IL-1) -induced keratinocyte growth factor (KGF) and GM-CSF in fibroblasts. These factors, in turn, adjust the balance between proliferation and differentiation of keratinocytes, ensuring proper architecture of the epidermis (Angel et al. 2002). Estrogens are known to regulate the proliferation of breast cancer cells and to alter their cytoarchitectural and phenotypic properties and one of the pathways used by this hormone is downregulating transcriptional repressors such as JunB (Frasor et al. 2003). On the other hand, okadaic acid (OA), an inhibitor of protein phosphatases 1 and 2A, induces differentiation in human MCF-7, AU-565, and MB-231 breast tumor cells by increasing the levels of early response genes junB, c-jun, and c-fos, and within a day's manifestation of differentiation (Kiguchi et al.1992). Altogether, the data support the concept that the genomic changes taking place in the parous breast are imprinted in the interlobular stroma and are an important determinant of the final signature of the parous breast against cancer.

Unifying Concepts

All the data discussed above support the mechanism postulated by Russo and Russo (I.H. Russo et al. 1991; J. Russo and I.H. Russo 1980, 1997) that pregnancy-induced protection is mediated by the induction of mammary gland differentiation driven by the hormonal milieu of pregnancy, which creates a specific genomic signature in the mammary gland that makes this organ permanently refractory to carcinogenesis (Fig. 2). It is also important to acknowledge that other explanations to the protective effect of pregnancy against carcinogenesis that are not completely exclusive have been reported, for example changes in the environment (Sinha et al. 1988) and or alterations in the immunological profile of the host (Thordarson et al. 1995). A further refinement of the mechanism of how pregnancy could affect cancer susceptibility through induction of differentiation of the mammary gland was first proposed by Russo and Russo, who postulated that the Lob 1 and the TEB found in the breast of nulliparous women or of young virgin rats, respectively, had not completed their differentiation into Lob 2, Lob 3, and Lob 4, retaining a high concentration of stem cells called Stem cells 1, which are susceptible to undergoing neoplastic transformation when exposed to a carcinogenic agent (J. Russo and I.H. Russo 1997) (Fig. 2). After the postmenopausal involution of the mammary gland, the architecture of the parous breast is similar to that of the nulliparous breast, containing predominantly Lob 1 composed of Stem cells 2, an epithelial cell population that is refractory to transformation. It was further postulated that the degree of differentiation acquired through early pregnancy permanently changes the genomic signature that differentiate the Lob 1 in early parous women from that of nulliparous women, shifting the Stem cell 1 to a Stem cell 2, which is refractory to carcinogenesis. These cells were called Stem cells 2 because after postlactational involution, the mammary epithelium remains capable of responding with proliferation and differentiation to the stimulus of a new pregnancy; however, these cells are refractory to carcinogenesis, even though they are stimulated to proliferate and to regenerate the whole mammary gland (Fig. 2). The Stem cell 2 is characterized by having a genomic signature that has been induced by the first cycle of differentiation (Table 1). During the last 8 years, supporting evidence for this mechanism has been generated by Russo and co-workers as well as by other researchers. Studies by Smith and co-workers (Boulanger et al. 2004; Henry et al. 2004; Wagner et al. 2002) using transgenic WAP-driven Cre and Rosa 26-fl-stop-fl-LacZ mice provided evidence of a new mammary epithelial cell population that originates from differentiated cells during pregnancy; 5%–10% of this parity-induced epithelium survives postlactational involution after the first pregnancy. With successive pregnancies, their percentage increases, reaching 60% of the total epithelium in multiparous females. The parity-induced mammary epithelial cells (PI-MEC) is equivalent to the Stem cells 2 postulated by Russo and Russo (1997), since these cells show the capacity for self-renewal and contribute to mammary outgrowth in transplantation studies. PI-MEC can function as alveolar progenitors in subsequent pregnancies, and it is thought that they may be related to differences in response to hormonal stimulation and carcinogenic agents observed between nulliparous and parous females (Boulanger et al. 2004; Henry et al. 2004; Wagner et al. 2002).

The crucial role of the number of mammary stem cells in breast cancer risk has also been recently postulated by Trichopoulos (2005): a number that may be reduced through the process of terminal differentiation after the first full-term pregnancy. Several authors have focused on finding molecular changes as a mechanism of the pregnancy-induced protection (D'Cruz et al. 2002; Ginger et al. 2001; Ginger and Rosen 2003; Medina and Smith 1999; Medina and Kittrel 2003; Srivastava et al. 1999; Trichopoulos et al. 2005). Russo and co-workers have found that the postpregnancy involuted mammary gland exhibits a genomic signature characterized by elevated expression of genes involved in the apoptotic pathways, such as testosterone repressed prostate message 2 (TRPM2), interleukin 1β-converting enzyme (ICE), bcl-XL, bcl-XS, p53, p21, and c-myc, which can be from three- to fivefold upregulated (Medina and Kittrell 2003; J. Russo and I.H. Russo 2004; Srivastava et al. 1999). The ac-

tivation of programmed cell death genes occurs through a p53-dependent process, modulated by c-myc and with partial dependence on the bcl2-family-related genes. In addition, inhibin A and B, heterodimeric nonsteroidal secreted glycoproteins with tumor suppressor activity, are also upregulated (I.H. Russo and J. Russo 1994; J. Russo and I.H. Russo 2004; Srivastava et al. 1999). Genes whose level of expression progressively increases with time of pregnancy reaching their highest levels between 21 and 42 days postpartum are those coding for a fragment of glycogen phosphorylase, AMP-activated kinase, bone morphogenetic protein 4, and vesicle-associated protein 1. The G/T mismatch-specific thymine DNA glycosylase gene is also increased fivefold in this model. These data indicate that the activation of genes involved in the DNA repair process, as found in the human breast (Table 1), is part of the signature induced in the mammary gland by pregnancy. These observations confirm previous findings that in vivo the ability of the cells to repair carcinogen-induced damage by unscheduled DNA synthesis and adduct removal is more efficient in the parous and animal mammary gland (Tay and Russo 1981a, b). The studies of Srivastava et al. (Srivastava et al. 1999; Sivaraman and Medina 2002) observed that p53 can be implicated in the protective effect of parity, which can be mimicked by treatment of virgin rats with estrogen and progesterone. Studies by Medina and Smith (1999) and Medina and Kittrell (2003) in the same hormonal model reported that the function of p53 is required for the hormone-mediated protection of DMBA-induced mammary tumorigenesis in mice. Genomic analysis of the mammary gland of virgin rats treated with estrogen and progesterone at doses that have been reported to mimic pregnancy, showed downregulation of certain growth-promoting molecules, whereas markers involved in cell cycle control or the modulation of transforming growth factor beta (TGF-β) signaling pathway were upregulated in the post-treatment involuted mammary gland. In this study, an unknown noncoding RNA (designated G.B7) and RbAp46, which has been implicated in a number of complexes involving chromatin remodeling, were found to be persistently upregulated in the lobules of the regressed glands (Ginger et al. 2001). Using gene profile analysis, D'Cruz and co-workers (2002) also observed downregulation of growth factors potentially involved in epithelial proliferation as well as persistent upregulation of TGF-β3 and several of its transcript targets in the involuted gland of parous rats and mice. The proposed model of parity-induced specific changes (J. Russo and I.H. Russo 1997) has been further confirmed by Ginger and Rosen, who reported that pregnancy induces multiple changes in the mammary epithelial cells, including nuclear accumulation of p53 and induction of whey acidic protein (WAP). During involution, a large component of the epithelium is eliminated through apoptosis, and a specific subpopulation of epithelial cells survives this process. The involuted mammary gland has persistent changes in gene expression, nuclear localization of p53, and an altered proliferative capacity in response to a carcinogen. Pregnancy would induce epigenetic changes, such as chromatin remodeling, DNA methylation/demethylation, and histone modifications, affecting cell fate in the parous mammary gland. All the genes that have been attributed to the Stem cell 2 seem to work in a different functional pathway from those described for the Stem cell 1 (Table 1). These data in the animal model demonstrate that the process of cell differentiation shifts the Stem cell 1 to Stem cell 2 (Fig. 2), cells that exhibit a specific genomic signature that could be responsible for the refractoriness of the mammary gland to carcinogenesis.

Acknowledgements

This work was supported by grant RO1-CA093599 from the National Cancer Institute, USA.

References

Aiyer AR, Honarpour N, Herz J et al (2005) Loss of Apaf-1 leads to partial rescue of the HAND2-null phenotype. Dev Biol 278:155–162

Angel P, Szabowski A (2002) Function of AP-1 target genes in mesenchymal-epithelial cross-talk in skin. Biochem Pharmacol 64:949–956

Ara J, Bannerman P, Shaheen F et al (2005) Schwann cell-autonomous role of neuropilin-2. J Neurosci Res 79:468–475

Ashley T, Plug A (1998) Caught in the act: deducing meiotic function from protein immunolocalization. Curr Top Dev Biol 37:201–239

Balogh GB, Heulings R, Mailo D et al (2006) Genomic Signature Induced by pregnancy in the human breast. International J Oncol 28:399–410

Ben-Zur T, Feige E, Motro B et al (2000) The mammalian Odz gene family: homologs of a Drosophila pair-rule gene with expression implying distinct yet overlapping developmental roles. Dev Biol 217:107–120

Bermingham NA, Hassan BA, Wang VY et al (2001) Proprioceptor pathway development is dependent on Math1. Neuron 30:411–422

Boulanger CA, Wagner KU, Smith GH (2004) Parity-induced mouse mammary epithelial cells are pluripotent, self-renewing and sensitive to TGF-beta1 expression. Oncogene 24.552–560

Boyum A, Fjerdingstad HB, Tennfjord VA et al (2004) Specific antibodies to mouse Sca-1- (Ly-6A/E) or Thy-1-positive haematopoietic progenitor cells induce formation of nitric oxide which inhibits subsequent colony formation. Eur J Haematol 73:427–430

Bulfone A, Menguzzato E, Broccoli V et al (2000) Barhl1, a gene belonging to a new subfamily of mammalian homeobox genes, is expressed in migrating neurons of the CNS. Hum Mol Genet 9:1443–1452

Bullejos M, Diaz de la Guardia R, Barragan MJ et al (2000) HMG-box sequences from microbats homologous to the human SOX30 HMG-box. Genetica 110:157–162

Byrd K, Corces VG (2003) Visualization of chromatin domains created by the gypsy insulator of Drosophila. J Cell Biol 162:565–574

Caggana M, Kilgallen J, Conroy JM et al (2001) Associations between ERCC2 polymorphisms and gliomas. Cancer Epidemiol Biomarkers Prev 10:355–360

Cassata G, Rohrig S, Kuhn F et al (2000) The Caenorhabditis elegans Ldb/NLI/Clim orthologue ldb-1 is required for neuronal function. Dev Biol 226:45–56

Chen J, Xu J, Ying K et al (2004) Molecular cloning and characterization of a novel human BTB domain-containing gene, BTBD10, which is down-regulated in glioma. Gene 340:61–69

Chen S, Corces VG (2001) The gypsy insulator of Drosophila affects chromatin structure in a directional manner. Genetics 159:1649–1658

Cremazy F, Berta P, Girard F (2001) Genome-wide analysis of Sox genes in Drosophila melanogaster. Mech Dev 109:371–375

Dai YS, Cserjesi P (2002) The basic helix-loop-helix factor, HAND2, functions as a transcriptional activator by binding to E-boxes as a heterodimer. J Biol Chem 277:12604–12612

Dai YS, Hao J, Bonin C et al (2004) JAB1 enhances HAND2 transcriptional activity by regulating HAND2 DNA binding. J Neurosci Res 76:613–622

Dawid IB, Toyama R, Taira M (1995) LIM domain proteins. C R Acad Sci III 318:295–306

D'Cruz CM, Moody SE, Master SR et al (2002) Persistent parity-induced changes in growth factors, TGF-beta3, and differentiation in the rodent mammary gland. Mol Endocrinol 16:2034–2051

De Martino SP, Errington F, Ashworth A et al (1999) sox30: a novel zebrafish sox gene expressed in a restricted manner at the midbrain-hindbrain boundary during neurogenesis. Dev Genes Evol 209:357–362

Dgany O, Wides R (2002) The Drosophila odz/ten-m gene encodes a type I, multiply cleaved heterodimeric transmembrane protein. Biochem J 363:633–643

Donnelly RP, Sheikh F, Kotenko SV et al (2004) The expanded family of class II cytokines that share the IL-10 receptor-2 (IL-10R2) chain. J Leukoc Biol 76:314–321

Endo K, Kawasaki S, Nakamura T et al (2004) The presence of keratin 5 as an IgG Fc binding protein in human corneal epithelium. Exp Eye Res 78:1137–1141

Essers J, Hendriks RW, Swagemakers SM et al (1997) Disruption of mouse RAD54 reduces ionizing radiation resistance and homologous recombination. Cell 89:195–204

Falke D, Fisher MH, Juliano RL (2004) Selective transcription of p53 target genes by zinc finger-p53 DNA binding domain chimeras. Biochim Biophys Acta 1681:15–27

Fiegel HC, Gluer S, Roth B et al (2004) Stem-like cells in human hepatoblastoma. J Histochem Cytochem 52:1495–1501

Frasor J, Danes JM, Komm B et al (2003) Profiling of estrogen up- and down-regulated gene expression in human breast cancer cells: insights into gene networks and pathways underlying estrogenic control of proliferation and cell phenotype. Endocrinology 144:4562–4574

Fukahi K, Fukasawa M, Neufeld G et al (2004) Aberrant expression of neuropilin-1 and -2 in human pancreatic cancer cells. Clin Cancer Res 10:581–590

Ghabrial A, Ray RP, Schupbach T (1998) Okra and spindle-B encode components of the RAD52 DNA repair pathway and affect meiosis and patterning in Drosophila cogenesis. Genes Dev 12:2711–2723

Ginger MR, Rosen JM (2003) Pregnancy-induced changes in cell-fate in the mammary gland. Breast Cancer Res 5:192–197

Ginger MR, Gonzalez-Rimbau MF, Gay JP et al (2001) Persistent changes in gene expression induced by estrogen and progesterone in the rat mammary gland. Mol Endocrinol 15:1993–2009

Ginis I, Luo Y, Miura T, Thies S, Brandenberger R, Gerecht-Nir S et al (2004) Differences between human and mouse embryonic stems cells. Dev Biol 269:360–380

Goyal RK, Lin P, Kanungo J et al (1999) Ajuba, a novel LIM protein, interacts with Grb2, augments mitogen-activated protein kinase activity in fibroblasts, and promotes meiotic maturation of Xenopus oocytes in a Grb2- and Ras-dependent manner. Mol Cell Biol 19:4379–4389

Haeryfar SM, Hoskin DW (2004) Thy-1: more than a mouse pan-T cell marker. J Immunol 173:3581–3588

Harris BZ, Venkatasubrahmanyam S, Lim WA (2002) Coordinated folding and association of the LIN-2, -7 (L27) domain. An obligate heterodimerization involved in assembly of signaling and cell polarity complexes. J Biol Chem 277:34902–34908

Hayashi K, Goodison S, Urquidi V et al (2003) Differential effects of retinoic acid on the growth of isogenic metastatic and non-metastatic breast cancer cell lines and their association with distinct expression of retinoic acid receptor beta isoforms 2 and 4. Int J Oncol 22:623–629

Henderson BE, Powell D, Rosario I et al (1974) An epidemiologic study of breast cancer. J Natl Cancer Inst 53:609–614

Henderson BE, Ross RK, Pike MC (1993) Hormonal chemoprevention of cancer in women. Science 259:633–638

Henry MD, Triplett AA, Oh KB et al (2004) Parity-induced mammary epithelial cells facilitate tumorigenesis in MMTV-neu transgenic mice. Oncogene 23:6980–6985

Hoatlin ME, Zhi Y, Ball H et al (1999) A novel BTB/POZ transcriptional repressor protein interacts with the Fanconi anemia group C protein and PLZF. Blood 94:3737–3747

Ito K, Fetten J, Khalili H et al (1997) Oligoclonality of CD8+ T cells in breast cancer patients. Mol Med 3:836–851

Iwase H (2003) Molecular action of the estrogen receptor and hormone dependency in breast cancer. Breast Cancer 10:89–96

Jang CY, Lee JY, Kim J (2004) RpS3, a DNA repair endonuclease and ribosomal protein, is involved in apoptosis. FEBS Lett 560:81–85

Johnson JD, Zhang W, Rudnick A et al (1997) Transcriptional synergy between LIM-homeodomain proteins and basic helix-loop-helix proteins: the LIM2 domain determines specificity. Mol Cell Biol 17:3488–3496

Jones MH, Hamana N, Nezu J et al (2000) A novel family of bromodomain genes. Genomics 63:40–45

Kelsey JL, Gammon MD, John EM (1993) Reproductive factors and breast cancer. Epidemiol Rev 15:36–47

Kiguchi K, Giometti C, Chubb CH et al (1992) Differentiation induction in human breast tumor cells by okadaic acid and related inhibitors of protein phosphatases 1 and 2A. Biochem Biophys Res Commun 189:1261–1267

Kirii Y, Magarian-Blander J, Alter MD et al (1998) Functional and molecular analysis of T cell receptors used by pancreatic- and breast tumor- (mucin-) specific cytotoxic T cells. J Immunother 21:188–197

Komitova M, Eriksson PS (2004) Sox-2 is expressed by neural progenitors and astroglia in the adult rat brain. Neurosci Lett 369:24–27

Kondoh H, Uchikawa M, Kamachi Y (2004) Interplay of Pax6 and SOX2 in lens development as a paradigm of genetic switch mechanisms for cell differentiation. Int J Dev Biol 48:819–827

Koopman P, Schepers G, Brenner S et al (2004) Origin and diversity of the SOX transcription factor gene family: genome-wide analysis in Fugu rubripes. Gene 328:177–186

Korioth F, Gieffers C, Maul GG et al (1995) Molecular characterization of NDP52, a novel protein of the nuclear domain 10, which is redistributed upon virus infection and interferon treatment. J Cell Biol 130:1–13

Kwon HJ, Breese EH, Vig-Varga E et al (2004) Tumor necrosis factor alpha induction of NF-kappaB requires the novel coactivator SIMPL. Mol Cell Biol 24:9317–9326

Lambe M, Hsieh CC, Chan HW et al (1996) Parity, age at first and last birth, and risk of breast cancer: a population-based study in Sweden. Breast Cancer Res Treat 38: 305–311

Leasure CS, Chandler J, Gilbert DJ et al (2001) Sequence, chromosomal location and expression analysis of the murine homologue of human RAD51L2/RAD51C. Gene 271:59–67

Levine A, Bashan-Ahrend A, Budai-Hadrian O et al (1994) Odd Oz: a novel Drosophila pair rule gene. Cell 77:587–598

Li S, Qiu F, Xu A et al (2004) Barhl1 regulates migration and survival of cerebellar granule cells by controlling expression of the neurotrophin-3 gene. J Neurosci 24:3104–3114

Lim Y, Lee SM, Kim M et al (2002) Complete genomic structure of human rpS3: identification of functional U15b snoRNA in the fifth intron. Gene 286:291–297

Lyamouri M, Enerly E, Lambertsson A (2002) Organization, sequence, and phylogenetic analysis of the ribosomal protein S3 gene from Drosophila virilis. Gene 294:147–156

MacMahon B, Cole P, Lin TM et al (1970) Age at first birth and breast cancer risk. Bull World Health Organ 43:209–221

Medina D, Kittrell FS (2003) p53 function is required for hormone-mediated protection of mouse mammary tumorigenesis. Cancer Res 63:6140–6143

Medina D, Smith GH (1999) Chemical carcinogen-induced tumorigenesis in parous, involuted mouse mammary glands. J Natl Cancer Inst 91:967–969

Miller CT, Yelon D, Stainier DY et al (2003) Two endothelin 1 effectors, hand2 and bapx1, pattern ventral pharyngeal cartilage and the jaw joint. Development 130:1353–1365

Miyagi S, Saito T, Mizutani K et al (2004) The Sox-2 regulatory regions display their activities in two distinct types of multipotent stem cells. Mol Cell Biol 24:4207–4220

Morikawa Y, Cserjesi P (2004) Extra-embryonic vasculature development is regulated by the transcription factor HAND1. Development 131:2195–2204

Murakami M, Kataoka K, Fukuhara S et al (2004) Akt-dependent phosphorylation negatively regulates the transcriptional activity of dHAND by inhibiting the DNA binding activity. Eur J Biochem 271:3330–3339

Nukaya I, Yasumoto M, Iwasaki T et al (1999) Identification of HLA-A24 epitope peptides of carcinoembryonic antigen which induce tumor-reactive cytotoxic T lymphocyte. Int J Cancer 80:92–97

Ohira M, Seki N, Nagase T et al (1998) Characterization of a human homolog (BACH1) of the mouse Bach1 gene encoding a BTB-basic leucine zipper transcription factor and its mapping to chromosome 21q22.1. Genomics 47:300–306

Osakabe K, Yoshioka T, Ichikawa H, Toki S (2002) Molecular cloning and characterization of RAD51-like genes from Arabidopsis thaliana. Plant Mol Biol Sep 50:71–81

Osaki E, Nishina Y, Inazawa J et al (1999) Identification of a novel Sry-related gene and its germ cell-specific expression. Nucleic Acids Res 27:2503–2510

Pai CY, Lei EP, Ghosh D et al (2004) The centrosomal protein CP190 is a component of the gypsy chromatin insulator. Mol Cell 16:737–748

Parnell TJ, Viering MM, Skjesol A et al (2003) An endogenous suppressor of hairy-wing insulator separates regulatory domains in Drosophila. Proc Natl Acad Sci U S A 100:13436–13441

Passegue E, Wagner EF, Weissman IL (2004) JunB deficiency leads to a myeloproliferative disorder arising from hematopoietic stem cells. Cell 119:431–443

Pei Y, Sherry DM, McDermott AM (2004) Thy-1 distinguishes human corneal fibroblasts and myofibroblasts from keratocytes. Exp Eye Res 79:705–712

Qin Q, Patil K, Sharma SC (2004) The role of Bax-inhibiting peptide in retinal ganglion cell apoptosis after optic nerve transection. Neurosci Lett 372:17–21

Recht J, Dunn B, Raff A et al (1996) Functional analysis of histones H2A and H2B in transcriptional repression in Saccharomyces cerevisiae. Mol Cell Biol 16:2545–2553

Russell MW, Kemp P, Wang L et al (1998) Molecular cloning of the human HAND2 gene. Biochim Biophys Acta 1443:393–399

Russo IH, Russo J (1994) Role of hCg and inhibition in breast cancer. International J Oncol 4:297–306

Russo IH, Medado J, Russo J (1989) Endocrine influences on mammary structure and development. In: Jones TC, Mohr U, Hunt RD 5eds) Integument and mammary gland laboratory animals. Springer-Verlag, Berlin Heidelberg New York, pp 252–266

Russo IH, Koszalka M, Russo J (1991) Comparative study of the influence of pregnancy and hormonal treatment on mammary carcinogenesis. Br J Cancer 64:481–484

Russo J, Russo IH (1980) Influence of differentiation and cell kinetics on the susceptibility of the rat mammary gland to carcinogenesis. Cancer Res 40:2677–2687

Russo J, Russo IH (1987a) Development of human mammary gland. In: Nevill MC, Daniel CW (eds) The mammary gland development, regulation, and function. Plenum, New York, pp 67–93

Russo J, Russo IH (1987b) Role of differentiation on transformation of human epithelial cells. In: Medina D (ed) Cellular and molecular biology of mammary cancer. Plenum, New York, pp 399–417

Russo J, Russo IH (1994) Toward a physiological approach to breast cancer prevention. Cancer Epidemiol Biomarkers Prev 3:353–364

Russo J, Russo IH (1997) Role of differentiation in the pathogenesis and prevention of breast cancer. Endocr Relat Cancer 4:1–15

Russo J, Russo IH (1998) Development of the human breast. In: Knobil E, Neill JD (eds) Encyclopedia of reproduction, Vol. 3. Academic, New York, pp 71–80

Russo J, Russo IH (1999) Cellular basis of breast cancer susceptibility. Oncol Res 11:169–178

Russo J, Russo IH (2004) Biological and molecular basis of breast cancer. Springer, Berlin Heidelberg New York

Russo J, Reina D, Frederick J et al (1988) Expression of phenotypical changes by human breast epithelial cells treated with carcinogens in vitro. Cancer Res 48:2837–2857

Russo J, Mills MJ, Moussalli MJ et al (1989) Influence of human breast development on the growth properties of primary cultures. In Vitro Cell Dev Biol 25:643–649

Russo J, Gusterson BA, Rogers AE et al (1990) Comparative study of human and rat mammary tumorigenesis. Lab Invest 62:244–278

Russo J, Rivera R, Russo IH (1992) Influence of age and parity on the development of the human breast. Breast Cancer Res Treat 23:211–218

Russo J, Calaf G, Russo IH (1993) A critical approach to the malignant transformation of human breast epithelial cells with chemical carcinogens. Crit Rev Oncog 4:403–417

Russo J, Romero AL, Russo IH (1994) Architectural pattern of the normal and cancerous breast under the influence of parity. Cancer Epidemiol Biomarkers Prev 3:219–224

Russo J, Ao X, Grill C et al (1999) Pattern of distribution of cells positive for estrogen receptor alpha and progesterone receptor in relation to proliferating cells in the mammary gland. Breast Cancer Res Treat 53:217–227

Russo J, Hu YF, Yang X et al (2000) Developmental, cellular, and molecular basis of human breast cancer. J Natl Cancer Inst Monogr 17–37

Russo J, Hu YF, Silva ID et al (2001a) Cancer risk related to mammary gland structure and development. Microsc Res Tech 52:204–223

Russo J, Lynch H, Russo IH (2001b) Mammary gland architecture as a determining factor in the susceptibility of the human breast to cancer. Breast J 7:278–291

Russo J, Moral R, Balogh GA, Mailo DA, Russo IH (2005) The protective role of pregnancy in breast cancer. Breast Cancer Res J 7:131–142

Salomon DS, Bianco C, Ebert AD et al (2000) The EGF-CFC family: novel epidermal growth factor-related proteins in development and cancer. Endocr Relat Cancer 7:199–226

Sancar A, Tang MS (1993) Nucleotide excision repair. Photochem Photobiol 57:905–921

Sanghavi SK, Shankarappa R, Reinhart TA (2004) Genetic analysis of Toll/Interleukin-1 Receptor (TIR) domain sequences from rhesus macaque Toll-like receptors (TLRs) 1–10 reveals high homology to human TLR/TIR sequences. Immunogenetics 56:667–674

Shen J, Samul R, Zimmer J et al (2004) Deficiency of neuropilin 2 suppresses VEGF-induced retinal neovascularization. Mol Med 10:12–18

Shen MM, Wang H, Leder P (1997) A differential display strategy identifies Cryptic, a novel EGF-related gene expressed in the axial and lateral mesoderm during mouse gastrulation. Development 124:429–442

Sinha DK, Pazik JE, Dao TL (1988) Prevention of mammary carcinogenesis in rats by pregnancy: effect of full-term and interrupted pregnancy. Br J Cancer 57:390–394

Sivaraman L, Medina D (2002) Hormone-induced protection against breast cancer. J Mammary Gland Biol Neoplasia 7:77–92

Srivastava P, Russo J, Russo IH (1997) Chorionic gonadotropin inhibits rat mammary carcinogenesis through activation of programmed cell death. Carcinogenesis 18:1799–1808

Srivastava P, Russo J, Russo IH (1999) Inhibition of rat mammary tumorigenesis by human chorionic gonadotropin associated with increased expression of inhibin. Mol Carcinog 26:10–19

Stevanovic M (2003) Modulation of SOX2 and SOX3 gene expression during differentiation of human neuronal precursor cell line NTERA2. Mol Biol Rep 30:127–132

Tay LK, Russo J (1981a) 7,12-dimethylbenz[a]anthracene-induced DNA binding and repair synthesis in susceptible and nonsusceptible mammary epithelial cells in culture. J Natl Cancer Inst 67:155–161

Tay LK, Russo J (1981b) Formation and removal of 7,12-dimethylbenz[a]anthracene–nucleic acid adducts in rat mammary epithelial cells with different susceptibility to carcinogenesis. Carcinogenesis 2:1327–1333

Thomachot MC, Bendriss-Vermare N, Massacrier C et al (2004) Breast carcinoma cells promote the differentiation of CD34+ progenitors towards 2 different subpopulations of dendritic cells with CD1a(high)CD86(-)Langerin- and CD1a(+)CD86(+)Langerin+ phenotypes. Int J Cancer 110:710–720

Thordarson G, Jin E, Guzman RC, Swanson SM, Nandi S, Tamalmantes F (1995) Refractoriness to mammary tumorigenesis in parous rats: it is caused by persistent changes in the hormonal environment or permanent biochemical alterations in the mammary epithelia? Carcinogenesis 16:2847–2853

Trapido EJ (1983) Age at first birth, parity, and breast cancer risk. Cancer 51:946–948

Trichopoulos D, Lagiou P, Adami HP (2005) Towards an integrated model for breast cancer etiology: the crucial role of the mammary tissue-specific stem cells. Breast Cancer Res 7:13–17

Troelstra C, van Gool A, de Wit J et al (1992) ERCC6, a member of a subfamily of putative helicases, is involved in Cockayne's syndrome and preferential repair of active genes. Cell 71:939–953

Tsuzuki T, Fujii Y, Sakumi K et al (1996) Targeted disruption of the Rad51 gene leads to lethality in embryonic mice. Proc Natl Acad Sci U S A 93:6236–6240

Vessey MP, McPherson K, Roberts MM et al (1985) Fertility in relation to the risk of breast cancer. Br J Cancer 52:625–628

Vig E, Green M, Liu Y et al (2001) SIMPL is a tumor necrosis factor-specific regulator of nuclear factor-kappaB activity. J Biol Chem 276:7859–7866

Vitale M, Pelusi G, Taroni B et al (2005) HLA class I antigen down-regulation in primary ovary carcinoma lesions: association with disease stage. Clin Cancer Res 11:67–72

Vorherr H (1974) The breast. New York, Academic

Wagner KU, Boulanger CA, Henry MD et al (2002) An adjunct mammary epithelial cell population in parous females: its role in functional adaptation and tissue renewal. Development 129:1377–1386

Watanabe Y, Toyoda R, Nakamura H (2004) Navigation of trochlear motor axons along the midbrain-hindbrain boundary by neuropilin 2. Development 131:681–692

Watts GS, Oshiro MM, Junk DJ et al (2004) The acetyl-transferase p300/CBP-associated factor is a p53 target gene in breast tumor cells. Neoplasia 6:187–194

Wei CC, Ho TW, Liang WG et al (2003) Cloning and characterization of mouse IL-22 binding protein. Genes Immun 4:204–211

Wellings SR, Jensen HM, Marcum RG (1975) An atlas of subgross pathology of the human breast with special reference to possible precancerous lesions. J Natl Cancer Inst 55:231–273

Wolk K, Kunz S, Witte E et al (2004) IL-22 increases the innate immunity of tissues. Immunity 21:241–254

Xu H, Firulli AB, Zhang X et al (2003) HAND2 synergistically enhances transcription of dopamine-beta-hydroxylase in the presence of Phox2a. Dev Biol 262:183–193

Yamaguchi Y, Narita T, Inukai N et al (2001) SPT genes: key players in the regulation of transcription, chromatin structure and other cellular processes. J Biochem (Tokyo) 129:185–191

Yamamoto M, Akira S (2004) TIR domain-containing adaptors regulate TLR-mediated signaling pathways]. Nippon Rinsho 62:2197–2203

Yang MY, Liu TC, Chang JG et al (2003) JunB gene expression is inactivated by methylation in chronic myeloid leukemia. Blood 101:3205–3211

Yuan L, Moyon D, Pardanaud L et al (2002) Abnormal lymphatic vessel development in neuropilin 2 mutant mice. Development 129:4797–4806

Zhou W, Liu G, Miller DP et al (2002) Gene-environment interaction for the ERCC2 polymorphisms and cumulative cigarette smoking exposure in lung cancer. Cancer Res 62:1377–1381

Zhou Y, Hagood JS, Murphy-Ullrich JE (2004) Thy-1 expression regulates the ability of rat lung fibroblasts to activate transforming growth factor-beta in response to fibrogenic stimuli. Am J Pathol 165:659–669

13 Estrogen Deprivation for Breast Cancer Prevention

Anthony Howell, Robert B. Clarke, Gareth Evans,
Nigel Bundred, Jack Cuzick, Richard Santen, Craig Allred

Recent Results in Cancer Research, Vol. 174
© Springer-Verlag Berlin Heidelberg 2007

Abstract

Estrogen deprivation (ED) either as a result of
a natural or artificial menopause or the use of
aromatase inhibitors in postmenopausal women
results in a reduction of the incidence of breast
cancer. Two major clinical trials of this approach
comparing anastrozole or exemestane with placebo are currently in progress to test their efficacy for prevention. Reduction of contralateral
breast lesions by at least 50% compared with
tamoxifen indicate this approach has promise.
The target lesion within the breast for ED is not
known but we argue that hyperplastic enlarged
lobular units (HELUs) as well as more advanced
lesions are good candidates. A major problem for
ED is de novo or acquired resistance to its effectiveness. We discuss potential mechanisms of resistance including high concentrations of tissue
estrogens, increase in growth factor, and signal
transduction pathways within the epithelial cell
and activation of paracrine pathways from breast
adipocytes, macrophages and fibroblasts. It may
be possible to increase effectiveness of ED by additional preventive agents or by lifestyle alterations.

Introduction

The importance of estrogen and one of its major receptors, estrogen receptor alpha (ERα),
on growth and development of the breast and
on tumour formation are well known (Key and
Pike 1988). In the absence of estrogen or ERα
(Boccinfuso and Korach 1997) the breast develops only minimally whilst excess estrogen or
increased expression or activation of ERα leads
to mammary epithelial cell proliferation and the
later development of premalignant and malignant lesions (Howell 1989). The importance of
estrogen is also apparent in animal models. For
example, transgenic mice with deregulated ERα
develop ductal hyperplasia, lobular hyperplasia
and ductal carcinoma in-situ (DCIS). Lesions
were not increased by estradiol administration,
indicating that receptor deregulation alone can
cause malignancy (Frech et al. 2005). In another
study, estrogen concentrations in the breast were
increased in aromatase enzyme transgenic mice,
leading to hyperplastic and dysplastic changes.
These were shown to be mediated by ERα since
no lesions developed in aromatase transgenic/
ERα knockout mice (Tekmal et al. 2005).

The majority of human breast cancers express
ERα (~70%) and a large proportion of these are
dependent upon estrogen since blocking estrogen binding to the receptor with agents such as
tamoxifen or reducing estrogen concentrations
(estrogen deprivation [ED]) by ovarian suppression or treatment with aromatase inhibitors results in tumour regression or stabilisation. ERα
blockade and ED are not only important for
breast cancer treatment but also for prevention
of the disease. Tamoxifen and raloxifene have
been the major approaches to prevention to date,
reducing the risk of ERα + ve breast cancers by
40% or more (Cuzick et al. 2003; Martino et al.
2004). However, there has been comparatively
little emphasis on ED as a method of breast cancer prevention. ED occurs naturally at the menopause, its effect may be enhanced by an early

menopause, either natural or artificial, and there is indirect evidence that further reduction of serum estradiol by modern aromatase inhibitors is effective (Cuzick 2005). Here we summarise data concerning the preventative effectiveness of the natural and early menopause and the use of AIs. It is also important for the future development of ED as a preventive strategy to define the target lesions in the breast which are prevented from progressing. Furthermore, we need to understand the mechanism of resistance to ED and how resistance may be prevented by additional therapeutic approaches.

The Effects of Estrogen Deprivation on Mammary Tumour Development

Estrogen deprivation occurs naturally at the menopause because of the cessation of ovarian function. This results in a reduction in the rate of increase of the incidence of breast cancer, producing an inflection on the age-incidence curve. In the absence of the menopause, we assume the age-incidence curve would continue to be log-linear, as it is in male breast cancer (Thomas 1993; Pike et al. 1983). Thus, the ED of the menopause reduces breast cancer risk, but this varies according to country (Fig. 1a). In the example shown, the approximate reductions in risk for a 65-year-old with a menopause at age 50 is 20% for a woman in Connecticut, 50% in Finland and 60% in a Japanese woman. Thus, the menopause is less preventive in the USA. We will explore the potential reasons for this resistance to ED later in this article.

An early menopause, whether natural or artificial, results in greater reductions in risk. Epidemiological studies indicate that a menopause between ages 35 and 45 is associated with an approximate risk reductions of 50%–80% compared with a natural menopause at age 50 (Hirayama and Wynder 1962; Feinleib 1968; Trichopoulos et al. 1972). Several studies have also indicated similar reductions in risk after oophorectomy to prevent ovarian cancer in women with germ line mutations in the breast cancer-associated genes *BRCA1* and *BRCA2* (Eisen et al. 2005 and references therein). Pike et al. (1997) estimated the reduction in risk of ovarian suppression at various

ages in nulliparous Californian women (Fig. 1b). For a woman aged 65, ovarian suppression at 40 was calculated to reduce risk by 40% compared with a natural menopause at age 50 and by 85% if ovarian suppression was initiated at age 30. Thus, the menopause itself reduces risk and there are additional decreases in risk if the menopause occurs early, either naturally or artificially.

In postmenopausal women, adrenal androgens are converted to estrogens by the enzyme aromatase, present in many tissues including the stroma and epithelium of the breast. Modern inhibitors of aromatase (AIs anastrozole, letrozole and exemestane) reduce postmenopausal estrogen levels in serum from 20–30 pM to around 1 pM – the limit of detection for sophisticated estradiol assays (Wang et al. 2005). In postmenopausal women, tissue estrogen concentrations may be much higher than in serum and there is evidence that these are markedly reduced by AIs. In studies conducted by Geisler (2003) in a group of 12 postmenopausal women, tumour estradiol concentrations were a mean of 217.9 fmol/g before and a mean of 18.4 fmol/g after 3 months of anastrozole. The concomitant change in plasma concentrations was from a mean of 24.2 pmol/l to 2.6 pmol/l.

Two trials (IBIS II: anastrozole vs placebo and MAP-3: exemestane vs placebo) are assessing the value of AIs for prevention for women at increased risk of breast cancer. Both are in the early phases of recruitment and thus we will not have randomised data on the effectiveness of AIs for primary prevention for some time. However, there have been multiple reported adjuvant trials which compare tamoxifen with an AI. In these, the AI used reduced contralateral breast cancer by approximately 50% compared with tamoxifen (Fig. 1c; Cuzick 2005). Since tamoxifen already reduces contralateral risk by 50%, these data suggest that AIs may reduce contralateral cancer risk by approximately 75%. This figure will be lower in a population of women not selected to have ERα+ve tumours (as is the case for adjuvant therapy), but the potential for AIs to reduce primary breast cancer by 60% or so is probable.

Thus, ED is a preventive strategy for breast cancer, the effectiveness of which varies according to age of withdrawal, extent of estrogen depletion and possibly country. The natural meno-

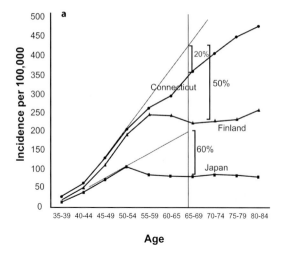

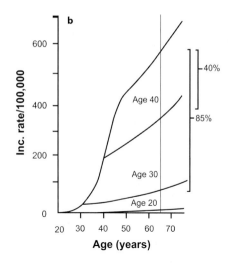

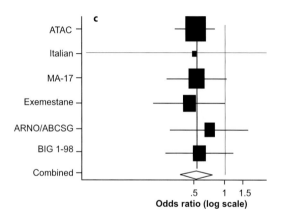

Fig. 1a–c Magnitude of the effects of estrogen withdrawal at the menopause by an early menopause and by aromatase inhibitors. **a** Menopause. Inflection of the age-incidence curve known as Clemmesen's hook. Assuming the age-incidence curve is linear in the absence of a menopause, the reduction of breast cancer depends on the country of residence. **b** Estimates by Pike et al. (1997) of the effects of a menopause at 40, 30 and 20 years in nulliparous California women. **c** Reduction of contralateral breast cancer in adjuvant trials of aromatase inhibitors (AIs) versus tamoxifen. The reduction by AIs is approximately 50% greater than tamoxifen (Cuzick 2005)

pause may reduce risk by 20%–60% compared with continuing menses, a menopause at age 40 may reduce risk by 50%–80% compared with a menopause at the age 50 and in postmenopausal women AIs may reduce risk by an estimated 60%. It is clear that ED is only partially successful for breast cancer prevention. It has no apparent effect on preventing ER-ve cancers, which may reflect escape of ER+ve lesions from estrogen dependence or it may be because they have a very different carcinogenic pathway. There is a need to improve the proportion of cancers prevented and we believe this will come from a better understanding of the target lesions for prevention within the breast and of the mechanisms of resistance to ED.

Targets for Estrogen Deprivation Within the Breast

Normal breast epithelium grows in response to estrogen during puberty and pregnancy and undergoes waves of proliferation and apoptosis during the menstrual cycle. Breast cancer arises from the epithelium or epithelial stem or precursor cells and there is general consensus that the site of origin is within the terminal duct lobular unit (TDLU). The question arises whether ED is effective because it results in quiescence of normal breast and prevents new lesions arising or does it act on pre-existing premalignant lesions within the breast or perhaps both? This question is not only of academic importance since if ED acts on pre-existing lesions it should be possible to predict the type of breast most appropriate for preventive approaches (mammographic density is an example) or even to detect early lesions by radiological or other imaging techniques.

Normal Breast Epithelium

Available evidence suggests that the normal breast is highly responsive to ED and shuts down proliferative activity within lobules. In premenopausal women, this phenomenon is exemplified by a marked decline in epithelial proliferation during the ED of the follicular phase of the menstrual cycle (Fig. 2a; Potten et al. 1988). The proliferative response of the breast declines before the menopause (Fig. 2a) and there is low proliferation in postmenopausal lobules (Fig. 2d). Low proliferative activity in postmenopausal lobules is surprising since many authors have demonstrated that the concentrations of estradiol and precursor steroids are similar in normal postmenopausal breast tissue and nipple aspirate fluid to the con-

centrations seen in tissue or fluid in premenopausal women (Blankenstein et al. 1992; Bonney et al. 1983; Chatterton et al. 2004; Pasqualini et al. 1996; Geisler 2003), although they are not as high as E_2 concentrations found in tumours. The requirement of the normal epithelium of the breast for relatively high concentrations of estradiol for proliferation are shown in the experimental result shown in Fig. 2b and c. Normal human epithelium obtained by biopsy was transplanted into immune deprived mice. Proliferation declined in the low estrogen environment of the mice. Estradiol pellets were implanted subcutaneously to give human follicular or luteal estradiol concentrations in the mice. Proliferation in the epithelium of the explants was measured by tritiated thymidine incorporation and progesterone receptor (PR) by immunochemistry. High follicular concentrations of estradiol (440 pml/l) only partially stimulated proliferation but maximally induced PR, indicating that cell cycle genes were more resistant to the inductive effects of estradiol than the PR (Clarke et al. 1997a; Fig. 2b, c).

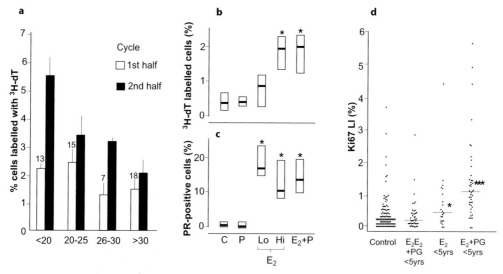

Fig. 2a–c Cell proliferation of normal human breast tissue. **a** Mean thymidine labelling index in the follicular and luteal phase of the menstrual cycle and the effect of age. **b** Differential effects of estradiol on proliferation and % cells +ve for progesterone receptor of normal human breast tissue transplanted into nude mice treated with estrogen pellets to give serum concentrations in the mouse equivalent to the follicular phase (*Lo*) and luteal (*Hi*) phase of the menstrual cycle. Follicular-phase estradiol only partially stimulates proliferation, whereas this is sufficient for maximal progesterone receptor stimulation. **c** Ki67 labelling of normal human epithelial breast tissue removed from postmenopausal women on no treatment and women treated with ERT or HRT for less than or more than 5 years * p < 0,05 *** p < 0,001

Some of the E_2 concentrations cited for normal breast tissue are equivalent to low-follicular-phase serum concentrations found in premenopausal women. Thus, in postmenopausal women, although tissue E_2 is high compared with plasma it may not be sufficiently high to stimulate proliferation. The relative resistance of the postmenopausal breast is indicated by breast biopsy data which show that estrogen replacement therapy does not appreciably affect the labelling index of postmenopausal breast epithelial cells even when given for more than 5 years (Fig. 2d; Dobson et al. 2000). In agreement with other groups, we find a small increase in proliferation when women are on combined estrogen and progestogen preparations (Hofseth et al. 1999). It is of interest that no histological differences could be detected between breasts from women taking and not taking HRT in a double-blind study, although differences have been reported in non-blinded studies (Hofseth et al. 1999; Fechner 1972) and increases in epithelial area were reported by Hofseth et al. (1999). The data summarised above indicate the normal breast lobule responds to ED by largely switching off proliferation and in the presence of ERT, PR is increased (Dobson et al. 2000; Hofseth et al. 1992) and there is also some increase in proliferation and possible histological change with prolonged use of HRT. Thus, we assume that the capacity to grow in the relatively low tissue estrogen environment of the menopause must occur within other epithelial structures of the breast.

Abnormal Breast Epithelium

A variety of abnormal epithelial structures have been described by pathologists. Perhaps one of the most thorough studies in this regard was performed by Wellings and his colleagues (Wellings et al. 1975; Wellings 1980). They sliced whole breasts either taken from women at autopsy with no history of breast malignancy or breasts containing a cancer or the breast contralateral to a cancer, both breasts being obtained at mastectomy. Whole breasts were cut into 2- to 3-mm sections and all observable lesions removed for histology. Wellings likened the list of abnormalities to the pathological equivalent of a differential

blood count (Table 1). One of the most common lesions found, particularly in the cancer associated and contralateral breasts, were lobule-like lesions which were greatly enlarged compared with a normal TDLU (Fig. 3). These were called atypical lobules type A (ALA) if the epithelial cells resembled those seen in ducts and ALB if the cells resembled those seen in the lobule. Wellings indicated that the range of epithelial atypia within ALA was from near normal (ALA type 1) to that approaching a diagnosis of DCIS (ALA type IV). ALA were found throughout the breast and because they showed a range of histological changes up to DCIS, Wellings considered ALA/B the precursors of cancer. In postmortem breasts, there were approximately 25–40 ALA per breast in young women, but these numbers declined markedly after the menopause (Fig. 4). Cancer-containing and contralateral breasts contained high numbers of ALA after the meno-

Table 1 The differential count of total lesions detected in breasts from controls at autopsy and cancer-containing and contralateral breasts. This study indicates the importance of the atypical lobule type A as showing a major difference between the two groups of breast (Wellings et al. 1975)

	Autopsy (183)	Cancer-associated (107)
Fibroadenoma	0.39	1.11
Persistent lobule	5.78	14.30
Large lobule	2.12	10.39
Hypersecretory lobule	1.87	1.39
Hyperplastic terminal duct	0.10	1.83
Atypical lobules type A	10.43	44.51
Atypical lobules type B	0.03	0.82
DCIS	0.08	5.45
LCIS	0.00	0.76
Hyperplastic duct	0.13	0.64
Duct papilloma	0.22	1.71
Sclerosing adenosis	1.85	1.83
Epithelial cyst	0.86	1.44
Stromal cyst	0.08	0.25
Apocrine cyst	4.50	14.96

Table 2 Characteristics of hyperplastic enlarged lobular units (HELU) according to the age they were removed from the breast (Lee et al. 2005)

	<50	50+	P
Estrogen receptor (% cells+ve)*			
TDLU	20	50	<0.001
HELU	70	90	0.13
Ki 67 (% cells+ve)			
TDLU	2.5	1.4	<0.036
HELU	6.5	4.1	<0.017
TUNEL (% cells+ve)			
TDLU	0.8	0.43	<0.001
HELU	0.23	0.19	0.41

N=324

* Average proportion occure representing one average proportion of positive cells (0 = none, 1 < 1/100, 2 = 1/100 to 1/10, 3 = 1/10 – 1/3, 4 = 1/3 – 2/3, and 5 ≥ 2/3)

pause and they were more likely to be associated with marked atypia (Fig. 4). The smaller normal TDLU rarely contained atypia again, suggesting that ALA/B were the origin of cancer.

Recently, Lee et al. (2005b) examined enlarged lobules derived from 324 breasts. They called these hyperplastic enlarged lobular units (HELU, Fig. 3) and examined the structures for expression of ERα, PR, proliferation (Ki 67) and apoptosis (Tunel, Table 2). The majority of cells in HELU were ERα + ve in contradistinction to normal TDLU. ERα+ve cells in normal TDLU increased from 20% before age 50 to 50% after age 50 (as expected), but in HELU 70% of cells on average were + ve for ERα in women under 50 and 90% in women over 50. Proliferation was higher in HELU, even after age 50 with a mean Ki 67 at 4.1%, and there was also a decline in apoptosis in HELU compared with TDLU. These data are important since they indicate that HELU are able

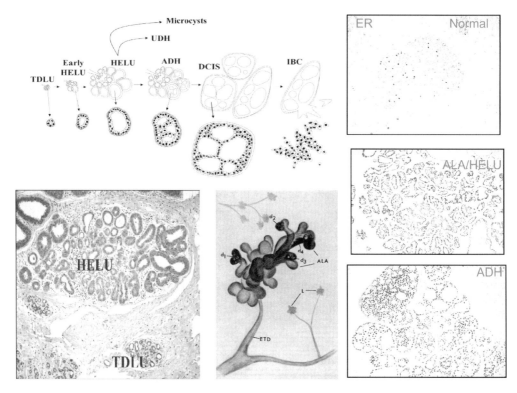

Fig. 3a–d Atypical lobules A (ALA)/hyperplastic enlarged lobular units (HELU). **a** Evolution of TDLU through HELU to invasive carcinoma. **b** Histological cross sections of a HELU and TDLU to indicate differences in size between the two types of structure. **c** Diagrams of ALA described by Wellings et al. (1975). **d** Estrogen receptor immunostaining to illustrate increase in the number of cells +ve between a normal TDLU (*upper box*), HELU (*middle box*) and ADH (*lower box*)

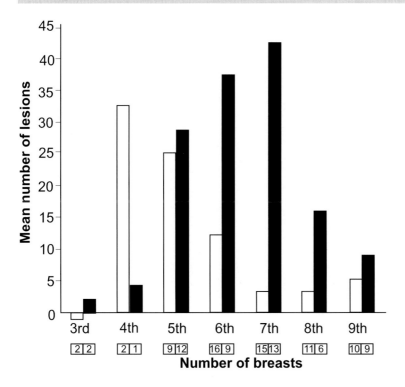

Fig. 4 Atypical lobules type A (ALA) in autopsy breasts and those containing or contralateral to a tumour. ALA in autopsy breasts contain fewer high-grade lesions and the numbers of ALA decline with age. In contradistinction, ALA from tumour or contralateral breasts are more likely to contain high-grade ALA and do not decline immediately after the menopause (Wellings et al. 1975)

to continue proliferating in the postmenopausal estrogen environment, which may be why such lesions are associated with DCIS and invasive malignancy.

Resistance to Estrogen Deprivation

Resistance Associated with Lifestyle Change?

Although ED at the menopause or associated with early menopause or treatment with AIs reduces the incidence of breast cancer, it is clear that only a proportion of tumours are prevented (Fig. 1). The protective effect of the menopause appears to be declining in many parts of the world, particularly in the West. Reduction is exemplified by data from the United States collected as part of the SEER programme. Figure 5a shows the age incident curves for breast cancer for the period 1973–1977 compared with those

from 1993–1995 for whites, blacks and other races (Karagas et al. 2000). Irrespective of ethnic group, there was a reduction in the angle of the age incidence curve at the menopause in the latter time period, indicating an increase in the numbers of postmenopausal breast cancers. This change may, in part, be related to differences in methods of cancer detection, but increases in postmenopausal breast cancer are also seen in non-screened populations. Yasui and Potter (1999) investigated the age incidence curves of receptor subtypes within a Danish series of cancers. They demonstrated that the proportion of ERα+PR+ tumours increased with age, whereas other phenotypes (ER+PR–, ER–PR+ and ER–PR–) either remained stable after the menopause or declined in relative number. The increase of ER+PR+ tumours with age is also seen in the Nurses Health Study. Thus, the major increase in breast cancer after the menopause is in the ER+PR+ phenotypes, which is more likely to

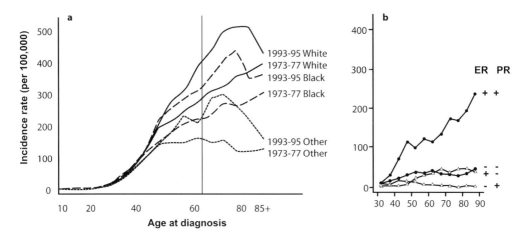

Fig. 5 **a** Age incidence curves from SEER in the United States for the period between 1973and 1977 compared with the period 1993–1995 for whites, blacks and other groups. The protective effect of the menopause appears to be declining with time (Karagas et al. 2000). **b** Receptor phenotype by age in the Nurses Health Study. *Black bar* ER+PR+, *crosshatched* ER+PR–, *empty* ER–PR– and *ticked* ER–PR–

respond to the endocrine environment after the menopause than the other three subtypes and may be the reason they are more common.

Several authors have investigated risk factors for breast cancer according to receptor phenotype. Many of the studies were small but the majority (*n*=31) were recently subjected to an overview analysis (Althuis et al. 2004). Reproductive factors such as late first birth and nulliparity were associated with ERα+ve rather than Era–ve tumours and early menarche was more consistently associated with ER+PR+ than ER–PR– tumours. Postmenopausal obesity was also more consistently associated with hormone receptor-positive tumours. There was no consistent association with oral contraceptive and hormone replacement therapy nor breast feeding, alcohol consumption, cigarette smoking, family history of breast cancer or premenopausal obesity. This important overview together with data indicating increasing ERα+PR+ tumours after the menopause suggests that changing reproductive factors and greater obesity may be responsible for the increases in postmenopausal breast cancer.

Changes in lifestyle have certainly occurred over the past 50 years, which could result in reduction in the effectiveness of natural ED and indicates a greater role for therapeutic intervention. These include changes in weight and physical activity and changes in reproductive habits.

For example, the incidence of obesity has undoubtedly increased during this time period as well as the reduction in physical activity. Obesity and lack of physical activity are associated with increases in plasma estradiol, which could affect proliferation of precursor lesions (Rinaldi et al. 2005; McTiernan et al. 2004). Changes in reproductive factors have been rapid in some populations. For example, in the Singapore Chinese the proportion of women having their first child at age 30–34 years increased from 19% in 1967 to 67% in 1989 (Chia et al. 2005).

Potential Cellular Mechanisms of Resistance to Estrogen Deprivation

Compared with normal TDLU, ERα+ve HELU, ADH, DCIS and invasive tumours have, on average, larger numbers of ER+ve cells and the question arises whether this alone might account for resistance to ED. However, other changes occur in premalignant and malignant ER+ve cells which also might account for resistance. Evidence from experiments on human TDLU (Clarke et al. 1997b) and in other species (Russo et al. 1999; Mallepell 2006) indicates that ERα+ve cells rarely divide but, in some way, signal to ER–ve cells to do so. A separation between sensor and effector cells has also been reported for

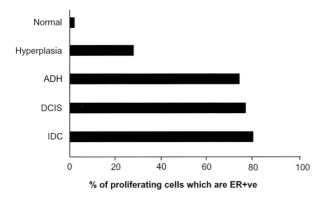

Normal
Hyperplasia
ADH
DCIS
IDC

0   20   40   60   80   100

% of proliferating cells which are ER+ve

Fig. 6 The proportions of proliferating cells in the normal breast and premalignant and malignant lesions which are proliferating. In normal TDLUs, few ERα+ve cells divide, whereas the majority of proliferating cells are ERα+ve in malignancy. Hyperplasia intermediate between normal and ADH/DCIS

prolactin receptor and PR (Brisken et al. 1998, 1999) and may be a protective mechanism to prevent uncontrolled proliferation. Other protective mechanisms reported in the rodent gland implicate transforming growth factor β (TGFβ) as a factor limiting ERα+ve cell proliferation (Ewan et al. 2005) and the need for ERα+ve regulated epithelial proliferation to have permissive signals to the stroma via production of amphiregulin which stimulates fibroblast EGFR and production of stromal growth factors (Wiesen et al. 1999; Luetteke et al. 1999). There is also evidence that ER+ve cells acquire the ability to proliferate in human premalignant and malignant lesions, which may be a mechanism whereby the ERα+ve cell can adapt and grow in a relatively low estrogen environment (Shoker et al. 1999; Clarke et al. 1997b). This may be because of the induction of amphiregulin since this important growth factor is increased in the estrogen stimulated normal human mammary gland and in HELU (Wilson et al. 2006; Lee et al. 2005b) On average, HELU were reported to have 27% of ERα+ve cells which were dividing (<5% in normal TDLU), and we have shown that hyperplasia of usual type ADH, DCIS and invasive cancer have increased numbers of these cells (Shoker et al. 2000, 1999; Lee et al. 2005a). It is of interest that treatment of the rodent mammary gland with the carcinogen MNU increases the numbers of ER+ve dividing cells (Sivaraman et al. 2001).

Another potential mechanism for resistance to ED is expansion of a resistant stem cell population within premalignant breast lesions. We have demonstrated that ERα+ve cells have some features of stem or precursor cells (Clarke et al. 2005) and cells which retain DNA radiolabel for long periods (a feature of stem cells) are ERα+ve (Clarke et al. 2005; Zeps et al. 1996). In normal tissue, homeostasis ERα+ve putative stem cells rarely divide, accounting for less than 4% of proliferating cells. However, a rare ERα+ve stem cell division event may be asymmetric, i.e. one daughter cell replacing the ERα+ve stem cell while the other daughter cell is a ERα-ve transit amplifying cell stimulated to further divide by the paracrine signals (discussed above) from the ERα+ve cells. Asymmetric cell division is often regulated by the Delta-Notch signalling pathway in development (Okano et al. 2005). We found that the ERα+ve putative stem cells expressed Musashi, a protein predicted to switch on the Notch signal only in the ERα+ve putative stem cell and not in the ERα-ve transit amplifying daughter cell (Clarke et al. 2003). In ERα+ve breast cancers, where the ERα+ve are highly proliferative, the Notch signalling pathway is highly activated, suggesting that the ERα+ve cells in cancers are symmetrically dividing and giving rise to two ERα+ve daughter cells (Clarke et al. 2003; Stylianou et al. 2006). We speculate that this may be an early event that occurs in HELU and causes expansion of the ERα+ve cell population via a signalling pathway that may be ED-resistant.

Thus, cellular mechanisms of resistance to ED may include changes in the proliferation status of the ERα+ve cells and its putative stem cell characteristics however. There is no doubt that most ERα+ve tumours in postmenopausal women are responding to the prevailing estradiol concentration since treatment with AIs preoperatively and preoperative withdrawal of HRT reduces cell proliferation within most ER+ve tumours (Dowsett et al. 2006; Prasad et al. 2003).

Molecular Changes in Response to Estrogen Deprivation

MCF-7 cells are a well-described breast cancer cell-line derived from a patient with a malignant pleural effusion. The cell line is ERα+ve and the ERα+ve cells are capable of dividing and thus experiments on this line may be seen as potentially modelling what happens in tumours and possibly premalignant lesions. In an important experiment, Masamura et al. (1994) showed that MCF-7 cells were able to adapt to a change in estrogen concentration. Wild type MCF-7 cells proliferate maximally at physiological concentrations of estradiol (about 10^{-9} M). When estrogen was removed from the medium, the cells ceased to divide for 3 months or so but then began to grow again (Fig. 7). A repeat of the estradiol dose response curve at this time indicated that the cells were growing in response to minute amounts of estrogen in the medium and proliferated maximally at 10^{-13} M concentrations (Fig. 7). These experiments were repeated by Martin et al. (2003) with similar results. Both groups have found that the MCF-7 cells respond to reduced estrogen by increasing nuclear ERα concentration and activity, activation of membrane ER alpha and

increased activity of growth factor receptors and activation of the PI3Kinase and MAPKinase signal transduction pathways (Martin et al. 2003; Santen et al. 2004, 2005). Sabnis et al. (2005) also showed increased growth factor receptor and signal transduction factor activity in their MCF-7 cells transfected with the gene for the aromatase enzyme and grown in estrogen-depleted conditions, but these cells were not sensitive to low estrogen. Other potential molecular mechanisms of increased cell sensitivity to estradiol include a reduction in NOD1 (da Silva Correia et al. 2006) and loss of nuclear PELP1 (Vadlamudi et al. 2005; Gururaj et al. 2006). Thus, it is possible that precursor lesions in the breast become sensitive to lower concentrations of estradiol, as demonstrated in tumour lines, although at present there is no experimental evidence for this phenomenon in this situation.

Other Potential Mechanisms of Resistance

The mechanisms of resistance outlined above involve an increase in the number of ER+ve cells, an increase in ER concentration and activation potentially at relatively low E_2 concentrations

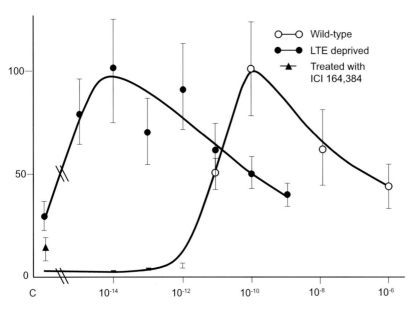

Fig. 7 Dose response curves for wild type MCF-7 compared with cells which were deprived of estrogen. *LTED* long-term estrogen-deprived cells (Masamura et al. 1994)

through signal transduction pathways within the cell. However, there is evidence that the ER may be activated by paracrine pathways from other cells in the breast including adipocytes, immune cells exemplified by macrophages and fibroblasts (Fig. 8). These cell types secrete adipokines, cytokines and growth factors which bind to cell surface receptors, and most have been reported to activate ER by various signal transduction pathways. Because of the difficulty of experiments involving premalignant lesions, most have been performed on ER+ve mammary tumour cell lines or primary tumours. Adipocytes secrete a large number of signalling molecules in response to the metabolic state of the body (Rajala and Scherer 2003). Supernatants from adipocytes or co-cultures with adipocytes stimulates mammary tumour cell line growth in-vitro (Iyengar et al. 2003, 2005; Manabe et al. 2003; Chamras et al. 1998). An important adipokine from the viewpoint of breast cancer is the polypeptide leptin which is secreted in response to increasing weight. Several studies have shown that leptin stimulates the growth of mammary tumours via its cell surface receptor, OB-Rb, and receptor-deficient mice do not develop oncogene-induced mammary tumours (Hu et al. 2002; Dieudonne et al. 2002; Cleary et al. 2004).

There is evidence that the ER is activated via the STAT and MAP kinase pathways by leptin (Yin et al. 2004; Catalano et al. 2004) and leptin stimulation can cause resistance to the pure antiestrogen fulvestrant (Garofalo et al. 2004). Leptin also alters the intracellular concentration of the energy-sensing enzyme complex AMP-activated protein kinase (AMPK). In energy-restricted states, AMPK increases in concentration and switches off cell growth via inhibition of the AKT/MTOR pathway (Hardie 2005). However, the opposite occurs in energy-replete states and is a potential mechanism whereby obesity may activate ER and mammary cell growth. Macrophages are found in tumours, premalignant lesions and the normal breast. They may be recruited, in part, because mammary epithelia secrete colony-stimulating factor. It is of interest that the breast does not develop in the absence of CSF and inhibition of CSF can cause tumour regression in experimental models (Lin et al. 2002; Aharinejad et al. 2004). Co-cultures of mammary tumour cells with macrophages stimulate growth via production of a variety of cytokines including tumour necrosis factor alpha (TNFα) (Hagemann et al. 2004). Cytokines via their epithelial cell surface receptors activate the transcription factor NFKβ which, in turn, can activate ER

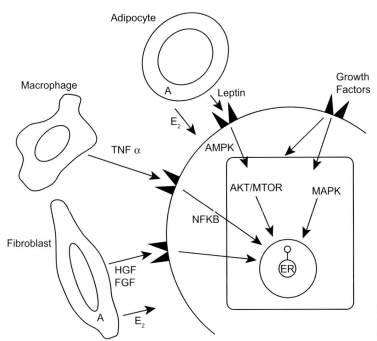

Fig. 8 Simplified view of potential pathways for activation of ERα. *A* aromatase

and stimulate growth and antiestrogen resistance (Hagemann et al. 2005; Rubio et al. 2006; Zhou et al. 2005; Biswas et al. 2005). Inhibition of NFKβ with the polyphenol parathenolide is reported to reverse resistance to antiestrogens (Riggins et al. 2005; de Graffenried et al. 2004). The NFKβ system is a potent tumour survival pathway in response to cytokine stimulation. Since estrogen is immunosuppressive through this pathway, ED alone may activate it. In chronic immunostimulated states such as rheumatoid arthritis, estrogen analogues with immunosuppressive but no growth factor activity are being developed (Keith et al. 2005).

Fibroblasts produce several growth factors capable of stimulating epithelial cell growth, some of which can be shown to activate the ER, including fibroblast growth factors (FGF) (McLeskey et al. 1998; Thottassery et al. 2004) and hepatocyte growth factor (HGF) (Rayala et al. 2006; Zhang et al. 2002). Numerous experiments concerning fibroblast epithelial interactions are summarised in recent reviews of Barcellos-Hoff and Medina (2005) and Haslam and Woodward (2003). Important experiments from the point of view of human fibroblast–epithelial interactions are those of Kuperwasser et al. (2004). They were able to grow normal and premalignant human mammary cells in immune-deprived mice where the mammary fat pad was humanised by transplantation of normal human mammary fibroblasts. Epithelial growth occurred in this system, particularly if the fibroblasts were irradiated before implantation and/or transfected with genes for HGF and TGFβ, indicating the importance of stroma for normal and premalignant epithelial cell growth. Thus, the secretions of adipocytes, macrophages and fibroblasts may induce epithelial proliferation by paracrine mechanisms and cause resistance to ED in postmenopausal women (Fig. 8). Some of this stimulation could be related to obesity, and recent studies indicating that obesity is associated with macrophage infiltration and activation may also be relevant to mammary tumour progression (Weisberg et al. 2003).

Treatment Strategies to Prevent Resistance to Estrogen Deprivation

The treatment strategies to reduce the known relative resistance to the ED of the menopause include premature ovarian suppression in premenopausal women and the use of potent AIs in postmenopausal women. Pike et al. (1999) suggested the use of luteinising hormone-releasing hormone analogues (LHRH) to cause ED with various types of add-back hormones to prevent flushes and bone loss (low-dose estradiol and low-dose androgens) and intermittent progesterone to protect the uterus. Spicer and Pike (2000) showed that this approach was feasible and we have conducted similar studies of 2 years of the LHRH agonist, goserelin, with add-back raloxifene (to protect bone) is feasible. However, large randomised trials will be required in order to determine whether temporary ovarian suppression will be effective for breast cancer prevention.

As judged by the reduction in contralateral breast cancer in adjuvant trials, the AIs look very promising as candidates to produce an estimated 60% reduction in breast cancer incidence in the moderate- to high-risk women being entered into the two major randomised trials of anastrozole and exemestane in progress at present. Whilst AIs have a better therapeutic ratio than tamoxifen, there are problems with hot flushes, joint aches and bone loss which need to be addressed.

Although contralateral breast cancer incidence is reduced markedly using AIs, we do not know whether this is a true preventive effect or a temporary suppression of subclinical premalignant/malignant change within the breast. Also, it is known that advanced and early breast cancer can become resistant to AIs, probably via some of the mechanisms discussed in Sect. 5 which implicate reactivation of ERα via enhanced growth factor and signal transduction pathways. In advanced breast cancer, there is great interest in adding various inhibitors of these pathways to prevent AI resistance but, at present, we do not have many data concerning the clinical effectiveness of this approach. A summary of clinical trials underway is given in a recent review by Johnston (2006). Two approaches may be particularly useful, ultimately for prevention. One is use of lapatinib, the dual EGFR/HER2 neu dual tyrosine kinase inhibitor which is showing promising single-agent activity with little toxicity. The other is the use of a combination of AI with the ERα downregulator fulvestrant. The combination of letrozole with fulvestrant is much more effective than either approach alone in inhibiting the growth of MCF-7 cells transfected with the aromatase enzyme in immunosuppressed mice (Jelovac et al. 2005).

A number of pathways stimulate the activity of the aromatase enzyme including prostaglandins IL6 and TNFα. Potentially this could cause resistance to aromatase inhibitors by increasing the substrate. Thus, there remains interest in attempting to reduce aromatase activity by inhibitors of prostaglandin synthesis via COX-2. Potentially TNFα and IL6 production by macrophages and adipocytes could be reversed by calorie restriction (as could several other pathways including NFKB and leptin). In this regard, it is of interest that a recent study examining gene expression profiles in subcutaneous abdominal fat in obese premenopausal women showed upregulation of multiple anti-inflammatory genes and downregulation of pro-inflammatory genes after a 1-month 800-calorie diet (Clement et al. 2004). We have recently reported that loss of 5% or more of body weight (and maintaining the loss) reduces premenopausal breast cancer by 40% and postmenopausal disease by 25% (Harvie et al. 2005). The difficulty of enforcing weight loss approaches is well known and there is increasing interest in calorie restriction (CR) mimetics such as 2 deoxyglucose and anti-diabetic agents such as metformin and the glitazones which act via the AMP kinase-AKT/MTOR energy sensing pathway, as an alternative to CR (Howell et al. 2005). NFKB activation is an important pathway for tumour promotion. Over 100 NFKB inhibitors are known and this is an active area of prevention research with such agents as parthenolide and resveratrol (Nakanishi and Toi 2005).

As shown in Fig. 8, most of the pathways described can result in ERα activation. Thus, general reviews on potential preventive agents acting by other mechanisms may be of interest for further reading (Manson et al. 2005; Shen and Brown 2003).

Future Directions

This review raised many more questions than it gives answers and highlights our relative lack of knowledge of the target for ED and the mechanism of effectiveness and resistance to this approach. As far as target lesions are concerned, we have highlighted the view that this may be the HELU since they are relatively common within the breast and show transitional histological features of near normality in some to approaching DCIS in others. Wellings has given us some indication that there are good HELU (or his ALA) which may regress after the menopause, whereas there may be breasts with bad HELU which have the propensity to continue proliferation after the menopause. However, tumours may arise directly from TDLU without having to go through a HELU phase and may arise by the known genotoxic effects of estrogen metabolites (Yager and Davidson 2006). We do not know whether they are responding to the predominant estradiol concentration or whether some or many of them have autonomous growth, nor do we know whether high tissue estradiol concentrations seen in tumours are found in HELU. Our knowledge of the potential mechanisms of resistance of potential target lesions for ED in the breast are derived from indirect epidemiological investigations, including changes in reproductive factors and weight and from studies of overt malignancy, particularly mammary tumour cell lines. It is likely that findings from these approaches and from animal studies of paracrine factors from other cell types will be relevant to the ED question, but this is by no means certain.

At present, potential ways to circumvent de novo and acquired resistance to ED is being pursued mainly in patients with advanced disease or with large primary tumours in the adjuvant situation. Some studies, including our own, are being performed by taking some sort of biopsy (perareolar FNA, ductal lavage or corecut) before and after an intervention. These are difficult studies because of the heterogeneity of the breast. If HELU are important we may not even be investigating the correct lesion. However, these approaches are possible and important. It is also possible to select lesions from the breast and transplant them for study in the nude mouse which may be a major important approach to defining mechanism and responsiveness to treatment in the future.

References

Aharinejad S, Paulus P, Sioud M et al. (2004) Colony-stimulating factor-1 blockade by antisense oligonucleotides and small interfering RNAs suppress growth of human mammary tumor xenografts in mice. Cancer Res 64:5378–5384

Althuis MD, Fergenbum JH, Garcia-Closas M et al. (2004) Etiology of hormone receptor-defined breast cancer: a systematic review of the literature. Cancer Epidemiol Biomarkers Prev 13:1558–1568

Barcellos-Hoff MH, Medina D (2005) New highlights on stroma-epithelial interactions in breast cancer. Breast Cancer Res 7:33–36

Biswas DK, Singh S, Shi O et al. (2005) Crossroads of estrogen receptor and NF-kappaB signalling. Sci STKE 288:pe27

Blankenstein MA, Szymczak J, Daroszewski J et al. (1992) Estrogens in plasma and fatty tissue from breast cancer patients and women undergoing surgery for non-oncological reasons. Gynecol Endocrinol 6:13–17

Bocchinfuso WP, Korach KS (1997) Mammary gland development and tumorigenesis in estrogen receptor knockout mice. J Mammary Gland Biol Neoplasia 2:323–334

Bonney RC, Reed MJ, Davidson K et al. (1983) The relationship between 17 beta-hydroxysteroid dehydrogenase activity and oestrogen concentrations in human breast tumours and in normal breast tissue. Clin Endocrinol 19:727–739

Brisken C, Parks S, Vass T et al. (1998) A paracrine role for the epithelial progesterone receptor in mammary gland development. Proc Natl Acad Sci U S A 95:5076–5081

Brisken C, Kaur S, Chavarria TE et al. (1999) Prolactin controls mammary gland development via direct and indirect mechanisms. Dev Biol 210:96–106

Catalano S, Mauro L, Marsico S et al. (2004) Leptin induces, via ERK1/ERK2 signal, functional activation of estrogen receptor alpha in MCF-7 cells. J Biol Chem 279:19908–19915

Chamras H, Bagga D, Elstner E et al. (1998) Preadipocytes stimulate breast cancer cell growth. Nutr Cancer 32:59–63

Chatterton RT Jr, Geiger AS, Mateo ET et al. (2004) Comparison of hormone levels in nipple aspirate fluid of pre and postmenopausal women: effect of oral contraceptives and hormone replacement. J Clin Endocrinol Metab 90:1686–1691

Chia K-S, Reilly M, Tan CS et al. (2005) Profound changes in breast cancer incidence may reflect changes into a westernized lifestyle: a comparative population-based study in Singapore and Sweden. Int J Cancer 113:302–306

Clarke RB, Howell A, Anderson E (1997a) Estrogen sensitivity of normal human breast tissue in vivo and implanted into athymic nude mice: analysis of the relationship between estrogen-induced proliferation and progesterone receptor expression. Breast Cancer Res Treat 45:121–133

Clarke RB, Howell A, Potten CS, Anderson E (1997b) Dissociation between steroid receptor expression and cell proliferation in the human breast. Cancer Res 57:4987–4991

Clarke RB, Anderson E, Howell A, Potten CS (2003) Regulation of human breast epithelial stem cells. Cell Prolif 36 [Suppl 1]:45–58

Clarke RB, Spence K, Anderson E et al. (2005) A putative human breast stem cell population is enriched for steroid receptor-positive cells. Dev Biol 277:443–456

Cleary MP, Juneja SC, Philips SC et al. (2004) Leptin receptor-deficient MMTV-TGF-alpha/Lepr(db)Lepr (db) female mice do not develop oncogene-induced mammary tumors. Exp Biol Med (Maywood) 229:182–193

Clement K, Viguerie N, Poitou C et al. (2004) Weight loss regulates inflammation-related genes in white adipose tissue of obese subjects. FASEB J 18:1657–1669

Cuzick J (2005) Aromatase inhibitors for breast cancer prevention. J Clin Oncol 23:1636–1643

Cuzick J, Powles T, Veronesi U et al. (2003) Overview of the main outcomes in breast cancer prevention trials. Lancet 361:296–300

Da Silva Correia J, Miranda Y, Austin-Brown N et al. (2006) Nod1-dependent control of tumor growth. Proc Natl Acad Sci U S A 103:1840–1845

De Graffenried LA et al. (2004) NF-kappa B inhibition markedly enhances sensitivity of resistant breast cancer tumor cells to tamoxifen. Ann Oncol 15:885–890

Dieudonne MN, Machinal-Quelin F, Serazin-Leroy V et al. (2002) Leptin mediates a proliferative response in human MCF7 breast cancer cells. Biochem Biophys Res Commun 293:622–628

Dobson RRH et al. (2000) The effects of prolonged HRT treatment in normal postmenopausal breast epithelium. Breast Cancer Res Treat 64:106

Dowsett M, Smith IE, Ebbs SR et al. (2006) Proliferation and apoptosis as markers of benefit in neo-adjuvant endocrine therapy of breast cancer. Clin Cancer Res 12:1024s–1030s

Eisen A, Lubinski J, Klijn J et al. (2005) Breast cancer risk following bilateral oophorectomy in BRCA1 and BRCA2 mutation carriers: an international case control study. J Clin Oncol 23:7491–7496

Ewan KB, Oketch-Rabah HA, Ravani SA et al. (2005) Proliferation of estrogen receptor-alpha-positive mammary epithelial cells is restrained by transforming growth factor-beta 1 in adult mice. Am J Pathol 167:409–417

Fechner RE (1972) Benign breast disease in women on estrogen therapy. Cancer 29:273–279

Feinleib M (1968) Breast cancer and artificial menopause: a cohort study. J Natl Cancer Inst 41:315–329

Frech MS, Halama ED, Tilli MT et al. (2005) Deregulated estrogen receptor α expression in mammary epithelial cells of transgenic mice results in the development of ductal carcinoma in-situ. Cancer Res 65:681–685

Garofalo C, Sisci D, Surmacz E (2004) Leptin interferes with the effects of the antiestrogen ICI 182,780 in MCF-7 breast cancer cells. Clin Cancer Res 10:6466–6475

Geisler J (2003) Breast cancer tissue estrogens and their manipulation with aromatase inhibitors and inactivators. J Steroid Biochem Mol Biol 86:245–253

Hagemann T, Robinson SC, Schulz M et al. (2004) Enhanced invasiveness of breast cancer cell lines upon co-cultivation with macrophages is due to TNF-alpha dependent up-regulation of matrix metalloproteases. Carcinogenesis 25:1543–1549

Hagemann T, Wilson J, Kulbe H et al. (2005) Macrophages induce invasiveness of epithelial cancer cells via NF-kB and JNK. J Immunol 175:1197–1205

Hardie DG (2005) New roles for the LKB1, AMPK pathway. Curr Opin Cell Biol 17:167–173

Harvie M, Howell A, Vierkant RA et al. (2005) Association of gain and loss of weight before and after menopause with risk of postmenopausal breast cancer in the IOWA women's health study. Cancer Epidemiol Biomarkers Prev 14:656–661

Haslam SZ, Woodward TL (2003) Host microenvironment in breast cancer development: epithelial-cell-stromal-cell interactions and steroid hormone action in normal and cancerous mammary gland. Breast Cancer Res 5:208–215

Hirayama T, Wynder EL (1962) A study of the epidemiology of cancer of the breast II. The influence of hysterectomy. Cancer 5:28–38

Hofseth, Raafat AM, Osuch JR et al. (1999) Hormone replacement therapy with estrogen or estrogen plus medroxyprogesterone acetate is associated with increased epithelial proliferation in the normal postmenopausal breast. J Clin Endocrinol Metab 84:4559–4565

Howell A (1989) Clinical evidence for the involvement of oestrogen in the development and progression of breast cancer. Proc R Soc Edin 95B:49–57

Howell A, Sims AH, Ong KR et al. (2005) Mechanisms of disease: prediction and prevention of breast cancer – cellular and molecular interactions. Nat Clin Prac Oncol 2:635–646

Hu X, Juneja SC, Maihle NJ, Cleary MP (2002) Leptin – a growth factor in normal and malignant breast cells and for normal mammary gland development. J Natl Cancer Inst 94:1704–1711

Iyengar P, Combs TP, Shah SJ et al. (2003) Adipocyte-secreted factors synergistically promote mammary tumourigenesis through induction of anti-apoptotic transcriptional programs and proto-oncogene stabilisation. Oncogene 22:6408–6423

Iyengar P, Espina V, Williams TW et al. (2005) Adipocyte-derived collagen VI affects early mammary tumor progression in vivo, demonstrating a critical interaction in the tumor/stroma microenvironment. J Clin Invest 115:1163–1176

Jelovac D, Macedo L, Goloubeva OG et al. (2005) Additive antitumor effect of aromatase inhibitor letrozole and antiestrogen fulvestrant in a postmenopausal breast cancer model. Cancer Res 65:5439–5444

Johnston SR (2006) Clinical efforts to combine endocrine agents with targeted therapies against epidermal growth factor receptor/human epidermal growth factor receptor 2 and mammalian target of Rapamycin in breast cancer. Clin Cancer Res 12:1061s–1068s

Karagas MR (2000) Cancers of the female reproductive system. Menopause biology pathology. Academic Press, London, pp 359–365

Keith JC Jr, Albert LM, Leathurby Y et al. (2005) The utility of pathway selective estrogen receptor ligands that inhibit nuclear factor-kappa B transcriptional activity in models of rheumatoid arthritis. Arthritis Res Ther 7:R427–R438

Key TJ, Pike MC (1988) The role of oestrogens and progestagens in the epidemiology and prevention of breast cancer. Eur J Cancer Clin Oncol 24:29–43

Kuperwasser C, Chavarria T, Wu M et al. (2004) Reconstruction of functionally normal and malignant human breast tissues in mice. Proc Natl Acad Sci U S A 101:4966–4971

Lee S et al. (2005a) Genetic alterations associated with early hyperplastic precursors of breast cancer. Breast Cancer Res Treat 94:24

Lee S et al. (2005b) Hormones, receptors and growth in hyperplastic enlarged lobular units: early potential precursors of breast cancer. Breast Cancer Res 8:1–9

Lin EY (2002) The macrophage growth factor CSF-1 in mammary gland development and tumor progression. J Mammary Gland Biol Neoplasia 7:147–162

Luetteke NC, Qiu TH, Fenton SE et al. (1999) Targeted inactivation of the EGF and amphiregulin genes reveals distinct roles for EGF receptor ligands in mouse mammary gland development. Development 126:2739–2750

Mallepell S, Krust A, Chambon P, Brisken C (2006) Paracrine signaling through the epithelial estrogen receptor α is required for proliferation and morphogenesis in the mammary gland. Proc Natl Acad Sci U S A 103:2196–2201

Manabe Y, Toda S, Miyazaki K et al. (2003) Mature adipocytes, but not preadipocytes, promote the growth of breast carcinoma cells in collagen gel matrix culture through cancer-stromal cell interactions. J Pathol 201:221–228

Manson MM, Farmer PB, Gescher A et al. (2005) Innovative agents in cancer prevention. Recent Results Cancer Res 166:257–275

Martin L-A, Farmer I, Johnston SR et al. (2003) Enhanced estrogen receptor (ER) α, ERBB2 and MARK signal transduction pathways operate during the adaptation of MCF-7 cells to long-term estrogen deprivation. J Biol Chem 278:30458–30468

Martino S, Cauley JA, Barrett-Conner E et al. (2004) Continuing outcomes relevant to Evista: breast cancer incidence in postmenopausal osteoporotic women in a randomised trial of raloxifene. J Natl Cancer Inst 96:1751–1761

Masamura S, Santner SJ, Heitjan DF, Santen RJ (1994) Estrogen deprivation causes estradiol hypersensitivity in human breast cancer cells. J Clin Endocrinol 80:2918–2925

McLeskey SW, Zhang L, El-Ashry D et al. (1998) Tamoxifen-resistant fibroblast growth factor-transfected MCF-7 cells are cross-resistant in vivo to the antiestrogen ICI 182,780 and two aromatase inhibitors. Clin Cancer Res 4:697–711

McTiernan A, Tworoger SS, Ulrich CM et al. (2004) Effect of exercise on serum estrogens in postmenopausal women: a 12 month randomised clinical trial. Cancer Res 64:2923–2928

Nakanishi C, Toi M (2005) Nuclear factor-kB inhibitors as sensitizers to anticancer drugs. Nat Rev 5:297–309

Okano H, Kawahara H, Toriya M et al. (2005) Function of RNA-binding protein Musashi-1 in stem cells. Exp Cell Res 306:349–356

Pasqualini JR, Chetrite G, Blacker C et al. (1996) Concentrations of estrone, estradiol and estrone sulfate and evaluation of sulfatase and aromatase activities in pre and postmenopausal breast cancer patients. J Clin Endocrinol Metab 81:1460–1464

Pike MC et al. (1997) A hormonal contraceptive approach to reducing breast and ovarian cancer risk: an update. Endocrinol Rel Cancer 4:125–133

Potten CS, Watson RJ, Williams GT et al. (1988) The effect of age and menstrual cycle upon proliferative activity of the normal human breast. Br J Cancer 58:163–170

Prasad R, Boland GP, Cramer A et al. (2003) Short term biologic response to withdrawal of hormone replacement therapy in patients with invasive breast carcinoma. Cancer 98:2539–2546

Rajala MW, Scherer PE (2003) Minireview: the adipocyte at the crossroads of energy homeostasis, inflammation and atherosclerosis. Endocrinology 144:3765–3773

Rayala SK, Hollander P, Balasenthil S et al. (2006) Hepatocyte growth factor-regulated tyrosine kinase substrate (HRS) interacts with PELPI and activates MAPK. J Biol Chem 281:4395–4403

Riggins RB, Zwart A, Nehra R, Clarke R (2005) The nuclear factor kappa B inhibitor parthenolide restores ICI 182,780 (Faslodex: fulvestrant)-induced apoptosis in antiestrogen-resistant breast cancer cells. Mol Cancer Ther 4:33–41

Rinaldi S, Key TJ, Peeters PH et al. (2005) Anthropometric measures, endogenous sex steroids and breast cancer risk in postmenopausal women: a study within the EPIC cohort. Int J Cancer 118:2832–2839

Rubio MF, Werbajh S, Cafferata EG et al. (2006) TNF-alpha enhances estrogen-induced cell proliferation of estrogen-dependent breast tumor cells through a complex containing nuclear factor-kappa B. Oncogene 25:1367–1377

Russo J, Ao X, Grill C, Russo IH (1999) Pattern of distribution of cells positive for estrogen receptor alpha and progesterone receptor in relation to proliferating cells in the mammary gland. Breast Cancer Res Treat 53:217–227

Sabnis GJ, Jelovac D, Long B, Brodie A (2005) The role of growth factor receptor pathways in human breast cancer cells adapted to long-term estrogen deprivation. Cancer Res 65:3903–3910

Shen Q, Brown PH (2003) Novel agents for the prevention of breast cancer: targeting transcription factors and signal transduction pathways. J Mammary Gland Biol Neoplasia 8:45–73

Shoker BS, Jarvis C, Clarke RB et al. (1999) Estrogen receptor-positive proliferating cells in the normal and precancerous breast. Am J Pathol 155:1811–1815

Shoker BS et al. (2000) Abnormal regulation of the estrogen receptor in benign breast lesions. J Clin Pathol 53:778–783

Sivaraman L, Hilsenbeck SG, Zhong L et al. (2001) Early exposure of the rat mammary gland to estrogen and progesterone blocks co-localisation of estrogen receptor expression and proliferation. J Endocrinol 171:75–83

Spicer DV, Pike MC (2000) Future possibilities in the prevention of breast cancer: luteinising hormone-releasing hormone agents. Breast Cancer Res 2:264–267

Stylianou S, Clarke RB, Brennan K (2006) Aberrant activation of notch signaling in human breast cancer. Cancer Res 66:1517–1525

Tekmal RR, Liu YG, Nair HB et al. (2005) Estrogen receptor alpha is required for mammary development and the induction of mammary hyperplasia and epigenetic alterations in the aromatase transgenic mice. J Steroid Biochem Mol Biol 95:9–15

Thomas DB (1993) Breast cancer in men. Epidemiol Rev 15:220–231

Thottassery JV, Sun Y, Westbrook L et al. (2004) Prolonged extracellular signal-regulated kinase 1/2 activation during fibroblast growth factor 1 or heregulin beta1-induced antiestrogen-resistant growth of breast cancer cells is resistant to mitogen-activated protein/extracellular regulated kinase kinase inhibitors. Cancer Res 64:4637–4647

Trichopoulos D, McMahon B, Cole P (1972) Menopause and breast cancer risk. J Natl Cancer Inst 48:605–613

Vadlamudi RK, Manavathi B, Balasenthil S et al. (2005) Functional implications of altered subcellular localization of PELP1 in breast cancer cells. Cancer Res 65:7724–7732

Wang S (2004) Recombinant cell ultrasensitive bioassay for measurement of estrogens in postmenopausal women. J Clin Endocrinol Metab 90:1407–1413

Weisberg SP, McCann D, Desai M et al. (2003) Obesity is associated with macrophage accumulation in adipose tissue. J Clin Invest 112:1796–1808

Wellings SR (1980) A hypothesis of the origin of human breast cancer from the terminal ductal lobular unit. Path Res Pract 166:515–535

Wellings SR, Jensen HM, Marcum RG (1975) An atlas of subgross pathology of the human breast with special reference to possible precancerous lesions. J Natl Cancer Inst 55:231–273

Wiesen JF, Young P, Werb Z, Cunha GR (1999) Signalling through the stromal epidermal growth factor receptor is necessary for mammary ductal development. Development 126:335–344

Yager JD, Davidson NE (2006) Estrogen carcinogenesis in breast cancer. N Eng J Med 354:270–282

Yasui Y, Potter JD (1999) The shape of age incidence curves of female breast cancer by hormone receptor status. Cancer Causes Control 10:431–437

Yin N, Wang D, Zhang H et al. (2004) Molecular mechanisms involved in the growth stimulation of breast cancer cells by leptin. Cancer Res 64:5870–5875

Zeps N (1996) Detection of a population of long-lived cells in mammary epithelium of the mouse. Cell Tissue Res 286:525–536

Zhang HZ, Bennett JM, Smith KG et al (2002) Estrogen mediates mammary epithelial cell proliferation in serum-free culture indirectly via mammary stroma-derived hepatocyte growth factor. Endocrinology 143:3427–3434

Zhou Y, Eppenberger-Castori S, Marx C et al (2005) Activation of nuclear factor-kappa B (NFkappaB) identifies a high-risk subset of hormone-dependent breast cancer. Int J Biochem Cell Biol 37:1130–1144

Part V   Prevention of Colorectal Cancers

14 Primary Dietary Prevention: Is the Fiber Story Over?

Cheryl L. Rock

Recent Results in Cancer Research, Vol. 174
© Springer-Verlag Berlin Heidelberg 2007

Abstract

Colorectal cancer is a major cause of morbidity in developed countries, and epidemiological and experimental research suggests that environmental factors, particularly diet, may play a key etiologic role. Among the various dietary factors that have been proposed to affect the risk and progression of colon cancer, dietary fiber has been of greatest interest, due to the effects of fiber on the function of the large bowel. Dietary fiber is a heterogeneous group of compounds, consisting of the remnants of plant cells resistant to hydrolysis by human alimentary enzymes. Several case–control studies and a few cohort studies have linked higher fiber intake to reduced risk for colorectal cancer, although the results of these observational studies have been inconsistent. In the large European Prospective Investigation into Cancer and Nutrition observational study, higher dietary fiber from foods was associated with an estimated 25% reduction in risk for large bowel cancer. However, no significant relationship between fiber intake (or major food sources of fiber) and risk for colorectal cancer was observed in a recently reported large pooled analysis of several cohort studies. Well-known limitations of observational studies, particularly relating to the collection and interpretation of dietary data, constrain conclusions from these studies. To date, intervention studies testing the relationship between dietary fiber and colon cancer have focused on whether fiber supplementation or diet modification can affect the risk for adenoma recurrence and growth in individuals with a history of adenomatous polyps. In four of these intervention studies, subjects in the intervention arm were prescribed dietary fiber supplements, and beneficial effects on adenoma recurrence were not observed over 3–5 years of follow-up. In a large randomized U.S. study, the Polyp Prevention Trial, the effect of prescribing diet modification (increased fiber and reduced fat intakes) was tested, and no effects on adenoma recurrence were observed, although dietary biomarker data suggest that the change in dietary intakes in the intervention arm was not substantial. The effect of increased dietary fiber intake on risk for colorectal cancer has not been adequately addressed in studies conducted to date. Longer-term trials and higher levels of fiber intake are strategies that have been suggested to increase knowledge in this area. Also, laboratory and clinical studies that continue to provide insight into biological mechanisms may help to better target intervention efforts.

Introduction

On a worldwide basis, cancer of the colon is the fourth most commonly diagnosed cancer, and incidence rates have been steadily increasing, especially in developed countries (WCRF/AICR 1997). In the U.S. alone, over 145,000 cases of colon and rectal cancer are currently diagnosed each year (Jemal et al. 2005). Results from ecologic and migrant studies have long suggested that diet is an important environmental factor that influences the risk and progression of colon cancer. Food provides nutrients and numerous other bioactive compounds, many of which have been specifically shown to have effects on cellular and molecular events and activities that have been identified in the development and progression of colon cancer (Milner 2004; Kris-Etherton et al. 2002; Rock 1998). As summarized in several reviews (Willett 1999, 2000; WCRF/AICR 1997), the continued accumulation of data on diet and cancer over the past several decades supports the concept that diet can affect risk and progression of colon cancer, although disentangling the effects of various foods, specific dietary constituents, and related lifestyle factors and characteristics (e.g., physical activity, obesity) that influence risk for colon cancer has proven to be very challenging.

Among the various dietary factors that have been proposed to affect the risk and progression of colon cancer, dietary fiber has probably been of greatest interest, due to the observed effects of fiber on the function of the large bowel. Dietary fiber reduces transit time, dilutes potential carcinogens, binds carcinogenic substances, stimulates bacterial anaerobic fermentation, and leads to the production of short-chain fatty acids that have favorable effects on cell growth regulation (Slavin 2003; Marlett et al. 2002). By definition, dietary fiber is a heterogeneous group of compounds, consisting of the remnants of plant cells resistant to hydrolysis by human alimentary enzymes: structural and storage polysaccharides and lignin (Marlett et al. 2002). Major sources of fiber in the diet include vegetables and fruit, whole grains, legumes, and nuts. All of these foods are complex, consisting of numerous bioactive constituents in addition to fiber, which can confound the interpretation of epidemiological studies. The interpretation of intervention studies testing whether fiber may have an effect on selected colon cancer-related outcomes also is complicated by the nature of the intervention, the time interval, the stage in the colon cancer continuum under study, and the magnitude and nature of change in fiber intake that is achieved. At this point, addressing whether or not the fiber story is over first requires a critical evaluation of problems and issues with the currently available data.

Key Issues

A major challenge in epidemiological research examining the link between nutritional factors, such as dietary fiber, and cancer risk are the well-known limitations in dietary assessment methodologies, as recently summarized (Prentice et al. 2004). Accurate assessment of diet has recognized limitations and constraints, even when the most well-developed and established dietary assessment methods are used. Improvements in food and dietary supplement databases used to assess status also are sorely needed to more accurately characterize actual intakes (Dwyer et al. 2003).

Most epidemiological observational studies relating dietary factors to cancer risk are conducted within a defined, specific population, using rather crude dietary assessment methodologies. As summarized by Prentice (2000), recent nutrient intakes may differ from those over the years or decades during the long process of the development of cancer, and nutrients (such as fiber) in the population under study may not be highly variable, which precludes identifying associations with cancer risk across a range of intakes. The diet is a complex mixture of foods and nutrients that are typically highly correlated, so estimating the relationship between cancer risk and a specific nutrient (such as fiber), while accommodating other dietary factors, is a challenging task even with the best analytical approaches (Prentice 2000). Most epidemiological studies involve collecting and reporting data on quantified nutrient intakes, but the nutrient or dietary factor in the analysis may be a surrogate or even simply an indicator of foods or a general dietary pattern. Assumptions regarding cause and effect also are not necessarily true. Whole grains, although a major source of dietary fiber, are also rich sources of compounds that exhibit hormonal and antioxidant activities (Slavin 2003): whole grains are not synonymous with fiber and may not even be the main source of fiber in an individual diet. Similarly, vegetables and fruit contribute a number of biologically active compounds to the diet, in addition to fiber. Evaluating and interpreting dietary data, whether expressed as intakes of specific foods or estimated nutrient intakes, cannot be approached simplistically. Also, the dietary pattern, or specifically, a high-fiber diet, is usually associated with lower level of red meat consumption, reduced likelihood of obesity, and greater likelihood of higher level of physical activity (Willett 1999), and evidence suggests that all of these factors may independently modify risk for colon cancer (WCRF/AICR 1997).

The identification of dietary biomarkers is currently considered an important research goal for nutritional epidemiology and cancer research (Prentice et al. 2004; Prentice 2003). In addition to being recognized as important to assess true exposure in observational epidemiological studies, dietary biomarkers are particularly meaningful in intervention studies. A specific dietary biomarker for fiber intake, which would verify and better characterize intake, has not been identified or established. As a marker of intake of vegetables and fruit (among the major sources of fiber in most diets), plasma or serum carotenoid concentrations have some utility in verifying intake of those dietary fiber sources. Plasma or serum carotenoid concentrations have been consistently shown to be a marker of vegetable and fruit intakes in observational studies, and tissue concentrations increase in response to feeding or prescribing these foods and in diet intervention studies that successfully promote increased vegetable and fruit intake (Rock et al. 2001; Polsinelli et al. 1998). Serum beta-sitosterol concentration is currently under study as a potential biomarker of intake of seeds, nuts, cereal, and legumes, which are other major sources of fiber (Muti et al. 2003). In the absence of a biomarker for fiber intake, estimated fiber intake in a free-living population should be assumed to be a crude estimate, which likely explains a great deal of the inconsistencies in the scientific literature.

To date, intervention studies testing the relationship between dietary fiber and colon cancer have focused on only one stage in the development and progression of colon cancer: whether fiber supplementation or diet modification can affect the risk for adenoma recurrence and growth in individuals with a history of adenomatous polyps, over a 2- to 5-year period of time (Asano and McLeod 2005). A finding of no effect in a study of this type does not address the possibility that a lifetime of high or low fiber intake, or differential fiber intake at another point in the cancer continuum, might affect risk for colon cancer.

Another issue with the relevant intervention studies to date relates to adherence with the prescribed regimen, and whether the degree of change in dietary intake (if that is the focus of

the intervention) was sufficient to promote biological changes relevant to colon cancer risk or progression. For example, in one study involving wheat bran supplementation, the median increase in fiber intake over baseline achieved in the intervention group was 7 g/day (MacLennan et al. 1995). In the large U.S. Polyp Prevention Trial (PPT), which aimed to promote an increase in fiber, fruit, and vegetable intakes, the absolute difference in daily fiber intake between the intervention and control groups over the 4-year period of the study was 6.9 g/1,000 kcal (Schatzkin et al. 2000), promoted in part by an increase in self-reported vegetable and fruit intake (Lanza et al. 2001). However, a worrisome finding that affects the interpretation of the results of this study is that the increase in serum carotenoid concentration (a biomarker of vegetable and fruit intake) in the intervention group was minimal, as discussed below.

Thus, several basic issues and considerations affect the interpretation of currently available data from studies to date that have addressed the question of whether dietary fiber plays a role in the risk and progression of colon cancer.

Recent Evidence from Epidemiological Observational Studies

As previously reviewed (WCRF/AICR 1997) reduced risk for colon cancer in association with higher fiber intake has been observed in most case–control studies. However, results from prospective cohort studies, in which dietary data are collected before the diagnosis of disease, are more inconsistent and generally do not identify a protective effect of dietary fiber (Willett 1999). Two notably large prospective epidemiological observational studies that have examined the relationship between risk for colorectal cancer and fiber intake reported results within the past few years, with opposite results and conclusions.

In the multi-center European Prospective Investigation into Cancer and Nutrition (EPIC) Study, data from 519,978 individuals, in whom 1,065 cases of colorectal cancer were identified during an average follow-up period of 4.5 years, were the focus of the analysis (Bingham et al. 2003). In that study, dietary fiber in foods was found to be inversely related to incidence of colorectal cancer (adjusted relative risk [RR] 0.75, 95% confidence interval [CI] 0.59–0.95, for highest vs lowest quintile), adjusted for age, weight, height, sex, non-fat energy intake, and energy from fat, and stratified by center. Analysis of relationships between colorectal cancer risk and intakes of specific foods did not reveal significant associations, although a protective effect from cereal fiber intake was marginally significant (p=0.06). The EPIC Study involves a very diverse study population recruited from ten European countries, so the range of consumption and heterogeneity of dietary intakes of food sources of fiber are notable. Country-specific questionnaires were used to assess dietary intakes, and 24-h dietary recalls were collected from 8% of the sample as an approach to calibrating the dietary questionnaires.

In a pooled analysis based on data from 13 prospective cohort studies, involving data collected from 725,628 men and women followed for 6–20 years across the studies, 8,081 colorectal cancer cases were identified, and the relationship between dietary fiber intake and colorectal cancer was examined (Park et al. 2005). In that study, a significant inverse association was found in the age-adjusted model (pooled RR, 0.84; 95%CI, 0.77–0.92, for highest vs lowest quintile). Adjusting for other risk factors (including age, body mass index, nondietary risk factors, multiple vitamin use, and energy intake) attenuated the association, although it remained significant. Adjustment for folate intake further attenuated the association, so that the relationship became nonsignificant, and further adjustment for red meat, milk, and alcohol intakes further weakened the association (RR, 0.94; 95%CI, 0.86–1.03, for highest vs lowest quintile). When risk was examined in relation to major food sources of fiber (whole grains and vegetables and fruit), significant associations were not identified. The dietary data used in this study were obtained via study-specific questionnaires with different levels of detail in queries for food choices relevant to fiber intake.

It would appear unlikely that epidemiological observational studies will find resolution on the issue of whether dietary fiber intake plays a role in the primary prevention of colorectal can-

cer, which may be attributable, at least in part, to the general constraints and limitations of this approach. Across these studies, differences in the populations under study, approaches used to collect and analyze the data (including the selection of covariates to include in multivariate analysis), and other study characteristics likely explain the divergent results.

Results from Intervention Studies and Clinical Trials

As noted above, intervention studies testing the relationship between dietary fiber and the risk and progression of colon cancer have focused on whether fiber supplementation or diet modification can affect adenoma recurrence and growth. The rationale for using recurrence of colorectal adenomas as the primary end point is that adenomatous polyps are considered precursors of most cancers of the large bowel (Einspahr et al. 1997), and a clinical trial testing the effect of fiber intake on incident colon cancer would require a large sample, a very long follow-up period, and considerable resources and support. However, it must be recognized that without specific knowledge of the critical points at which diet may affect the development of colon cancer, the focus of intervention studies to date may not appropriately test for effects of dietary fiber on risk for colon cancer.

As summarized in two recent comprehensive reviews (Asano and McLeod 2005; Faivre and Bonithon-Kopp 2002), four studies have tested the effect of fiber supplementation (wheat bran or ispaghula husk) on polyp recurrence, although one of these studies (DeCosse et al. 1989) was excluded from the Cochrane Review because it did not meet the requirement for predefined outcomes. Another notable characteristic of that study is that while subjects in only one treatment arm were prescribed supplemental wheat bran, subjects in both arms were prescribed supplemental vitamin C and alpha-tocopherol. In three of the studies, the subjects were individuals who had a previous adenoma; in the study by DeCosse et al. (1989), the subjects had been diagnosed with familial polyposis. In these studies, the amount of wheat bran prescribed ranged from 11 to 22.5 g/day, and in the study involving supplementation with ispaghula husk (Bonithon-Kopp et al. 2000), the amount prescribed was 3.5 g/day. The length of follow-up ranged from 3 to 5 years. No effect on adenoma recurrence was observed in the studies involving wheat bran supplementation (Alberts et al. 2000; MacLennan et al. 1995; DeCosse et al. 1989), and a significant increase in adenoma recurrence was observed in association with ispaghula husk supplementation in the study that tested that intervention (Bonithon-Kopp et al. 2000).

The effect of diet modification to promote increased fiber intake on adenoma recurrence has been examined in two studies reported to date. In one of these studies (McKeown-Eyssen et al. 1994), the goal for subjects in the intervention arm was to achieve 50 g/day fiber intake and less than 20% energy from fat. After 12 months of dietary counseling, the intervention group reported an average of 35 g/day fiber intake and 25% energy from fat, while the control group reported an average of 16 g/day fiber intake and 35% energy from fat. In the total study sample of 201 subjects, no significant effect on adenoma recurrence was observed at the 2-year follow-up time point, although nonsignificant differential effects were suggested in the analysis of gender subgroups.

The effect of increasing intakes of fiber (with the goal of 18 g/1,000 kcal) and vegetables and fruit (aiming for five to eight servings/day), concurrent with reduced fat intake (20% energy from fat), on adenoma recurrence at 4 years following randomization was the focus of the PPT (Schatzkin et al. 2000). The PPT was a large randomized trial involving 2,079 study participants, and those assigned to the intervention group received over 50 h of dietary counseling. The absolute difference between the self-reported daily intakes of the intervention and control groups over the 4-year period was 9.7% energy from fat, 6.9 g/1,000 kcal dietary fiber, and 1.1 servings/1,000 kcal vegetables and fruit (Lanza et al. 2001). As noted above, however, the intervention group exhibited only a minimal increase in total serum carotenoid concentration (approximately 5%), despite reporting substantially increased carotenoid intake in association with reported increased intake of vegetables and fruit.

The difference between the control and intervention groups for this dietary biomarker was statistically significant, but the minimal change that was observed is not consistent with the dietary intakes that were reported.

Do the intervention studies conducted to date resolve the question of whether dietary fiber intake plays a role in primary prevention? Issues such as the timing in the cancer continuum, the length of follow-up in the studies, the nature of the intervention, and the degree of change in intake that was actually achieved all affect how confidently one can answer that question. The need for longer-term trials and higher levels of dietary fiber intake in the intervention has been suggested (Asano and McLeod 2005). Also, laboratory and clinical studies that continue to provide insight about biological mechanisms may help to better target intervention efforts, if future studies are to be conducted with a more in-depth knowledge base.

Conclusions

At this point, reviews of the scientific literature on the health benefits of fiber intake have uniformly agreed on the general recommendation that increased fiber intake, relative to current average intakes in developed countries, is well founded (Food and Nutrition Board 2002; Marlett et al. 2002). Current dietary recommendations in the U.S. advise fiber intakes of 38 and 25 g/day for men and women, respectively, aged 19–50 years, and 30 and 21 g/day for men and women aged 51 years and older, based on thorough review of evidence relating fiber to optimal health and disease prevention (Food and Nutrition Board 2002). Nutritional surveys conducted over the past decade suggest that median fiber intake ranges from 16.5 to 17.9 g/day for men and 12.1 to 13.8 g/day for women in the U.S., so the levels of intake that are currently recommended represent a considerable increase for most individuals. The rationale for this recommendation is based on the consistent evidence relating increased fiber intake to lower risk for common gastrointestinal problems (e.g., constipation, diverticulosis, diverticulitis) and cardiovascular disease, recognizing that the specific link between fiber intake and risk for colon cancer has not been as established as with these other conditions.

Another relevant benefit of dietary fiber that has been observed in both epidemiological and experimental studies is that this dietary constituent is a key feature of a diet that is low in energy density. Current evidence strongly supports the concept that a low-energy density diet, which is characterized by high dietary fiber intake, may play a critical role in promoting weight control and in preventing adult weight gain (Liu et al. 2003; Burton-Freeman 2000). Obesity is a nutritional factor that appears to promote a considerable increase in risk for several types of cancer, including colon cancer (Calle et al. 2003). Finally, fiber-rich foods, such as vegetables and fruits, whole grains, legumes and nuts, are all good sources of essential nutrients and other bioactive compounds that exhibit numerous biological activities that promote normal cell growth regulation and function (Slavin 2003; Marlett et al. 2002).

On the basis of current evidence, the definitive relationship between dietary fiber intake and risk and progression of colon cancer cannot be resolved at this time. However, increased fiber intake remains a dietary strategy that may contribute (indirectly, if not directly) to reduced risk and progression of cancer.

References

Alberts DS, Martinez ME, Roe DJ, Guillen-Rodriguez JM, Marshall JR, van Leeuwen JB et al (2000) Lack of effect of a high-fiber cereal supplement on the recurrence of colorectal adenomas. N Engl J Med 342:1156–1162

Asano TK, McLeod RS (2005) Dietary fibre and the prevention of colorectal adenomas and carcinomas (Cochrane Review), The Cochrane Library, Issue 4, Wiley, Chichester

Bingham SA, Day NE, Luben R, Ferrari P, Silmani N, Norat T et al (2003) Dietary fibre in food and protection against colorectal cancer in the European Prospective Investigation into Cancer and Nutrition (EPIC): an observational study. Lancet 361:1496–1501

Bonithon-Kopp C, Kronborg O, Glacosa A, Rath U, Faivre J, the European Cancer Prevention Organisation Study Group (2000) Calcium and fiber supplementation in prevention of colorectal adenoma recurrence: a randomized intervention trial. Lancet 356:1300–1336

Burton-Freeman B (2000) Dietary fiber and energy regulation. J Nutr 130 [Suppl]:272S–275S

Calle EE, Rodriguez C, Walker-Thurmond K, Thun MJ (2003) Overweight, obesity and mortality from cancer in a prospectively studied cohort of U.S. adults. N Engl J Med 348:1625–1638

DeCosse JJ, Miller HH, Lesser ML (1989) Effect of wheat fiber and vitamin C and E on rectal polyps in patients with familial adenomatous polyposis. J Natl Cancer Inst 81:1290–1297

Dwyer J, Picciano MF, Raiten DJ, Members of the Steering Committee (2003) Food and dietary supplement databases for what we eat in America-NHANES. J Nutr 133 [Suppl]:624S–634S

Einspahr JG, Alberts DS, Gapstur SM, Bostick RM, Emerson SSD, Gerner EW (1997) Surrogate endpoint biomarkers as measures of colon cancer risk and their use in cancer chemoprevention trials. Cancer Epidemiol Biomarkers Prev 6:37–48

Faivre J, Bonithon-Kopp C (2002) Effect of fiber and calcium supplementation on adenoma recurrence and growth. IARC Sci Publ 156:457–461

Food and Nutrition Board, Institute of Medicine (2002) Dietary reference intakes for energy, carbohydrate, fiber, fat, fatty acids, cholesterol, protein, and amino acids. National Academy, Washington, DC

Jemal A, Murray T, Ward E, Samuels A, Tiwari RC, Ghafoor A et al (2005) CA Cancer J Clin 55:10–30

Kris-Etherton PM, Hecker KD, Bonanome A, Coval SM, Binkoski AE, Hilpert KF et al (2002) Bioactive compounds in foods: their role in the prevention of cardiovascular disease and cancer. Am J Med 113 [Suppl]:71S–88S

Lanza E, Schatzkin A, Daston C, Corle D, Freedman L, Ballard-Barbash R et al (2001) Implementation of a 4-y, high-fiber, high-fruit-and-vegetable, low-fat dietary intervention: results of dietary changes in the Polyp Prevention Trial. Am J Clin Nutr 74:387–401

Liu S, Willett WC, Manson JE, Hu FB, Rosner B, Colditz G (2003) Relation between changes in intakes of dietary fiber and grain products and changes in weight and development of obesity among middle-aged women. Am J Clin Nutr 78:920–927

MacLennan R, Macrae FA, Bain C, Battistutta D, Chapuis P, Gratten H (1995) Randomized trial of intake of fat, fiber and beta carotene to prevent colorectal adenomas. J Natl Cancer Inst 87:1760–1766

Marlett JA, McBurney MI, Slavin JL (2002) Position of the American Dietetic Association: health implications of dietary fiber. J Am Diet Assoc 102:993–1000

McKeown-Eyssen G, Brigh-See E, Dion P, Bruce WR, Jazmajl V (1994) A randomized trial of a low-fat high-fibre diet in the recurrence of colorectal polyps. J Clin Epidemiol 47:525–536

Milner JA (2004) Molecular targets for bioactive food components. J Nutr 134 [Suppl]:2492S–2498S

Muti P, Awad AB, Schunemann H, Fink CS, Hovey K, Freudenheim JL et al (2003) A plant-food-based diet modifies the serum beta-sitosterol concentration of hyperandrogenic postmenopausal women. J Nutr 133:4252–4255

Park V, Hunter DJ, Spiegelman D, Bergkvist L, Berrino F, van den Brandt PA et al (2005) Dietary fiber intake and risk of colorectal cancer. JAMA 294:2849–2857

Polsinelli ML, Rock CL, Henderson SA, Drewnowski A (1998) Plasma carotenoids as biomarkers of fruit and vegetable servings in women. J Am Diet Assoc 98:194–196

Prentice RL (2000) Future possibilities in the prevention of breast cancer. Fat and fiber and breast cancer research. Breast Cancer Res 2:268–276

Prentice RL (2003) Dietary assessment and the reliability of nutritional epidemiology reports. Lancet 362:182–183

Prentice RL, Willett WC, Greenwald P, Alberts D, Bernstein L, Boyd NF et al (2004) Nutrition and physical activity and chronic disease prevention: research strategies and recommendations. J Natl Cancer Inst 96:1276–1287

Rock CL (1998) Nutritional factors in cancer prevention. Hematol Oncol Clin N Am 12:975–991

Rock CL, Moskowitz A, Huizar B, Saenz CC, Clark JT, Daly TL et al (2001) High vegetable and fruit diet intervention in premenopausal women with cervical intraepithelial neoplasia. J Am Diet Assoc 101:1167–1174

Schatzkin A, Lanza E, Corle D, Lance P, Iber F, Caan B et al (2000) Lack of effect of a low-fat, high-fiber diet on the recurrence of colorectal adenomas. N Engl J Med 342:1149–1155

Slavin J (2003) Why whole grains are protective: biological mechanisms. Proc Nutr Soc 62:129–134

Willett WC (1999) Goals for nutrition in the year 2000. CA Cancer J Clin 49:331–352

Willett WC (2000) Diet and cancer. Oncologist 5:393–404

World Cancer Research Fund in Association with American Institute for Cancer Research (WCRF/AICR) (1997) Food, nutrition and the prevention of cancer: a global perspective. American Institute for Cancer Research, Washington, DC

15 Prevention and Early Detection of Colorectal Cancer – New Horizons

Gad Rennert

Recent Results in Cancer Research, Vol. 174
© Springer-Verlag Berlin Heidelberg 2007

Abstract

Colorectal cancer is potentially one of the most preventable malignancies. Nutritional awareness (low fat, low red meat, high fruits and vegetables) and regular physical activity have major potential for primary prevention of this malignancy, while early detection technologies have the potential of both influencing mortality from colorectal cancer as well as enhancing primary prevention through detection and removal of lesions that could potentially develop into cancer. While the potential for prevention is large, its materialization is far from being optimal. The large-scale lifestyle changes in the population necessary to reduce colorectal cancer rates are hard to achieve, and most of the early detection technologies are either invasive or otherwise nonappealing to the population. Thus, without abandoning the proven prevention methods, new avenues need to be investigated to deal with this malignancy, which carries both high morbidity and high mortality. Such new avenues can now be followed, both in prevention and detection. Chemoprevention, or the use of medications to prevent disease, has now been extensively explored in colorectal cancer. Some of these interventions, such as supplemental fibers, have failed to demonstrate the anticipated effect, while others such as calcium supplementation have been shown to reduce formation of premalignant lesions, polyps, or adenomas. Data accumulating in recent years have suggested that aspirin, nonsteroidal anti-inflammatory drugs, and selective COX-II inhibitors all have a potential to reduce both colorectal cancer and colorectal adenomas. Issues of safety and therapeutic indexes have recently come up as barriers to the use of COX-II inhibitors, and have again drawn attention to aspirin as a potential drug of choice. Association studies have also shown a major potential role for statins in colorectal cancer prevention. New methodologies in cancer detection involve the introduction of colonography or virtual colonoscopy, and the development of methods of detection of genetic somatic mutations in feces or peripheral blood. While radiological techniques currently avoid the need for premedication and are less invasive, they currently still require similar gut cleansing to colonoscopy, can also lead to perforation, are costly, and carry a non-negligible exposure to radiation. Genetic analysis of the stool for mutations in tumor cells is evolving as a promising technique, struggling to achieve both high sensitivity and high specificity with the right combination of mutations sought. With all of these developments taking place, the near future will undoubtedly bring about the expected reduction in colorectal cancer mortality.

Background

Colorectal cancer is among the most common cancers in the developed world with increasing incidence rates. Lifestyle factors typical to developed countries are therefore implicated as the major cause of colorectal cancer (Potter and Hunter 2002). While many promising new treatments for colorectal cancer have been introduced in recent years, it remains one of the more lethal tumors, with only about 50% of the patients surviving for 5 years or more. Late stage at diagnosis is one of the reasons for the poor outcome. Primary prevention and early detection are therefore of major importance in the fight against this disease.

The Unconsummated Potential

Colorectal cancer is considered to be a preventable malignancy. Consuming a diet high in vegetables and fruits, low in red meat and possibly low in fat, engaging in regular physical activity, and avoiding obesity have all been demonstrated to be related to reduced risk for colorectal cancer in a variety of association studies (Wallace et al. 2005; Frezza et al. 2006; Rapp et al. 2005; Chao et al. 2005; Larrson et al. 2005; Bingham 2006). Studies have also demonstrated a negative association between the consumption of calcium and dairy products and folic acid and the risk of colorectal cancer (Slattery et al. 2004a; Larsson et al. 2005). A large variety of early detection technologies offer potential for both reduced mortality from colorectal cancer, as well as for primary cancer prevention through detection and removal of polyps and adenomas that could potentially develop into cancer (Canadian Task Force 2001). The current most commonly used technologies for early detection are tests for the detection of occult blood in stool (with a variety of products of varying sensitivity) and lower gastrointestinal tract endoscopy (sigmoidoscopy and colonoscopy).

Materializing the Potential – What Are the Facts?

While the potential for prevention is large, its materialization is far from being optimal. As a result, there is a continuous increase in the incidence of colorectal cancer in many Western countries. Meaningful lifestyle changes by the population at large, necessary for reduction in colorectal cancer rates, are hard to achieve, and most of the early detection technologies are either invasive or otherwise nonappealing to the population, leading to low performance. Thus, without deserting the proven prevention methods, new avenues need to be explored to deal with this common and deadly malignancy.

New Horizons in Chemoprevention

Chemoprevention, or the use of medications to prevent disease, has been extensively explored in colorectal cancer in recent years. Some of these interventions, such as supplemental fibers, have failed to demonstrate the anticipated effect (Park et al. 2005; Rennert 2002; Bingham 2006). A recent randomized controlled study in women failed to demonstrate a preventive effect of a low-fat diet (Beresford et al. 2006). These failures occurred in spite of massive supportive data for the protective effects of these approaches gained in observational studies and raise a variety of questions about the validity of results of various study methods (Rennert 2006). Other interventions such as calcium supplementation have been shown to slightly reduce formation of premalignant lesions, polyps, or adenomas (Baron et al. 1999; Grau et al. 2005).

What Drugs for Chemoprevention?

Chemopreventive drugs for an average risk population must be proven efficacious and safe. Data accumulating in recent years have suggested that aspirin, nonsteroidal anti-inflammatory drugs and possibly also selective COX-II inhibitors, all have a potential to reduce colorectal cancer and colorectal adenomas in average and high-risk populations (Thun et al. 2002; Hull 2005). Such data came from association case–control and cohort studies (Poynter et al. 2005; Chan et al. 2005; Sansbury et al. 2005; Slattery et al. 2004b), and from randomized controlled studies (RCTs) (Baron et al. 2003; Sandler et al. 2003; Benamouzig et al. 2003; Phillips et al. 2002) (Table 1) and were supported by laboratory studies (Charames and Bapat 2006; Din et al. 2004; Boon et al. 2004; Reddy et al. 2005). Two randomized trials have not demonstrated a preventive effect of these drugs against CRC (Cook et al. 2005; Gann et al. 1993). Issues of safety and therapeutic indexes have recently come up as barriers to the use of COX-II inhibitors (Bresalier et al. 2005; Solomon et al. 2005), and have again drawn attention to aspirin as a potential drug of choice.

Table 1 Studies evaluating the effects of aspirin on colorectal adenomas and carcinomas prevention

Author	Ref journal	Study type	Target population	N	Aspirin dosage	End-point	Follow-up time	Aspirin effect
Baron et al. 2003	N Eng J Med	RCT	Previous adenoma	1,121	81	Adenoma recurrence	3 years	0.81 (0.69–0.96)
					325			0.96 (0.81–1.13)
Sandler et al. 2003	N Eng J Med	RCT	Previous CRC	635	325	Adenoma formation	12.8 months (mean)	0.65 (0.46–0.91)
Cook et al. 2005	JAMA	RCT	Healthy women (WHS)	39,876	100 QOD	CRC	10 years	0.97 (0.77–1.24)
Chan et al. 2005	JAMA	Cohort	NHS/healthy	82,911	325 (14+ pills/week)	CRC	10+ years	0.77 (0.67–0.88) 0.47 (0.31–0.71)
Benamouzig et al. 2003	Gastroenterology	RCT	Previous adenoma	272	160	Adenoma formation	1 year	0.85 (0.57–1.26)
					300			0.61 (0.37–0.99)
Gann et al. 1993	J Natl Cancer Inst	RCT	PHS Physician Health Study	22,071	325 QOD	CRC adenomas	5 years	1.15 (0.80–1.65) 0.86 (0.68–1.10)

RCT randomized controlled trial, CRC colorectal cancer, WHS, QOD

What Doses? What Side Effects?

There is insufficient data to decide if a full dose (325 mg) or a low-dose (75–100 mg) of aspirin is needed to achieve a preventive effect. Baron et al. (2003) found low-dose aspirin to reduce the risk of adenoma recurrence, while Sandler et al. (2003) found the high dose, and not the low dose, effective.

Randomized controlled trials of low-dose aspirin in males and females have shown only a slightly increased risk of hemorrhage compared to control groups (Wald and Law 2003; Cook et al. 2005). If low-dose aspirin is proven effective in colorectal cancer prevention, the low side effects profile will make it highly attractive for population-wide prevention. A recent association study has also shown a major potential role for statins in colorectal cancer prevention (Poynter et al. 2005), but randomized controlled trials conducted for the purpose of secondary prevention of coronary heart diseases have failed to show such an effect (Jacobs et al. 2006), as did a recent meta analysis (Dale 2006). In practical terms, low-dose aspirin and statins are already commonly used for the purpose of cardiovascular disease prevention (Ajani et al. 2006; Teeling et al. 2005). It is there-fore only a matter of time before their preventive effect on colorectal cancer incidence is expected to be seen and no further targeted action will be needed to encourage the population to use them against colorectal cancer.

New Horizons in Early Detection

New technologies in cancer detection include the introduction of colonography or virtual colo-noscopy and the development of genetic meth-ods to detect tumor-related mutations in feces or peripheral blood.

Colonography/Virtual Colonoscopy

These modern radiological techniques employ advanced CT technology to detect polyps and tu-mors in the colon. Pickhardt et al. (2003) demon-strated that high-quality performance of virtual colonoscopy can achieve a detection rate or sen-sitivity comparable to that of optic colonoscopy (Fig. 1). This was achieved using a flythrough technique coupled with a 2D multidetector with narrow collimation and employing the Viatronix

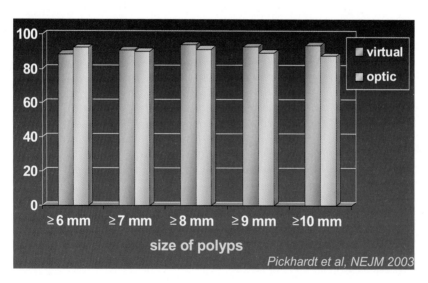

Fig. 1 Sensitivity of virtual colonoscopy compared to optic colonoscopy (using flythrough technique and 2D multide-tector with 1.25–2.50 mm collimation and Viatronix V3D)

V3D software. It is important to emphasize that employing less than optimal technology yields a detection outcome that is inferior to that of optic colonoscopy (Mulhall et al. 2005). The noninvasiveness and lack of need for premedication of this technique make it an attractive option for mass screening. Nevertheless, currently available technology still requires intensive colon cleansing, which is disliked by the population, requires insufflation that can lead to perforation if not carefully monitored, and involves a high cost, similar to optic colonoscopy. Modern tagging techniques, which will render colon cleansing unnecessary and make the examination prep-free, will undoubtedly improve its appeal to the population. Two deficiencies of the virtual colonoscopy over optic colonoscopy are exposure to radiation, at a current magnitude of 5–10 mSv or two to three times the annual natural background exposure, and the lack of ability to remove or biopsy a polyp or a lesion when identified, thus requiring an intervening optic colonoscopy. It is therefore plausible that in the future virtual colonoscopy will be more suitable for screening average risk population with a low pretest probability of disease (adenomas, cancers) and therefore low probability of need for biopsies. At the same time,

symptomatic and high-risk people, with higher pretest probability for findings, should continue to be offered optic colonoscopy. If a decision to incorporate periodic virtual colonoscopy into a routine screening program is made, major attention needs to be paid to assuring high-quality testing with multidetector scanners, flythrough technology, and narrow collimation, while controlling for radiation level and cost.

Stool Genetics

Genetic analysis of the stool for mutations in tumor cells is evolving as a promising colorectal cancer screening technique. While the genetic background of sporadic colorectal cancer formation is well described (Fearon and Vogelstein 1999; Bodmer 2006) (Fig. 2), the optimal panel of mutations to be sought in a stool sample that will reach high sensitivity and specificity for adenoma and cancer detection is still undetermined (Davies et al. 2005; Brenner and Rennert 2005). Most studies have evaluated mutations in APC, p53 and k-ras, representing the classical *WNT*-pathway, while others have added mutations in the MSI pathway such as BAT26 or MLH1. In

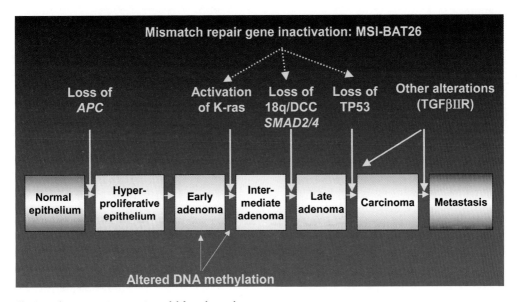

Fig. 2 Multi-step carcinogenesis model for colorectal tumors

addition, more generalized markers of DNA integrity and methylation such as long DNA or DNA integrity assay have been added (Imperiale et al. 2004; Tagore et al. 2003; Koshiji et al. 2002; Rengucci et al. 2001; Dong et al. 2001; Ahlquist et al. 2000). These approaches have yielded sensitivity varying between 51.6% and 100% for cancers and 10.5% and 81.8 for adenomas, with specificity of 86.7% and 100% for carcinomas. The most sensitive were the least specific (Table 2). However, caution should be practiced at this stage, as all the above-mentioned studies have only involved between 22 and 52 cancers each. This genetic approach carries a major appeal as it is easy to perform, is noninvasive, and does not carry any noticeable risk. If it can be performed with modest cost and if the need for bulks of stool can be avoided, it will carry an even higher appeal for population screening. It has been shown that stool can be recovered from FOBT cards and analyzed for k-ras (Lev 2000) to significantly improve the positive predictive value of the FOB test itself (Rennert et al. 2006). An approach based on test cards rather than bulks of feces might carry an even higher appeal to the population.

Summary

CRC is highly preventable, with a combination of lifestyle changes, chemoprevention with simple drugs, and adenoma identification through screening. Mortality can be further reduced by early detection of cancer using common screening technologies such as FOBT or endoscopy.

Due to their high use for other indications, the effect of commonly used drugs is expected to be seen even without organized interventions.

Virtual colonoscopy and fecal DNA tests are very promising technologies that, in the near future, will enhance detection of premalignant neoplasms and lead to prevention of colorectal cancer.

Table 2 Studies evaluating screening for colorectal tumors employing stool-based DNA markers

DNA markers	Number of CRCs detected	CRC sensitivity (%)	Number of adenomas detected	Adenoma sensitivity (%)	Number of false-positive controls	CRC specificity (%)
21 Mutations in APC, TP53 and KRAS; BAT26 and long DNA	16/31	51.6	110/1,051	10.5	79/1423	94.4
21 Mutations in APC, TP53 and KRAS; BAT26 and DNA-integrity assay	33/52	63.5	16/28	57.1	8/212	96.2
15 Mutations in APC, TP53 and KRAS; BAT26 and long DNA	20/22	90.9	9/11	81.8	2/28	93
7 Mutations in TP53 and KRAS; 5 MSI markers	31/46	67.4	Not performed	N/A	0/18	100
3 Mutations in TP53 and KRAS; BAT26	36/51	70.6	Not performed	N/A	Not performed	N/A
Loss of heterozygosity at the microsatellite loci APC, TP53, DCC, MLH1, D9S162, IFNα and D9S171	30/30	100	Not performed	N/A	2/15	86.7

Davies et al. 2005

References

Ahlquist DA, Skoletsky JE, Boynton KA, Harrington JJ, Mahoney DW, Pierceall WE, Thibodeau SN, Shuber AP (2000) Colorectal cancer screening by detection of altered human DNA in stool: feasibility of a multitarget assay panel. Gastroenterology 119:1219–1227

Ajani UA, Ford ES, Greenland KJ, Giles WH, Mokdad AH (2006) Aspirin use among U.S. Adults behavioral risk factor surveillance system. Am J Prev Med 30:74–77

Baron JA, Beach M, Mandel JS, van Stolk RU, Haile RW, Sandler RS, Rothstein R, Summers RW, Snover DC, Beck GJ, Bond JH, Greenberg ER (1999) Calcium supplements for the prevention of colorectal adenomas. Calcium Polyp Prevention Study Group. N Engl J Med 340:101–107

Baron JA, Cole BF, Sandler RS, Haile RW, Ahnen D, Bresalier R, McKeown-Eyssen G, Summers RW, Rothstein R, Burke CA, Snover DC, Church TR, Allen JI, Beach M, Beck GJ, Bond JH, Byers T, Greenberg ER, Mandel JS, Marcon N, Mott LA, Pearson L, Saibil F, van Stolk RU (2003) A randomized trial of aspirin to prevent colorectal adenomas. N Engl J Med 348:891–899

Benamouzig R, Deyra J, Martin A, Girard B, Jullian E, Piednoir B, Couturier D, Coste T, Little J, Chaussade S (2003) Daily soluble aspirin and prevention of colorectal adenoma recurrence: one-year results of the APACC trial. Gastroenterology 125:328–336

Beresford SAA, Johnson KC, Ritenbaugh C et al. (2006) Low-fat dietary pattern and risk of colorectal cancer. JAMA 295:643–654

Bingham S (2006) The fibre-folate debate in colo-rectal cancer. Proc Nutr Soc 65:19–23

Bodmer WF (2006) Cancer genetics: colorectal cancer as a model. J Hum Genet 51:391–396

Boon EM, Keller JJ, Wormhoudt TA, Giardiello FM, Offerhaus GJ, van der Neut R, Pals ST (2004) Sulindac targets nuclear beta-catenin accumulation and Wnt signalling in adenomas of patients with familial adenomatous polyposis and in human colorectal cancer cell lines. Br J Cancer 90:224–229

Brenner DE, Rennert G (2005) Fecal DNA biomarkers for the detection of colorectal neoplasia: Attractive, but is it feasible? J Natl Cancer Inst 97:1107–1109

Bresalier RS, Sandler RS, Quan H, Bolognese JA, Oxenius B, Horgan K, Lines C, Riddell R, Morton D, Lanas A, Konstam MA, Baron JA; Adenomatous Polyp Prevention on Vioxx (APPROVe) Trial Investigators (2005) Cardiovascular events associated with rofecoxib in a colorectal adenoma chemoprevention trial. N Engl J Med 352:1092–1102

Canadian Task Force on Preventive Health Care (2001) Colorectal cancer screening. Recommendation statement from the Canadian Task Force on Preventive Health Care. CMAJ 165:206–208

Chan AT, Giovannucci EL, Meyerhardt JA, Schernhammer ES, Curhan GC, Fuchs CS (2005) Long-term use of aspirin and nonsteroidal anti-inflammatory drugs and risk of colorectal cancer. JAMA 294:914–923

Chao A, Thun MJ, Connell CJ, McCullough ML, Jacobs EJ, Flanders WD, Rodriguez C, Sinha R, Calle EE (2005) Meat consumption and risk of colorectal cancer. JAMA 293:172–182

Charames GS, Bapat B (2006) Cyclooxygenase-2 knockdown by RNA interference in colon cancer. Int J Oncol 28:543–549

Cook NR, Lee IM, Gaziano JM, Gordon D, Ridker PM, Manson JE, Hennekens CH, Buring JE (2005) Low-dose aspirin in the primary prevention of cancer: the Women's Health Study: a randomized controlled trial. JAMA 294:47–55

Dale KM, Coleman CI, Henyan NN, Kluger J, White CM (2006) Statins and cancer risk: a meta-analysis. JAMA 295:74–80

Davies RJ, Miller R, Coleman N (2005) Colorectal cancer screening: prospects for molecular stool analysis. Nat Rev Cancer 5:199–209

Din FV, Dunlop MG, Stark LA (2004) Evidence for colorectal cancer cell specificity of aspirin effects on NF kappa B signalling and apoptosis. Br J Cancer 91:381–388

Dong SM, Traverso G, Johnson C, Geng L, Favis R, Boynton K, Hibi K, Goodman SN, D'Allessio M, Paty P, Hamilton SR, Sidransky D, Barany F, Levin B, Shuber A, Kinzler KW, Vogelstein B, Jen J (2001) Detecting colorectal cancer in stool with the use of multiple genetic targets. J Natl Cancer Inst 93:858–865

Fearon ER, Vogelstein B (1990) A genetic model for colorectal tumorigenesis. Cell 61:759–767

Frezza EE, Wachtel MS, Chiriva-Internati M (2006) Influence of obesity on the risk of developing colon cancer. Gut 55:285–291

Gann PH, Manson JE, Glynn RJ, Buring JE, Hennekens CH (1993) Low-dose aspirin and incidence of colorectal tumors in a randomized trial. J Natl Cancer Inst 85:1220–1224

Grau MV, Baron JA, Barry EL, Sandler RS, Haile RW, Mandel JS, Cole BF (2005) Interaction of calcium supplementation and nonsteroidal anti-inflammatory drugs and the risk of colorectal adenomas. Cancer Epidemiol Biomarkers Prev 14:2353–2358

Hull MA (2005) Cyclooxygenase-2: how good is it as a target for cancer chemoprevention? Eur J Cancer 41:1854–1863

Imperiale TF, Ransohoff DF, Itzkowitz SH, Turnbull BA, Ross ME (2004) Fecal DNA versus fecal occult blood for colorectal cancer screening in an average-risk population. N Engl J Med 351:2704–2714

Jacobs EJ, Rodriguez C, Brady KA, Connell CJ, Thun MJ, Calle EE (2006) Cholesterol-lowering drugs and colorectal cancer incidence in a large United States cohort. J Natl Cancer Inst 98:69–72

Koshiji M, Yonekura Y, Saito T, Yoshioka K (2002) Microsatellite analysis of fecal DNA for coilorectal cancer detection. J Surg Oncol 80:34–40

Larsson SC, Giovannucci E, Wolk A (2005) A prospective study of dietary folate intake and risk of colorectal cancer: modification by caffeine intake and cigarette smoking. Cancer Epidemiol Biomarkers Prev 14:740–743

Larsson SC, Rafter J, Holmberg L, Bergkvist L, Wolk A (2005) Red meat consumption and risk of cancers of the proximal colon, distal colon and rectum: the Swedish Mammography Cohort. Int J Cancer 113:829–834

Lev Z, Kislitsin D, Rennert G, Lerner A (2000) Utilization of K-ras Mutations Identified in Stool DNA for the Early Detection of Colorectal Cancer. J Cell Biochem 34 [Suppl]:35–39

Mulhall BP, Veerappan GR, Jackson JL (2005) Meta-analysis: computed tomographic colonography. Ann Intern Med 142:635–650

Park Y, Hunter DJ, Spiegelman D, Bergkvist L, Berrino F, van den Brandt PA, Buring JE, Colditz GA, Freudenheim JL, Fuchs CS, Giovannucci E, Goldbohm RA, Graham S, Harnack L, Hartman AM, Jacobs DR Jr, Kato I, Krogh V, Leitzmann MF, McCullough ML, Miller AB, Pietinen P, Rohan TE, Schatzkin A, Willett WC, Wolk A, Zeleniuch-Jacquotte A, Zhang SM, Smith-Warner SA (2005) Dietary fiber intake and risk of colorectal cancer: a pooled analysis of prospective cohort studies. JAMA 294:2849–2857

Phillips RK, Wallace MH, Lynch PM, Hawk E, Gordon GB, Saunders BP, Wakabayashi N, Shen Y, Zimmerman S, Godio L, Rodrigues-Bigas M, Su LK, Sherman J, Kelloff G, Levin B, Steinbach G; FAP Study Group (2002) A randomised, double blind, placebo controlled study of celecoxib, a selective cyclooxygenase 2 inhibitor, on duodenal polyposis in familial adenomatous polyposis. Gut 50:857–860

Pickhardt PJ, Choi JR, Hwang I, Butler JA, Puckett ML, Hildebrandt HA, Wong RK, Nugent PA, Mysliwiec PA, Schindler WR (2003) Computed tomographic virtual colonoscopy to screen for colorectal neoplasia in asymptomatic adults. N Engl J Med 349:2191–2200

Potter JD, Hunter D (2002) Colorectal cancer. In: Adami HO, Hunter D, Trichopoulos D (eds) Textbook of cancer epidemiology. Oxford University Press, Oxford, pp 188–211

Poynter JN, Gruber SB, Higgins PDR, Almog R, Bonner JD, Rennert HS, Low M, Greenson JK, Rennert G (2005) Statins and the Risk of Colorectal Cancer. N Engl J Med 352:2184–2192

Rapp K, Schroeder J, Klenk J, Stoehr S, Ulmer H, Concin H, Diem G, Oberaigner W, Weiland SK (2005) Obesity and incidence of cancer: a large cohort study of over 145,000 adults in Austria. Br J Cancer 93:1062–1067

Reddy BS, Patlolla JM, Simi B, Wang SH, Rao CV (2005) Prevention of colon cancer by low doses of celecoxib, a cyclooxygenase inhibitor, administered in diet rich in omega-3 polyunsaturated fatty acids. Cancer Res 65:8022–8027

Rengucci C, Maiolo P, Saragoni L, Zoli W, Amadori D, Calistri D (2001) Multiple detection of genetic alterations in tumors and stool. Clin Cancer Res 7:590–593

Rennert G (2002) Dietary intervention studies and cancer prevention. Eur J Cancer Prev 11:419–425

Rennert G (2006) Are we taking the right approach in planning chemoprevention studies? Nat Clin Pract Oncol 3:464–465

Rennert G, Brenner D, Rennert HS, Lev Z (2006) K-ras in stool from test cards improves the positive predictive value of FOBT. Cancer Epidemiol Biomarkers Prev (submitted)

Sandler RS, Halabi S, Baron JA, Budinger S, Paskett E, Keresztes R, Petrelli N, Pipas JM, Karp DD, Loprinzi CL, Steinbach G, Schilsky R (2003) A randomized trial of aspirin to prevent colorectal adenomas in patients with previous colorectal cancer. N Engl J Med 348:883–90

Sansbury LB, Millikan RC, Schroeder JC, Moorman PG, North KE, Sandler RS (2005) Use of nonsteroidal antiinflammatory drugs and risk of colon cancer in a population-based, case-control study of African Americans and Whites. Am J Epidemiol 162:548–558

Slattery ML, Neuhausen SL, Hoffman M, Caan B, Curtin K, Ma KN, Samowitz W (2004a) Dietary calcium, vitamin D, VDR genotypes and colorectal cancer. Int J Cancer 111:750–756

Slattery ML, Samowitz W, Hoffman M, Ma KN, Levin TR, Neuhausen S (2004b) Aspirin, NSAIDs, and colorectal cancer: possible involvement in an insulin-related pathway. Cancer Epidemiol Biomarkers Prev 13:538–545

Solomon SD, McMurray JJ, Pfeffer MA, Wittes J, Fowler R, Finn P, Anderson WF, Zauber A, Hawk E, Bertagnolli M Adenoma prevention with celecoxib (APC) study investigators (2005) Cardiovascular risk associated with celecoxib in a clinical trial for colorectal adenoma prevention. N Engl J Med 352:1071–1080

Tagore KS Lawson MJ, Yucaitis JA, Gage R, Orr T, Shuber AP, Ross ME (2003) Sensitivity and specificity of a stool DNA multitarget assay panel for the detection of advanced colorectal neoplasia. Clin Colorectal Cancer 3:47–53

Teeling M, Bennett K, Feely J (2005) The influence of guidelines on the use of statins: analysis of prescribing trends 1998–2002. Br J Clin Pharmacol 59:227–232

Thun MJ, Henley SJ, Patrono C (2002) Nonsteroidal anti-inflammatory drugs as anticancer agents: mechanistic, pharmacologic, and clinical issues. J Natl Cancer Inst 94:252–266

Wald NJ, Law MR (2003) A strategy to reduce cardiovascular disease by more than 80%. BMJ 326:1419

Wallace K, Baron JA, Karagas MR, Cole BF, Byers T, Beach MA, Pearson LH, Burke CA, Silverman WB, Sandler RS (2005) The association of physical activity and body mass index with the risk of large bowel polyps. Cancer Epidemiol Biomarkers Prev 14:2082–2086

Part VI Prevention of Skin and Brain Tumors

16

New Perspectives on Melanoma Pathogenesis and Chemoprevention

Frank L. Meyskens, Jr., Patrick J. Farmer, Sun Yang, Hoda Anton-Culver

Recent Results in Cancer Research, Vol. 174
© Springer-Verlag Berlin Heidelberg 2007

Abstract

Epidemiologic studies implicate ultraviolet radiation (sunlight) as an etiologic agent for the pathogenesis of melanoma. However, the experimental evidence is less convincing. We present information from recent experimental findings that elevation of reactive oxygen species follows from melanin serving as a redox generator, and that this may play an important role in the etiology and pathogenesis of cutaneous melanoma. These observations offer a new paradigm for the development of preventive (and therapeutic) approaches to this disease.

Introduction

The incidence of melanoma has increased rapidly in the last few decades. Fortunately, early detection and prompt surgical intervention has increased 5-year survival in 1970 from 50% to nearly 90% today. Nevertheless, the morbidity from this disease is considerable and the years of productive life lost still high. Epidemiologic and experimental data has confirmed that ultraviolet light radiation (UVR) is etiologic for most cases of non-melanoma skin cancer. However, the relationship and correlation of UVR and melanoma is much more complex. Its definitive involvement in the direct etiology and pathogenesis of the disease is problematic and requires a better mechanistic understanding and/or reconsideration of its involvement (Berwick et al. 2005).

Epidemiologic data suggests that "at best" UVR accounts for only 40%–50% of the attributable risk for melanoma. The data is not simple, and unlike non-melanoma skin cancer, the risk is not correlated with cumulative UVR exposure, but rather, intermittent exposure, especially serious sunburns earlier in life. Also, intensive "sun sense" campaigns have not led to a decrease in the incidence of melanoma, although evidence does suggest that regular exposure to sunlamps may indeed be harmful.

Implicating UVR is also difficult at a molecular level as UVR-signature mutations, although uniformly found in non-melanoma skin cancer, are rarely detected in benign nevi, dysplastic nevi, or in primary or advanced melanoma cells. Furthermore, direct transformation of human melanocytes with UVR has not been successfully accomplished, despite many attempts to do so. Recent studies of the distribution of BRAF mutations in primary melanomas suggest that there are at least two pathways: one in which chronic sun damage is not associated with BRAF mutation and a second in which BRAF mutations occurred in melanomas that developed in skin that was not sun-damaged . (Curtin et al. 2005). In neither case were classical UVR mutations in the BRAF gene evident. However, the development of a transgenic mouse model that, after UVR exposure at the neonatal stage, does lead to melanomas that simulate the human disease pathologically may help elucidate the etiologic and pathogenic role of this carcinogen (Ha et al. 2005; Wolnicka-Glubisz and Noonan 2006). However, this model is highly engineered (hepatocyte growth factor and stem cell factor have been introduced) and its direct relevance to understanding the pathogenesis of human melanoma remains to be established.

In toto, this data suggests several distinct possibilities: UVR's transforming effect on DNA is mediated by reactive oxygen species (ROS) or other molecules; UVR works indirectly to transform melanocytes via a paracrine effect; UVR works in concert with a yet to be identified co-carcinogen; or that the epidemiologic results are spurious and UVR is not involved at all in melanoma pathogenesis.

Developing a New Paradigm for Melanoma Etiology and Pathogenesis

The adverse results of the β-carotene and lung cancer prevention trials in which this nutrient (although at pharmacologic doses) led to more, rather than fewer, lung cancers in heavy smokers (Omenn et al. 1994) led me to reconsider the role of antioxidants in carcinogenesis, especially in melanoma genesis. One of the unique features of melanocytes is that they produce the unique differentiation product melanin whose major function has always been presumed to be protection against UVR. There are several unique features about melanin and its synthesis that merit comment:

- Hydrogen peroxide is generated and consumed during the synthesis of melanin.
- Melanin synthesis occurs in a complex and poorly understood complex organelle, the melanosome, which has many lysosomal properties.
- Melanin functions as an antioxidant in normal melanocytes.

For some time, it has been recognized that abnormalities of melanin synthesis lead to a range of benign pigmentary diseases. There is also available considerable descriptive data that has suggested melanosomes are abnormal in melanoma cells and became progressively deranged during the pathogenic process (Rhodes et al. 1988). However, the functional consequences of these abnormalities for transformation have been largely ignored.

Redox Status of Melanocytes and Melanoma Cells

We initially asked a simple question: How do melanocytes respond to oxidative stress? (Meyskens et al. 1997). The conclusions from our studies are summarized as follows, and illustrated in Fig. 1. Melanoma were exposed to a low dose of H_2O_2 generated by adding titered amounts of glucose oxidase to the medium, and with a fixed dose of glucose, a predictable amount of H_2O_2 was generated. (Using UVR-B as the source of ROS was too complex as it produces many cellular effects including direct DNA damage.) The intracellular oxidative response was determined by luminol-enhanced chemiluminescence, a crude signal for superoxide/peroxide flux. The results were surprising, in that no fluorescence signal was apparent in several non-melanin-containing cell lines. In normal human melanocytes (NHM), a small signal was initially generated, but rapidly suppressed over a few minutes. In contrast, a large and continuous chemiluminescence response was seen in all melanoma cell lines tested. The signal was quickly abrogated by added exogenous catalase in both melanocytes and melanoma cells. However, when exogenous superoxide dismutase was added, the luminescence signal was mildly decreased in melanocytes but greatly enhanced in all melanoma cells tested. We postulated that melanoma cells contain a potential generator of superoxide anion that was not found in melanocytes or other cells.

Further studies using various redox-sensing probes indicated that melanoma cells have increased intracellular ROS at all stages of the cell cycle compared to melanocytes, implicating that the elevation was largely due to superoxide anion (Meyskens et al. 2001). Subsequently, an electrochemical model of eumelanin (dihydroxyindole polymerized on a graphite surface) (Gidanian et al. 2002) and was used to measure ROS generation, as measured by spin trapping molecules of superoxide and hydroxyl radicals. It was demonstrated that exposure of synthetic eumelanin to oxygen led to that the generation of ROS, markedly enhanced by the addition of transition metals (Farmer et al. 2003). Previous speciation characterization had suggested that an

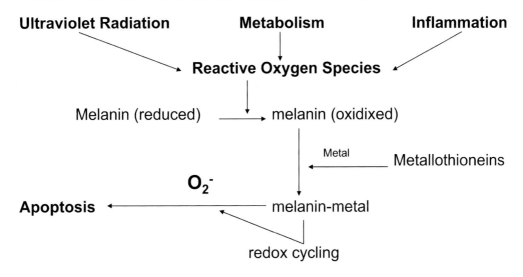

Fig. 1 The altered state of melanin during melanomagenesis. Melanin is normally in a reduced antioxidant state. Exposure to ROS leads to an oxidized condition which facilitates binding of transition metals (and other compounds such as polyphenol chlorinated biphenyls). Metal uptake into the cell is closely regulated by a family of metallothioneins. This situation sets up the oxidized melanin as a redox generator, which leads to increasing intracellular oxidative stress, a widespread adaptive response including TF upregulation, cell death, a high rate of cellular turnover and secondary intrinsic drug resistance (see Meyskens et al. 2001)

oxidized species within the melanin, a quinone imine, could serve as a powerful metal chelator (Spoganicz 2002), and this might then enhance the pro-oxidant generation of ROS. Importantly, the ROS generated by the synthetic melanin behaved in the same manner as the melanoma cell lines, in that exogenous catalase quenched the signal but superoxide dismutase greatly enhanced the signal (Farmer 2003); and using the EPR and DNA clipping assays, the similar phenomenon as described above was demonstrated with intact melanoma cells, reconfirming the initial luminescence experiments. These results suggested that melanin in melanocytes became pro-oxidant during the transformation process; utilizing the idea that metals may enhance this behavior, we have designed a number of lipophilic chelators (Farmer et al. 2005) as candidate chemotherapeutic drugs.

Part and parcel of our observations has been documentation of the constitutive upregulation of redox-sensitive transcription factors-TFs (AP-1 and NF-KB) in melanomas (Meyskens et al. 1999; McNulty et al. 2001, 2004; Yang et al.

2004; Yang and Meyskens 2005). A surprising result was that enhancement of oxidative stress led to further TFs upregulation. We therefore wondered what addition of an antioxidant would do and fortuitously chose PDTC as the antioxidant. Much to our surprise, PDTC produced apoptosis in the melanoma cells, even at very low concentrations. With the realization that PDTC is both an antioxidant and chelator, we tested a series of chelators on melanoma cell growth. Antioxidants had little effect but transition metal chelation produced a strong apoptotic effect. One such compound, disulfiram, was readily available, as it has been used for over 50 years, as an anti-alcohol aversion drug and was found to be active as an antimelanoma therapy at nanomolar concentrations (Cen et al. 2002, 2004). Based on these and other studies, we have now initiated a phase II trial of disulfiran plus arsenical trioxide for patients with advanced melanoma disease.

Based on these findings, we postulated that the etiology and pathogenesis of melanoma is a redox-driven process that offered opportunities for understanding the etiology and pathogenesis of the disease as well as providing entry points and targets for developing new therapies (Meyskens et al. 2004).

A remarkable feature of this phenomenon is that melanosomes themselves become more and more abnormal and melanin particles are released extracellularly during the progression of melanoma genesis (Jimbow et al. 1989; Rhodes et al. 1988). Our preliminary data indicate that these abnormal melanosomes are a potent source of intra- and extracellular superoxide anion.

Epidemiologic Evidence for Metal Involvement in Melanin Etiology and Pathogenesis

There is a considerable amount of occupational epidemiology that suggests that high exposure to metals or polyphenol chlorinated biphenyls (PCPs) is a risk factor for melanoma (Austin and Reynolds 1986; Loomis et al. 1997). Relative risks for printers, lithographers, electrical utility, and semiconductor workers are consistently elevated (1.5–4.0), and in many studies a dose and time exposure effect are evident (i.e., Loomis et al. 1997). Dietary studies also implicate excessive alcohol ingestion as a risk factor (RR above 2.0) (Millen et al. 2204), probably working through its metabolite acetaldehyde, which results in increased ROS. In contrast, broad dietary studies suggest that dietary antioxidants are protective against melanoma development (RR = 0.7).

No genetic studies of metallothioneins that regulate metal uptake or their polymorphisms and melanoma risk have yet been reported. However, one large study of this enzyme has shown that MT expression is an unfavorable prognostic sign and can identify those thin melanomas (<1.5 mm) that are aggressive (Weinlich et al. 2005).

Upregulation of Transcription Factors in the Pathogenesis of Melanoma

We have shown that AP-1 and NF-kB are elevated early in the pathogenic process, are protective against apoptosis-inducing events, and respond to redox stress by further upregulation in response to increased ROS. We have recently focused on the multifunctional protein apurinic/apyrimidinic endonuclease/redox effector 1 (APE/Ref-1), which functions in both the third step in base excision repair and also reduces a wide range of TFs so that they can bind to DNA sites and effect their action (Yang et al. 2005). We have recently shown that the polyphenoic antioxidant resveratrol binds to the redox pocket of Ref-1 and slows melanoma growth. We are in the process of designing a number of inhibitors based on this lead compound and by using an iterative structure–function approach and three-dimensional software modeling.

Conclusions

Our studies of the role of reactive oxygen species in melanoma genesis have led us to several conclusions. During the process of transformation and progression of the cutaneous melanocyte:

1. Melanin is converted from an antioxidant to a pro-oxidant, takes on properties of a metal chelator, becomes a redox generator, and produces large amounts of superoxide anion.
2. Intracellular oxidative stress increases markedly during pathogenesis and produces a cascade of adaptive responses with transcriptional factor activation including AP-1, Ref-1, and APE/Ref-1 that lead to drug resistance.
3. An understanding of these events provides a new scientific basis for developing novel preventive (see Meyskens et al. 1994) and therapeutic approaches (see Meyskens et al. 2001) to melanoma management (see Meyskens 2003).

References

Austin DF, Reynolds P (1986) Occupation and malignant melanoma of the skin. Recent Results Cancer Res 102:98–107

Berwick M, Armstrong BK, Ben-Porat L, Fine J, Kricker A, Eberle C, Barnhill R (2005) Sun exposure and mortality from melanoma. J Natl Cancer Inst 97:195–199

Cen D, Gonzalez R, Buckmeier J, Kahlon R, Tohidian NB, Meyskens FL Jr (2002) Disulfiram induces apoptosis in human melanoma cells: a redox-related process. Mol Cancer Ther 1:197–204

Cen D, Brayton D, Shahandeh B, Meyskens FL Jr (2004) Farmer PDisulfiram facilitates intracellular Cu uptake and induces apoptosis in human melanoma cells. J Med Chem 47:6914–6920

Curtin JA, Fridlyand J, Kageshita T, Patel HN, Busam KJ, Kutzner H, Cho KH, Aiba S, Brocker EB, LeBoit PE, Pinkel D, Bastian BC (2005) Distinct sets of genetic alterations in melanoma. N Engl J Med 353:2135–2147

Farmer PJ, Gidanian S, Shahandeh B, Di Bilio AJ, Tohidian N, Meyskens FL Jr (2003) Melanin as a target for melanoma chemotherapy: Pro-oxidant effect of oxygen and metals on melanoma viability. Pigment Cell Res 16:273–279

Farmer PJ, Brayton D, Moore C, Williams D, Shahandeh B, Cen D, Meyskens FL Jr (2005) Targeting melanoma via metal-based stress. In: Sessle JL, Doctrow SR, McMurray TJ, Lippard SJ (eds) Medicinal inorganic chemistry. 903:400–414

Gidanian S, Farmer PJ (2002) Redox behavior of melanins: direct electrochemistry of dihydroxyindolemelanin and its Cu and Zn adducts. J Inorg Biochem 89:54–60

Ha L, Noonan FP, De Fabo EC, Merlino G (2005) Animal models of melanoma. J Investig Dermatol Symp Proc 10:86–88

Jimbow K, Horikoshi T, Takahashi H, Akutsu Y, Maeda K (1989) Fine structural and immunohistochemical properties of dysplastic melanocytic nevi: comparison with malignant melanoma. J Invest Dermatol 92 [Suppl]:304S–309S

Loomis D, Browning SR, Schenck AP, Gregory E, Savitz DA (1997) Cancer mortality among electric utility workers exposed to polychlorinated biphenyls. Occup Environ Med 54:720–728

Meyskens FL Jr (2003) Management of Human Melanoma: What has the last decade wrought? Oncologist 8:448–450

Meyskens FL Jr, Chau V, Tohidian N, Buckmeier J (1997) Luminol enhanced Chemiluminescent response of human melanocytes and melanoma cells to Hydrogen Peroxide Stress. Pigment Cell Res 10:184–189

Meyskens FL Jr, Buckmeier JA, Tohidian NB (1999) Activation of nuclear factor-κB in human metastatic melanoma cells and the effect of oxidative stress. Clin Cancer Res 5:1197–1202

Meyskens FL Jr, McNulty SE, Buckmeier JA, Tohidian NB, Spillane TJ, Kahlon RS, Gonzalez RI (2001) Aberrant redox regulation in human metastatic Melanoma cells compared to normal melanocytes. Free Radical Biol Med 31:799–808

Meyskens FL Jr, Farmer P, Anton-Culver H (2004) Etiologic pathogenesis of melanoma: a unifying hypothesis for the missing attributable risk. Clin Cancer Res 10:2581–2583

McNulty S, Tohidian NB, Meyskens FL Jr (2001) Rel A, p50 and inhibitor of kappa B alpha are elevated in human metastatic melanoma cells and respond aberrantly to ultraviolet light B. Pigment Cell Res 14:456–465

McNulty S, del Rosario R, Cen D, Meyskens FL Jr, Yang S (2004) Comparative expression of NFkB proteins in melanocytes of normal skin vs. benign intradermal naevus and human metastatic melanoma biopsies. Pigment Cell Research 17:173–180

Millen AE, Tucker MA, Hartge P, Halpern A, Elder DE, Guerry D 4th, Holly EA, Sagebiel RW, Potischman N (2004) Diet and melanoma in a case-control study. Cancer Epidemiol Biomarkers Prev 13:1042–1051

Omenn GS, Goodman G, Grizzle J, Thornquist M, Meyskens FL Jr et al (1991) CARET, the β-carotene and retinol efficacy trial to prevent lung cancer in asbestos-exposed workers and in smokers. Anti-Cancer Drugs 2:79–86

Rhodes AR, Seki Y, Fitzpatrick TB, Stern RS (1988) Melanosomal alterations in dysplastic melanocytic nevi. A quantitative, ultrastructural investigation. Cancer 61:358–369

Weinlich G, Eisendle K, Hassler E, Baltaci M, Fritsch PO, Zelger B (2006) Metallothionein – overexpression as a highly significant prognostic factor in melanoma: a prospective study on 1270 patients. Br J Cancer 94:835–841

Wolnicka-Glubisz A, Noonan FP (2006) Neonatal susceptibility to UV induced cutaneous malignant melanoma in a mouse model. Photochem Photobiol Sci 5:254–260

Yang S, McNulty S, Meyskens FL Jr (2004) During human melanoma progression AP-1 binding pairs are altered with loss of c-Jun in vitro. Pigment Cell Res 17:74–83

Yang S, Meyskens FL Jr (2005) Alteration in activating protein 1 (AP-1) composition correlate with phenotypic differentiation changes induced by resveratrol in human melanoma. Mol Pharmacol 67:298–308

17 Vitamin D – An Emerging Issue in Skin Cancer Control. Implications for Public Health Practice Based on the Australian Experience

Craig Sinclair

Recent Results in Cancer Research, Vol. 174
© Springer-Verlag Berlin Heidelberg 2007

Abstract

Over recent years, the evidence has been accumulating that vitamin D has a positive impact on our health. This is likely to have an impact on the future of our public health advice related to skin cancer prevention. This paper explores, from a public health perspective based on Australian experience, how skin cancer prevention messages need to be managed in light of new information about vitamin D and in particular, the times when sun protection advice should be provided. Conclusions are drawn in relation to how the vitamin D message can be complementary to the sun protection message and explores what health practitioners should do in light of artificial tanning sunbeds being a potential source of vitamin D.

Introduction

Exposure to ultraviolet radiation accounts for around 99% of non-melanoma skin cancers and 95% of melanomas in Australia (Armstrong 2000). On the other hand, there is very good evidence that exposure to sunlight enhances vitamin D levels that can have an impact on improving bone and musculoskeletal health for older people who are vitamin D-deficient (Weathererall 2000; Bischoff et al. 2003). This paradox creates a significant challenge for those working in public health to ensure an appropriate balance is communicated to the general public that takes into account the risks and benefits of sun exposure.

With Australia having one of the highest rates of skin cancer in the world, prevention campaigns have been part of the Australian public health landscape since the early 1980s. Slogans such as Slip! Slop! Slap! and SunSmart have a very high public profile and there is considerable policy and practice in place that reinforces sun protective behaviour (Montague et al. 2001).

The Cancer Council Victoria has the longest standing and best evaluated program in Australia where there has been population monitoring of sun protective behaviour and attitudes since 1987. Over this time there has been a significant reduction in the desire to tan, improved use of sun protective items such as hats and sunscreen and a significant reduction in sunburn rates (Hill et al. 1993; Dobbinson et al. 2002). The benefit of these campaigns has been a reduction in non-melanoma skin cancer rates in younger age groups (Staples et al. 2006).

The improvement in sun protection policies and practices has come about largely because of a long standing integrated health promotion intervention that utilises mass media as the primary method to communicate to the general population combined with community-based interventions. Given this success, it is not too surprising that the media have been very responsive to research reports that highlight the benefits of vitamin D that may run counter to well-established skin cancer prevention messages.

Vitamin D Deficiency

In recent years, research has identified findings that were showing high levels of mild (between 25 and 50 nmol/l) vitamin D deficiency in the general populations in the southern states of Australia over winter months. Any levels less than 50 nmol/l can lead to increased parathyroid hormone secretion and high bone turnover (Working Group of the Australian and New Zealand Bone and Mineral Society 2005). In a Geelong (Victoria 37°S) study by Pascoe et al., it was shown that 43% of females over the winter months were mildly vitamin D-deficient and 8% of 20- to 59-year-old women were regarded as moderately to severely vitamin D-deficient (less than 25 nmol/l) (Pasco et al. 2001). In addition to this, 80% of dark-skinned veiled women were noted as being vitamin D deficient. Older people who are institutionalised or housebound are also at a particularly high risk of vitamin D deficiency (Flicker et al. 2003; Sambrook et al. 2002). Vitamin D deficiency is not just confined to adults: in a Tasmanian (42°S) study, it was found that 10% of healthy 8-year-olds (mean age) were found to be mildly deficient during the winter months (Jones et al. 1999).

Vitamin D production decreases during winter when the intensity of ultraviolet radiation is lower. The body can rely on tissue stores of vitamin D for between 30 and 60 days, assuming vitamin D levels are adequate prior to winter (Grover and Moreley 2001). In most cases, any vitamin D reduction during winter is corrected in summer when more sunlight is received with more time spent outdoors. While this correction may occur, it is still important to prevent deficiency during winter, as fracture rates increase with deficiency, particularly with older adults (Weathererall 2000).

Key Outcomes from a Joint Position Statement

In 2004, Osteoporosis Australia were raising concerns in the media about vitamin D deficiency at the same time that new research by Hughes et al. was coming out about possible benefits of sun exposure in reducing non-Hodgkin lymphoma (Huges et al. 2004). Given the significant media attention centred around possible or real benefits of sun exposure, the Cancer Council Victoria considered it was necessary to develop a position statement with the Australasian College of Dermatologists (ACOD), Osteoporosis Australia (OA), Australia and New Zealand Bone and Mineral Society (ANZBMS) and the Cancer Council Australia (CCA) to ensure consistent information was being provided to the general public.

On 15 July 2004, the Cancer Council Victoria and the National Cancer Control Initiative hosted an expert meeting with representatives from relevant disciplines to investigate whether there was a basis for a common understanding relating to the risks and benefits of sun exposure. A report from that meeting was published along with a number of key recommendations that had unanimous support from all parties (Cancer Control Research Institute 2004). In addition, following the meeting a position statement was approved and released in March 2005 that had the approval of the ACOD, OA, ANZBMS and the CCA (The Cancer Council Australia 2005). The process of reaching agreement with each of the parties was critical in ensuring consistency in the messages being delivered to the media around the vitamin D issue and to provide confidence to the general community that there was consistent health advice from each of the key agencies.

The position statement resulted in a number of key outcomes directly related to skin cancer control. Essentially it was agreed that:

- A balance is required between avoiding increases in skin cancer and maintaining adequate vitamin D levels.
- Sun protection messages needed to shift away from the notion that people have to protect themselves against the sun at all times.
- Skin cancer campaigns need to note that there are benefits and harms associated with sun exposure and that a balance between the two needs to be achieved. This had not been a general perspective of skin cancer prevention messages to date.
- Sun protection messages should refrain from messages that relate to encouraging people to stay indoors, instead they should be about en-

couraging people to take the right precautions when they are outside.

- Sun protection should only be applicable when the ultraviolet index is greater than 3.

The Relationship Between Sun Exposure and Other Diseases

There is in Australia unanimous agreement by the ACOD, OA, ANZBMS, and CCA that there is high-level evidence for the harmful effects of sun exposure in terms of skin cancer and for the beneficial effects of sun exposure in maintaining adequate vitamin D levels to protect against bone fracture (Trivedi et al. 2003). However, all parties agree that substantially more evidence is required before conclusions can be drawn between sun exposure and a possible beneficial effect with other cancers such as breast, prostate, bowel, or non-Hodgkin lymphoma and autoimmune diseases such as multiple sclerosis. The biological pathways underlying these empirically observed observations are still not clear and in some instances the epidemiological evidence is equivocal. It was agreed by all parties that it is not appropriate to make statements about a protective effect of UV radiation exposure for these diseases because substantially more studies with good individual exposure measures by season is required.

How Much Sun Exposure Is Enough?

The most difficult factor in coming to an agreed position statement has been to determine what would be a reasonable level of sun exposure necessary for healthy bone growth and development that will not add to a substantial risk of skin cancer. It was clear amongst OA, ANZBMS and the ACOD that we are still a long way from having sufficient evidence to suggest where this point should be exactly. This difficultly stems almost entirely from the limitation and paucity of existing research. This issue is also compounded because skin type, age and culturally related clothing practices vary the ability to absorb vitamin D through UV exposure.

Recognising the limitations of existing evidence, a very pragmatic approach was adopted in Australia. Based on evidence relating to bone gracture and vitamin D, it was agreed that one-third of a minimal erythemal dose (MED) to 15% of the body, (e.g. the face, arms and hands) on most days of the week would be sufficient to maintain adequate vitamin D absorption to reduce osteoporosis risk (Newson et al. 2004). In practice this equates in the Australian context to only 10 min sun exposure either side of the peak UV period on most days of the week over summer and 2–3 h per week sun exposure during the winter months. This level was acceptable to the ACOD, as it was considered that the general population were already likely to be exceeding these recommendations as part of their normal day-to-day activity, even if they were always adopting sun protective measures during periods of high ultraviolet (UV) radiation. In addition, all parties agreed that the benefit of some sunlight is far greater for general good health than it is detrimental for skin cancer.

Therefore there is no recommendation that people should deliberately expose themselves to the sun to enhance their vitamin D levels. The only exception are those people who are at high risk of being vitamin D-deficient and when controlled sun exposure outside the peak UV periods may be beneficial to their health if supplementation was not available.

Times of the Year and Times of the Day When Sun Protection Should Be Applied

The Global UV index released by the World Health Organization (WHO) in 2002 is a very useful tool to determine when sun protection is required and equally when it is not necessary (WHO 2002). According to the Global UV index that is now the international standard for UV measurement, sun protection should be promoted when the UV index is 3 or above.

Figure 1 provides an example of the appropriate times of the year when we should be communicating the sun protection message. For example, Melbourne (Australia 38°S) shows that between the winter months of May and August inclusive, it is unlikely that sun protection will

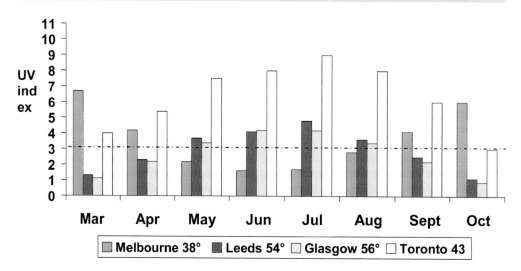

Fig. 1 Average UV levels per month by city. UV data for Melbourne, Leeds and Glasgow sourced from Gies et al. (2004)

be necessary unless people will be near highly reflective surfaces such as snow and water, or at high altitudes. In the northern hemisphere over the summer months, it shows that the appropriate time for Leeds UK at 54°N would be that sun protection advice should be reinforced between the months of May and August inclusive. For Glasgow, Scotland at 56°N it would be for a similar duration, in Toronto, Canada at 43°N, sun protection campaigns would be appropriate for at least between March and October inclusive.

The UV Index can also be a useful tool to determine what time of the day that sun protection in required. In Australia, the Bureau of Meteorology in conjunction with the Cancer Councils have been illustrating for the first time the UV index in terms of a peak value for the day as well as the times of day when sun protection is required (see Fig. 2). This provides very useful information for the general public to guide their behaviour.

People with dark skin who wear veils, particularly in pregnancy or for elderly or infirm people, those with malabsorption syndromes, organ transplant patients and those with personal risk factors of skin cancer will require a tailored health management plan that is likely to include vitamin D supplementation.

Is Increased Physical Activity a Key Part of the Solution?

Of significant note is that mildly deficient vitamin D levels (between 25 and 50 nmol/l) in the general population has been only during winter periods. Notably, children who were obese had lower vitamin D levels and higher levels of vitamin D were seen in adolescent boys who participated in sport (Jones et al. 1999, 2005). Therefore, by encouraging people to be more physically active outdoors in winter months, we will not only be increasing their vitamin D levels, but also importantly contributing to their overall good health. Increasing levels of physical activity will not be a solution, however, at latitudes where little if any UV is present over winter months.

Vitamin D Deficiency and Sun Protection: Are the Messages Complementary?

Vitamin D deficiency in the Australian context in the general population is largely confined to winter months in southern states when the sun protection message is not a relevant public health message. When the Global UV index is in the moderate to extreme range, undertaking

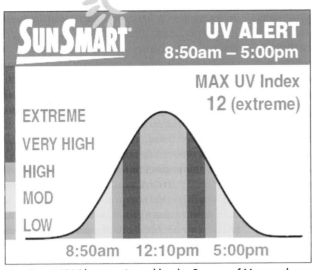

SunSmart UV Alert was issued by the Bureau of Meteorology

Fig. 2 UV Index as issued by the Australian Bureau of Meteorology

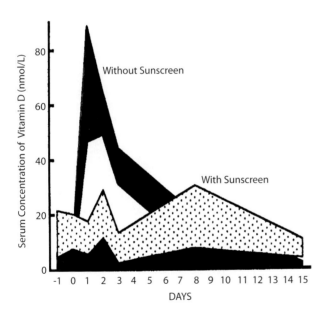

Fig. 3 Circulating concentrations of vitamin D after a single exposure to one minimal erythemal dose of simulated sunlight either with a sunscreen, with a sun protection factor of 8, or a topical placebo cream. Matsouka et al. (1987)

sun protection measures such as regular sunscreen application is unlikely to increase osteoporosis risk (Farrerons et al. 2001; Marks 1999). A study by Matsouka et al. (Fig. 3) showed that while sunscreen use initially reduced vitamin D absorption, this effect was dissipated after 7 days (Matsuoka et al. 1987).

Artificial Tanning Sunbeds and Vitamin D

The size of the artificial tanning sunbed industry and the number of people who use them represent a significant challenge to those working in skin cancer control. The sunbed industry is based on the glorification of a tan, the antithesis of the objectives of those working in skin cancer prevention. In the United States, the sunbed industry continues to grow with a $1 billion a year turnover and 30 million patrons visiting sunbeds annually (Spencer and Amonette 1995; Levine et al. 2005). This growth in patronage has also been seen in Europe where it has gone from less than 5% of the adult population in Belgium, France and Germany in 1980 to 33% by 1995 (Autier et al. 1994).

In December 2005, a significant outcome was achieved by Canada's largest sunbed provider in an agreement with the Canadian Competition Bureau that allows the company to promote that vitamin D can be maintained or increased as a result of a tanning session in which the tanning equipment incorporates UVB irradiance. This outcome could possibly have a significant flow-on effect in other countries by allowing artificial tanning operators to claim a health benefit that they may not have been able to do in the past.

This is a concern because sunbeds emit high levels of a known carcinogen that makes regular sunbed use a risk factor for skin cancer (Gallagher et al. 2005; Young 2004). Despite any possible benefit that UVB-emitting sunbeds might have in terms of increasing vitamin D levels, there use must continue to be discouraged because of the well-known detrimental effects of their use. The WHO have clear directions in terms of what should be expected in terms of regulations or a code of practice for operators (WHO 2003). This includes restricting access to those under the age of 18, ensuring warning notices are placed in all cubicles and in the foyer area, ensuring all new clients to the establishment sign a consent form as well as ensuring all operators are adequately trained.

Conclusion

With appropriate refinements of the sun protection message, sun protection programs do not have to compete with the human need for vitamin D, the two messages can be quite complementary. In terms of key recommendations for going forward, every opportunity should be made to promote the Global UV Index to those responsible for delivering sun protection campaigns to guide when sun protective behaviour

should be encouraged as well as when it may not be required.

In terms of public health, we must continue to raise public awareness of potential negative health effects from excessive sun exposure during periods when UV is in the moderate to extreme range. In periods when the UV level is low (<3), it will be important to not encourage sun protective behaviour, except near highly reflective surfaces or high altitudes. In high latitude countries with very low UV levels for a significant proportion of the year, the increased use of vitamin D fortification in food and supplementation for high-risk individuals should be considered.

Further research is required to understand the relationship between vitamin D and risk of cancer and autoimmune diseases and to determine how much sun exposure is necessary to achieve adequate vitamin D levels. This information will help determine the right balance between the need for vitamin D vs the known benefits of sun protection.

In terms of artificial tanning sunbeds, despite any possible vitamin D benefit that may be derived from machines that emit UVB, their use should continue to be discouraged due to the intensity of the output of a well-known carcinogen and the lack of controls that govern their use.

Skin cancer prevention has been proven to reduce skin cancer rates, and given the significant morbidity and mortality associated with the disease, it is important that investments in skin cancer prevention remain a high public health priority.

References

Armstrong BK (2004) How sun exposure causes skin cancer. In: Hill D, Elwood JM, English DR (eds) Prevention of skin cancer. Kluwer, Dordrecht

Autier P, Dore JF, Lejeune F et al (1994) Cutaneous malignant melanoma and exposure to sunlamps or sunbeds. An EORTC multicenter case-control study in Belgium, France and Germany. Int J Cancer 58:809–813

Bischoff HA, Stahelin HB, Dick W et al (2003) Effects of vitamin D and calcium supplementation on falls: a randomised controlled trial. J Bone Miner Res 18:343–351

Cancer Control Research Institute of the Cancer Council of Victoria (2004) Sun and Health. http://www.ncci.org.au/pdf/Sun%20and%20Health/wshop_report.pdf. Cited 23 August 2006

Dobbinson S, Hill D, White V (2002) Trends in sun protection: Use of sunscreen, hats and clothing over the past decade in Melbourne, Australia. UV radiation and its effects—an update 2002. Proceedings of a workshop, 26–28 March 2002, Christchurch, New Zealand. National Institute of Water and Atmospheric Research (NIWA), the Royal Society of New Zealand

Farrerons J, Barnadas M, Lopez-Navidad A, Renau A, Rodriguez J, Yoldi B, Alomar A (2001) Sunscreen and risk of osteoporosis in the elderly: a two-year follow-up. Dermatology 202:27–30

Flicker L, Mead K, MacInnis RJ et al (2003) Serum vitamin D and falls in older women in residential care in Australia. J Am Geriatr Soc 51:1533–1538

Gallagher RP, Spinelli JJ, Lee TK (2005) Tanning beds, sunlamps, and risk of cutaneous malignant melanoma. Cancer Epidemiol Biomarkers Prev 14:562–566

Gies P, Roy C, Javorniczky J, Henderson S, Lemus-Deschamps L, Driscoll C (2004) Global Solar UV Index: Australian measurements, forecasts and comparison with the UK. Photochem Photobiol 79:32–39

Grover S, Morley R (2001) Vitamin D deficiency in veiled or dark skinned pregnant women. Med J Aust 175:251–252

Hill D, White V, Marks R, Borland R (1993) Changes in sun-related attitudes and behaviours, and reduced sunburn prevalence in a population at high risk of melanoma. Eur J Cancer Prev 2:447–456

Hughes A-M, Armstrong BK, Vajdic C, Turner J, Grulich A, Fritschi L, Milliken S, Kaldor J, Benke G, Kricker A (2004) Sun exposure may protect against non-Hodgkin lymphoma: a case-control study. Int J Cancer 112:865–871

Jones G, Blizzard C, Riley M, Parameswaran V, Greenaway T, Dwyer T (1999) Vitamin D levels in prepubertal children in Southern Tasmania: prevalence and determinants. Eur J Clin Nutr 52:824–829

Jones G, Dwyer T, Hynes K, Parameswaran V, Greenaway TM (2005) Vitamin D insufficiency in adolescent boys in Northwest Tasmania: prevalence, determinants and relationship to bone turnover markers. Osteoporos Int 16:636–641

Levine JA, Sorace M, Spencer J, Siegel DM (2005) The indoor UV tanning industry: a review of skin cancer risk, health benefit claims, and regulation J Am Acad Dermatol 53:1038–1044

Marks R (1999) Sunscreens and vitamin D levels. J Am Acad Dermatol 40:497

Matsuoka LY, Ide L, Wortsman J, MacLaughlin JA, Holick MF (1987) Sunscreens suppress cutaneous vitamin D3 synthesis. J Clin Endocrinol Metab 64:1165–1168

Montague M, Borland R, Sinclair C (2001) Slip Slop Slap and SunSmart. 1980–2000. Skin cancer control and 20 years of population based campaigning. Health Educ Behav 28:290–305

Nowson CA, Diamond TH, Pasco JA, Mason RS, Sambrook PN, Eisman JA (2004) Vitamin D in Australia. Issues and recommendations. Aust Fam Physician 33:133–138

Pasco JA, Henry MJ, Nicholson GC, Sanders KM, Kotowicz MA (2001) Vitamin D status of women in the Geelong Osteoporosis Study: association with diet and casual exposure to sunlight. Med J Aust 175:401–405

Sambrook PN, Cameron ID, Cumming RG et al (2002) Vitamin D deficiency is common in frail institutionalised older people in northern Sydney [letter]. Med J Aust 176:560

Spencer J, Amonette R (1995) Indoor tanning: risks, benefits and future trends. J Am Acad Dermatol 33:288–298

Staples M, Elwood M, Burton R, Williams J, Marks R, Giles G (2006) Non-melanoma skin cancer in Australia: the 2002 national survey and trends since 1985. Med J Aust 184:6–10

The Cancer Council Australia (2005) Risks and and benefits of sun exposure: position statement. http://www.cancer.org.au/documents/Risks_Benefits_Sun_Exposure_MAR05.pdf. Cited 23 August 2006

Trivedi DP, Doll R, Khaw KT (2003) Effect of four monthly oral vitamin D3 (cholecalciferol) supplementation on fractures and mortality in men and women living in the community: randomised double blind controlled trial. BMJ 326:469

Weathererall M (2000) A meta-analysis of 25 hydroxyvitamin D in older people with fracture of the proximal femur. N Z Med J 113:137–140

WHO (2002) Global Solar UV Index: a practical guide. WHO. http://www.who.int/uv/publications/globalindex/en/index.html. Cited 23 August 2006

WHO (2003) Artificial tanning sunbeds: risk and guidance. http://www.who.int/uv/publications/sunbed-
publ/en. Cited 23 August 2006

Working Group of the Australian and New Zealand
Bone and Mineral Society, Endocrine Society of
Australia and Osteoporosis Australia (2005) Vi-
tamin D and adult bone health in Australia and
New Zealand: a position statement Med J Aust
182:281–285

Young AR (2004) Tanning devices-fast track to skin
cancer? Pigment Cell Res 17:2–9

18 Are Gliomas Preventable?

Victor A. Levin

Recent Results in Cancer Research, Vol. 174
© Springer-Verlag Berlin Heidelberg 2007

Abstract

Gliomas are a family of primary central nervous system tumors of variable malignancy that are derived from supporting glia (astrocytes, oligodendrocytes, ependymal cells) or their progenitors/stem cells. There are two potential strategies to prevention: preventing gliomas from forming and preventing lower-grade gliomas from developing into higher-grade gliomas. Each would lower time-dependent mortality. Each also depends on an understanding of what causes gliomas so that these factors can be modulated. In this presentation, I will discuss primary prevention, chemoprevention, and screening. I will first focus on the known chromosomal, genetic, and protein changes associated with the different histologic varieties of glioma and the environmental, hereditary, and infectious/viral factors that may promote glioma development and malignant progression. I will discuss a number of clinical scenarios that eventuate from the known genetic patterns of these tumors and the changes in genetic patterns that reflect malignant progression. The basic thinking is that if one could prevent specific gene mutations and/or deletions or gains of specific chromosomes that lead to the development of low-grade (WHO 2) gliomas, then theoretically this would reduce the occurrence of high-grade (WHO 3 and 4) gliomas and hence the almost certain death that now is the fate of most patients with these tumors. In the case of de novo WHO 3 and 4 tumors, being able to prevent or counter specific gene mutations and/or the deletion of specific chromosomes would in itself reduce the occurrence of these gliomas and increase survival. Alternatively, a curative treatment for low-grade glioma that prevents these chromosomal/gene changes would prevent some glioblastomas (WHO 4) from forming and would have the same desired effect on survival. Obviously, for the latter to be achieved, we must also be able to diagnose and treat low-grade gliomas earlier.

Introduction

In this article, I will examine the prevention of gliomas from three perspectives: primary prevention, chemoprevention, and screening. Prevention strategies today aim to reduce a cancer focus by altering a known or highly suspect pathway that leads to the cancer or by removing or controlling a precancerous lesion(s). Examples of each are well-known to those involved in cancer prevention. However, to cite a few examples, one strategy to reducing the risk of carcinoma of the lung is behavioral and involves attempting to convince smokers to stop smoking and young people not to start smoking. In the case of colon cancer, a preventive strategy is to identify and remove the precancerous colon polyps by colonoscopy (with a special focus on patients with familial adenomatous polyposis or hereditary non polyposis colon/colorectal cancer) and thereby prevent the development of carcinoma of the colon. Yet another preventive strategy is to reduce exposure to DNA-damaging agents such as ultraviolet radiation to the skin by wearing protective clothing, applying sunscreens, and reducing exposure to lower the risk of melanoma and other skin cancers in light-skinned people. In other cancers, being vigilant for a premalignant marker helps to protect against cancer, as is the case for highly dysplastic oral leukoplakia that can progress to oropharyngeal squamous cell carcinoma. Other prevention approaches exploit our knowledge of the risks related to certain foods and environmental chemicals and radionuclides. Some strategies draw on science and pseudo-science, such as is the case for diet and vitamin ingestion to fortify body defenses with antioxidant chemicals and vitamins to prevent DNA damage and possible cancer. This is currently an imprecise and potentially risky approach, as shown for beta carotene ingestion, which proved to heighten the risk of lung cancer in smokers (Littman et al. 2004).

All these various strategies are based on an understanding of the risk factors that lead to or exacerbate specific cancers in humans. In fact, without that knowledge, there can be no prevention strategies. Such strategies do not exist for a specific family of central nervous system (CNS) malignancies, the gliomas, because the risk factors are currently incompletely understood. Gliomas are believed to derive from glial cells that support neuronal function in the CNS, in particular the precursors of astrocytes, oligodendrocytes, and ependymal cells or their progenitors/stem cells. Typically, these tumors are named on the basis of their most common elements—astrocytoma, oligodendroglioma, ependymoma, or a mixture of lineages, such as the oligoastrocytoma. They are graded in malignancy from WHO 1 to WHO 4. I will discuss here the status and the feasibility of prevention strategies for the infiltrative WHO 2 to WHO 4 tumors.

Primary Prevention

To first determine whether a prevention strategy can even be formulated for gliomas, I will first discuss the etiology for gliomas. I will focus on the known chromosomal, genetic, and protein changes associated with the different histologic varieties of glioma and the environmental factors, hereditary syndromes, and infectious/viral agents that have been implicated in the development of gliomas.

Genetic and Molecular Factors

Much is known today about the chromosomal deletions and gene mutations that occur in astrocytomas and oligodendrogliomas as they become more malignant. These genetic and associated protein changes are summarized in Table 1. To date, chromosomal deletions (Chr 1p, 9p, 10p, 10q, 11p, 13q, 19q, 22q) and either cell surface receptor amplification (EGFR, PDGFR) or receptor ligand overexpression (PDGFα, PDGFβ, IGFBP2) predominate, with regulators of cell cycle and DNA damage repair/apoptosis (p53, Rb, CDK4, MDM 2, CDKN2A, CDKN2B) a close second. Critical to the prevention of these cancers is thus being able to prevent the accumulation of chromosomal alterations. To date, this has not been achievable in mammalian systems, let alone in humans. It is possible, however, to target receptors with antibodies and receptor kinase domains with small molecules and thereby thwart the malignant effect of these defective molecules. These two approaches have led to the introduction of many drugs into clinical use and the approval of at least four new drugs for the treatment of non-glioma cancers. Unfortunately, targeting an amplified receptor with small-molecule drugs can be problematic from a conservation of mass perspective, since there are now many more sites for the drug to bind to and potentially too few drug molecules to sufficiently block the amplified receptor and hence have any marked effect on the malignant phenotype. Other approaches are being considered as a means of circumventing this problem, one of which are RNAi constructs that inhibit protein production.

Environmental Factors

Epidemiology studies have provided clues to environmental factors that can lead to the formation of gliomas, but there remain few definitive observations with respect to environmental or occupational causes of glioma (El-Zein et al. 2002). Although brain tumors can be experimentally induced in a high proportion of rodents by exposure to chemicals such as nitrosoureas, the association between chemical exposure and

Table 1 Chromosomal and protein changes observed in different grades of gliomas (Kleihues et al. 2002; Kleihues and Ohgaki 2000; Louis and Cavenee 2001)

Histology	Chromosomal	Protein
Astrocytoma (WHO 2)	p53 Mutation (>65%)	PDGFα
	Chr 17p loss (30%–44%)	PDGFαR overexpression (~60%)
	Chr 22q loss	Expression of invasion-associated molecules
Anaplastic astrocytoma (WHO 3)	CDKN2A & CDKN2B deletion/ chr 9p loss	CDK4 amplification
	Rb mutation/Chr 13q loss (~25%)	
	Chr 19p loss (~50%)	
	Chr 11p loss	
Glioblastoma (WHO 4)	PTEN mutation (~30%)	CDK4 amplification
	Chr 10q loss	EGFR amplification (~40%) & overexpression (~60%)
	Chr 10p loss	MDM 2 amplification (<10%) & overexpression (~50%)
	Chr 22q loss	IGFBP2 overexpressed
	CDKN2A & CDKN2B deletion/ chr 9p loss/ p16 deletion (30%–40%)	Nestin
	Rb mutation/Chr 13q loss	PDGFαR amplification (<10%)
		DCC loss of expression (~50%)
Oligodendroglioma	Chr 1p loss (60%–70%)	
	Chr 19q loss (50%–80%)	
Ependymoma	Chr 22 loss (25%–50%)	

brain tumors is limited to a few occupations and scenarios. Attempts have been made to determine whether there is a higher-than-expected incidence of brain tumors in people exposed to pesticides, herbicides, and fertilizers (Musicco et al. 1988; Preston-Martin 1996; Zahm and Devesa 1995), but the results are not uniformly convincing (Carreon et al. 2005; Lee et al. 2005; Loyant et al. 2005; Musicco et al. 1982). There also has been a variable reported association of petrochemical exposure in the workplace or nearby residential areas with a higher incidence of gliomas, but this appears to be more the case for white collar than blue collar workers (Austin and Schnatter 1983; Beall et al. 2001; Moss 1985; Neuberger et al. 2003; Olin et al. 1987; Teta et al. 1991). Thus, at this time, aside from a known association between vinyl chloride and gliomas, there are few

common chemical or environmental threads among these observations (Moss 1985; Teta et al. 1991).

Environmental exposure to electromagnetic fields has been widely discussed as a causative factor in childhood cancers as well as in adult gliomas. However, a relationship between electromagnetic field exposure and the occurrence of glial tumors has been refuted (Floderus et al. 1993; Gurney et al. 1996; Kheifets et al. 1999; Tynes and Haldorsen 1997), as has a relationship between cellular telephone use and the development of gliomas (Inskip et al. 2001).

Some unexplained observations are that gliomas are more common in right-handed males and whites (Chen et al. 2001). In addition, they may be more prevalent in higher socioeconomic groups (Carozza et al. 2000; Grayson 1996) and less common in those with autoimmune diseases or a prominent history of allergies (Schlehofer et al. 1999). Thus, the sum of environmental evidence is certainly not a great deal to build a prevention strategy on.

Hereditary Syndromes

At this juncture, we know of a few heritable causes of glioma and many genetic changes associated with malignant progression from grade WHO 2 to WHO 4. The clearest risk factor is a hereditary tumor syndrome. The most common hereditary tumor syndrome associated with CNS tumors are the neurofibromatoses. Neurofibromatosis type 1 (NF1) is an autosomal dominant disorder affecting 1 in 3,000 individuals that causes intracranial and extracranial benign Schwann cell tumors. Optic gliomas and other astrocytomas also occur at a significantly higher frequency in patients with NF1. Certainly, if NF1 could be eliminated or better treated at an early stage in these people, we might be able to reduce the number of gliomas that form or even prevent any gliomas from forming.

In some families with Li-Fraumeni syndrome, there is a gene mutation in p53 on chromosome 17p, and in glioma patients, there is a higher frequency of germline p53 mutations, especially in those with multifocal glioma, glioma and another primary malignancy, and a family history of cancer (Kyritsis et al. 1994, 1995, 1996). Abrogating p53 mutations would also be expected to reduce some lower- and mid-grade gliomas.

Infectious/Viral Associations

While viruses have been directly implicated in the development of gliomas in rats, dogs, and monkeys, the number and breadth of studies conducted to understand their role in the development of gliomas in humans are quite limited, probably because of the difficulties in designing meaningful studies for this group. This is because, in all cases, direct CNS injection of the virus is required. In rats, the avian sarcoma virus produces glial tumors; in dogs, the Rous sarcoma virus leads to gliosarcomas; and in owl monkeys,

a human polyoma virus (JC virus) produces glial neoplasms. Although a direct association between virus exposure and CNS tumors has not been established in humans, there are some hints from family studies and school and community clusters that this may be an important factor (Wrensch et al. 1997). However, it is extremely difficult to pinpoint mutations caused by a virus to validate this hypothesis.

Efforts to implicate the contamination of polio vaccine with simian virus 40 (SV40) as a putative cause for at least a subset of gliomas in adults or children failed to produce data in support of this (Engels et al. 2002; Rollison et al. 2005). In addition, since the JC virus has been found to exist in cancer-free subjects, its connection to tumorigenesis does not appear strong. It has, however, been cited as an etiologic agent in a case of pleomorphic xanthoastrocytoma (Martin et al. 1985) and in oligodendrogliomas (Rencic et al. 1996), but the association has not been confirmed.

Sometimes it is what we do not find that provides some unexpected insight. Such was the case for Wrensch et al. (1997), who found that adults in the San Francisco Bay area with gliomas were significantly *less likely* to have had either chickenpox or shingles than controls and less likely than controls to have antibody to varicella zoster virus, the agent causing chickenpox and shingles.

Regardless, from a clinical perspective, many of the family and geographic groupings of glioma patients implicate a viral etiology. Similarly, there are also hints of a viral influence in gliomatosis cerebri, an uncommon pattern of glioma growth characterized by widely dispersed glioma growth infiltrating multiple cerebral lobes and extending into gray matter. Unfortunately, studies into a viral cause of gliomas to date have not pointed the way to a logical prevention strategy based on infectious/viral agents.

Chemoprevention

Certainly if medical/pharmaceutical scientists find a method to prevent DNA damage and loss of chromosome and chromatin, then we all could expect to live longer without cancer. Short of that, we need therapeutic strategies to decrease the rate of transformation of WHO 2 tumors to more malignant phenotypes. This might be as easy as chronic dosing with a drug such as alpha-difluoromethylornithine (DFMO) (Levin et al. 1992) or a combination of new signal transduction inhibitors.

In scientific and lay publications, there are and likely will continue to be proposals to modify our nutrition to include a greater number of substances to counter mutation, chromosomal changes, and exposure to carcinogens, out of the belief that this will reduce the types of chromosomal changes and gene mutations that we associate with cancers and, by extension, the malignant progression of gliomas. Unfortunately, there is no clear path to follow at this time that would justify a prevention trial and so we will leave this area for the time and focus on other potential opportunities in screening strategies.

Screening

If prevention is defined as preventing death at the expected time from a given disease, then the early diagnosis and treatment of gliomas would benefit from screening efforts. This is certainly the case with breast cancer and mammographic screening. While there is no straightforward strategy for preventing gliomas, one could argue that, regardless of etiology, if low-grade gliomas (WHO 2) could be diagnosed at an early stage and effectively treated, then possibly the number of WHO 3 and WHO 4 gliomas that form and the time to formation could be positively affected. Even if mid-grade gliomas (WHO 3) could be diagnosed earlier, this might reduce mortality in patients with this family of tumors. This mammography corollary is possible today because of the widespread availability of magnetic resonance imaging (MRI) in much of the world.

However, let us first consider the pros and cons of prevention screening for gliomas using MRI. Let us assume that the non-contrast FLAIR (fluid-attenuated inversion recovery) MRI sufficed to screen for non-contrast-enhanced WHO 2 tumors as well as contrast-enhancing WHO 3 and 4 tumors. To estimate the potential cost and benefit that might accrue to such a screening program for gliomas, we need to make some assumptions about the disease process and the potential gains yielded by early diagnosis. Table 2 summarizes some of these variables and the approximate numerical values for the United States based on recent tumor registry information (Anonymous 2005; Davis and Preston-Martin 1999; Levin et al. 2000, 2001, 2003; Ohgaki and

Table 2 Factors important to the consideration of MRI screening for the prevention of gliomas (Anonymous 2005; Davis and Preston-Martin 1999; Levin et al. 2000, 2001, 2003; Ohgaki and Kleihues 2005)

	Value	Total cases in U.S. for 1 year	Percent population
WHO 2 mean age at presentation	34		
WHO 3 mean age at presentation	40–42		
WHO 4 mean age at presentation	51–53		
Incidence (/100,000), WHO 3, 4 at 40 years	2.49	6,723	0.15%
Incidence (/100,000), WHO 3, 4 at 50 years	5.62	15,174	0.48%
Incidence WHO 2 at 40 years[a]	1.26	3,402	0.08%
Incidence WHO 2 at 50 years[a]	1.19	3,213	0.10%
Population at 40 years	4,378,800.00		1.62%
Population at 50 years	3,145,200.00		1.16%
Cost of axial FLAIR MRI	$250		
U.S. population	270,000,000		

[a]May be an overestimate

Kleihues 2005). From a treatment perspective, the complete surgical removal of a glioma is the most efficacious approach and the one most likely to lead to long-term survival for patients with WHO 2 tumors (Bauman et al. 1999; Fisher et al. 2001; Keles et al. 2001; Sakata et al. 2001;

Schiffer et al. 1997; Shaw et al. 1993; Winger et al. 1989). However, this group may constitute only approximately 13% of patients (see Table 3). This raises the question of whether an early diagnosis in the remaining patients could lead to a greater certainty of cure compared with those diagnosed

Table 3 Basis for values for "total" or gross total resection (GTR) by histology

Histology	GTR	95% resection	5-year survival	Reference
Low-grade	16.9%		88%	Nomura 2003
Low-grade		20%	75%	Nomura 2003
Astrocytoma/oligodendroglioma	12%–13%		85%–89%	Nomura 2003
Low-grade	8%–10%			Estimate of MDACC neurosurgery colleagues
LG Modeling value =	13%			
Anaplastic astrocytoma		24%–28%		Levin et al. 2003
Anaplastic astrocytoma	7.1%		46%	Nomura 2003
Anaplastic oligodendroglioma	12.4%		100%	Nomura 2003
Anaplastic oligodendroglioma		24%	61%	Nomura 2003
AA/AO/AOA	3%–5%			Estimate of MDACC neurosurgery colleagues
AG Modeling value =	6%			
Glioblastoma	7.4%		18%	Nomura and Japan 2003
Glioblastoma		35%–38%		Levin et al. 2000
Glioblastoma		22%	11%	Nomura 2003
Glioblastoma	19%			Simpson et al. 1993
GBM	5%–10%			Estimate of MDACC neurosurgery colleagues
GBM Modeling value =	11%			

Table 4 Estimated cases of de novo WHO 3 and WHO 4 tumors compared to those resulting from transformation from a lower grade

Age	WHO 2	Transformed WHO 3[a]	de novo WHO 3	Transformed WHO 4	de novo WHO 4[b]
40	3,402	1,701	538	1,345	3,139
50	3,213	1,607	3,446	3,036	7,085

This table was computed from values in Table 2, such that at age 40 years there will be ~3,402 WHO 2 tumors and ~6,723 WHO 3–4 tumors. Further, it is assumed that the ratio of WHO 3:WHO 4 tumors = 1:2 and that 70% of WHO 4 tumors will be de novo

[a]This was computed based on a 50% transformation rate from WHO 2 to higher-grade tumors (Muller et al. 1977a, b)

[b]This was taken as 70% (Kleihues and Ohgaki 1999)

when they become symptomatic and/or more malignant. This question, of course, cannot be answered since we do not know how many or how long WHO 2 tumors go undiagnosed during a normal lifetime, if indeed any do. In addition, even for patients with WHO 2 tumors, age at diagnosis and the dose and benefit of radiation therapy and/or chemotherapy are somewhat disputed today (Fisher et al. 2001; Levin 1996; Levin et al. 2001; Prados et al. 1997; Shaw et al. 2002).

Another issue is that while glioma progression from WHO 2 to WHO 3 and, ultimately, to WHO 4 is well appreciated, it is also clear that WHO 4 tumors can occur de novo in about 70% of cases (Kleihues and Ohgaki 1999). WHO 3 tumors can also occur de novo, though the percentage of cases is less well known. In Table 4, I used an estimate of 50% for de novo cases at ages 40 and

50 years (Muller et al. 1977a, b). Figure 1 shows a flow schema of this thinking and Fig. 2 depicts the expected cases in each category. The reality is that the majority of WHO 2 gliomas could transform to a more malignant phenotype (≥WHO 3) during the patient's lifetime, which indicates the potential value of screening with MRI.

Table 5 is a summary of the hypothetical subsets and costs for only the subset of patients who undergo true gross total resection (GTR). Clearly, it would be a costly undertaking to screen all 40-year-old patients in the United States to find the approximately 1,000 patients with WHO 2 to WHO 4 gliomas that theoretically would be helped by GTR. The cost for a one-time screen at age 40 would be in excess of $1 billion and produce a cost for quality-adjusted year of life gained of approximately $79,000–$118,000, depending

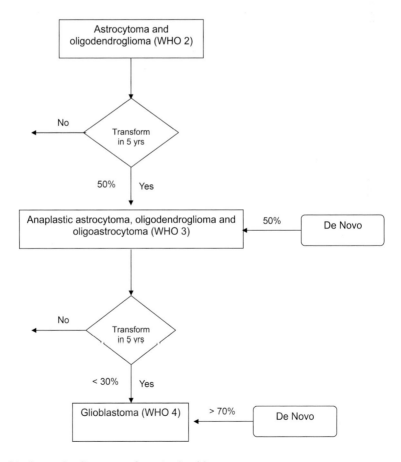

Fig. 1 Flow chart of tumor histology and malignant transformation (grade)

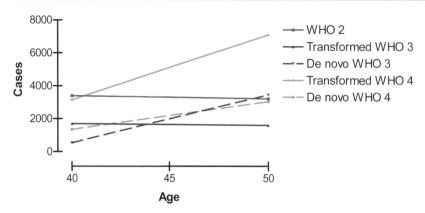

Fig. 2 Projected distribution and number of different grades of glioma in the U.S. based on Table 4

Table 5 Calculation of the cost/quality year gained for patients benefiting from MRI screening at ages 40 and 50 years by virtue of being a candidate for a true total resection of tumor

	% Patients GTR	Patients at 40 years	Average increase in life	QOL	Quality years gained	Patients at 50 years	Average increase in life	QOL	Quality years gained
WHO 2	13%	442	30	0.9	11,941	418	20	0.9	7,518
WHO 3	6%	133	10	0.8	1,065	303	5	0.8	1,213
WHO 4	11%	493	2	0.8	789	1,113	1	0.8	891
Subtotal		1069			13,795	1,834			9,622
% Age group		0.024%				0.058%			
Cost for testing age group once		$1,094,700,000				$786,300,000			
Cost/quality year gained		$79,354				$81,721			

on expectations for the number of quality years gained. Recall also that this is only for a one-time screen at age 40. How often should people over 40 years of age be screened? If we were to screen a new group of 40-year-olds each year for 5 years and re-screen the original 40-year-old group on the 5th year, the total cost in the United States would exceed $6.5 billion dollars.

Another question to consider regarding screening is whether there would be additional benefits to some patients who are diagnosed earlier and, therefore, might have a longer and less symptomatic life as a result. To place a numerical value on this, however, is next to impossible at this time.

For a cost comparison, colorectal cancer screening costs between $10,000 and $40,000 for each quality-adjusted year of life gained and cervical cancer screening with Pap smears costs around $15,000 and higher per quality-adjusted year of life (Saha et al. 2001). Thus, while MRI screening for asymptomatic glioma patients does not appear to be a reasonable cost-effective undertaking at this time, especially given the palliative nature of most treatments today, this would certainly change if a greater number of WHO 2 tumors could be treated for cure and patients with WHO 3 tumors could expect a median 15-year progression-free survival.

Acknowledgements

I would like to thank Beth Notzon for editorial assistance and Dr. Bernard Levin for helpful discussion and constructive advice regarding prevention strategies.

References

Anonymous (2005) Central Brain Tumor Registry of United States Special Data Analysis (December 15, 2005)

Austin SG, Schnatter AR (1983) A cohort mortality study of petrochemical workers. J Occup Med 25:304–312

Bauman G, Lote K, Larson D, Stalpers L, Leighton C, Fisher B, Wara W, Macdonald D, Stitt L, Cairncross JG (1999) Pretreatment factors predict overall survival for patients with low-grade glioma: A recursive partitioning analysis. Intl J Radiat Oncol Biol Phy 45:923–929

Beall C, Delzell E, Rodu B, Sathiakumar N, Lees PS, Breysse PN, Myers S (2001) Case–control study of intracranial tumors among employees at a petrochemical research facility. J Occup Environ Med 43:1103–1113

Carozza SE, Wrensch M, Miike R, Newman B, Olshan AF, Savitz DA, Yost M, Lee M (2000) Occupation and adult gliomas. Am J Epidemiol 152:838–846

Carreon T, Butler MA, Ruder AM, Waters MA, Davis-King KE, Calvert GM, Schulte PA, Connally B, Ward EM, Sanderson WT, Heineman EF, Mandel JS, Morton RF, Reding DJ, Rosenman KD, Talaska G, Cancer B (2005) Gliomas and farm pesticide exposure in women: the Upper Midwest Health Study. Environ Health Perspect 113:546–551

Chen P, Aldape K, Wiencke JK, Kelsey KT, Miike R, Davis RL, Liu J, Kesler-Diaz A, Takahashi M, Wrensch M (2001) Ethnicity delineates different genetic pathways in malignant glioma. Cancer Res 61:3949–3954

Davis FG, Preston-Martin S (1999) Epidemiology. Incidence and survival. In: Bigner DD, McLendon RE, Bruner JM (eds) Russell and Rubinstein's pathology of tumors of the nervous system. Arnold, London, pp 7–11

El-Zein R, Minn Y, Wrensch M, Bondy ML (2002) Epidemiology of brain tumors. In: Levin VA (ed) Cancer in the nervous system. Oxford University Press, Oxford, pp 252–268

Engels EA, Sarkar C, Daniel RW, Gravitt PE, Verma K, Quezado M, Shah KV (2002) Absence of simian virus 40 in human brain tumors from northern India. Int J Cancer 101:348–352

Fisher BJ, Leighton CC, Vujovic O, Macdonald DR, Stitt L (2001) Results of a policy of surveillance alone after surgical management of pediatric low grade gliomas. Int J Radiat Oncol Biol Phys 51:704–710

Floderus B, Persson T, Stenlund C, Wennberg A, Ost A, Knave B (1993) Occupational exposure to electromagnetic fields in relation to leukemia and brain tumors: a case-control study in Sweden. Cancer Causes Control 4:465–476

Grayson JK (1996) Radiation exposure, socioeconomic status, and brain tumor risk in the US Air Force: a nested case-control study. Am J Epidemiol 143:480–486

Gurney JG, Mueller BA, Davis S, Schwartz SM, Stevens RG, Kopecky KJ (1996) Childhood brain tumor occurrence in relation to residential power line configurations, electric heating sources, and electric appliance use. Am J Epidemiol 143:120–128

Inskip PD, Tarone RE, Hatch EE, Wilcosky TC, Shapiro WR, Selker RG, Fine HA, Black PM, Loeffler JS, Linet MS (2001) Cellular-telephone use and brain tumors. N Engl J Med 344:79–86

Keles GE, Lamborn KR, Berger MS (2001) Low-grade hemispheric gliomas in adults: a critical review of extent of resection as a factor influencing outcome. J Neurosurg 95:735–745

Kheifets LI, Sussman SS, Preston-Martin S (1999) Childhood brain tumors and residential electromagnetic fields (EMF). Rev Environ Contam Toxicol 159:111–129

Kleihues P, Ohgaki H (1999) Primary and secondary glioblastomas: from concept to clinical diagnosis. Neuro-oncol 1:44–51

Kleihues P, Ohgaki H (2000) Phenotype vs genotype in the evolution of astrocytic brain tumors. Toxicol Pathol 28:164–170

Kleihues P, Louis DN, Scheithauer BW, Rorke LB, Reifenberger G, Burger PC, Cavenee WK (2002) The WHO classification of tumors of the nervous system. J Neuropathol Exp Neurol 61:215–225; discussion 226–219

Kyritsis AP, Bondy ML, Xiao M, Berman EL, Cunningham JE, Lee PS, Levin VA, Saya H (1994) Germline p53 gene mutations in subsets of glioma patients. J Natl Cancer Inst 86:344–349

Kyritsis AP, Bondy ML, Hess KR, Cunningham JE, Zhu D, Amos CJ, Yung WK, Levin VA, Bruner JM (1995) Prognostic significance of p53 immunoreactivity in patients with glioma. Clin Cancer Res 1:1617–1622

Kyritsis AP, Xu R, Bondy ML, Levin VA, Bruner JM (1996) Correlation of p53 immunoreactivity and sequencing in patients with glioma. Mol Carcinog 15:1–4

Lee WJ, Colt JS, Heineman EF, McComb R, Weisenburger DD, Lijinsky W, Ward MH (2005) Agricultural pesticide use and risk of glioma in Nebraska, United States. Occup Environ Med 62:786–792

Levin VA (1996) Controversies in the treatment of low-grade astrocytomas and oligodendrogliomas. Curr Opin Oncol 8:175–177

Levin VA, Prados MD, Yung WK, Gleason MJ, Ictech S, Malec M (1992) Treatment of recurrent gliomas with eflornithine. J Natl Cancer Inst 84:1432–1437

Levin VA, Uhm JH, Jaeckle KA, Choucair A, Flynn PJ, Yung WKA, Prados MD, Bruner JM, Chang SM, Kyritsis AP, Gleason MJ, Hess KR (2000) Phase III randomized study of postradiotherapy chemotherapy with alpha-difluoromethylornithine-procarbazine, N-(2-chloroethyl)-N'-cyclohexyl-N-nitrosurea, vincristine (DFMO-PCV) versus PCV for glioblastoma multiforme. Clin Cancer Res 6:3878–3884

Levin VA, Leibel SA, Gutin PH (2001) Neoplasms of the central nervous system. In: DeVita VTJ, Hellman S, Rosenberg SA (eds) Cancer: principles and practice of oncology. Lippincott-Raven, Philadelphia, pp 2100–2160

Levin VA, Hess KR, Choucair A, Flynn PJ, Jaeckle KA, Kyritsis AP, Yung WK, Prados MD, Bruner JM, Ictech S, Gleason MJ, Kim HW (2003) Phase III randomized study of postradiotherapy chemotherapy with combination alpha-difluoromethylornithine-PCV versus PCV for anaplastic gliomas. Clin Cancer Res 9:981–990

Littman AJ, Thornquist MD, White E, Jackson LA, Goodman GE, Vaughan TL (2004) Prior lung disease and risk of lung cancer in a large prospective study. Cancer Causes Control 15:819–827

Louis DM, Cavenee WK (2001) Molecular biology of central nervous system neoplasms. In: DeVita VTJ, Hellman S, Rosenberg SA (eds) Cancer: principles and practice of oncology. Lipincott-Raven, Philadelphia, pp 2091–2099

Loyant V, Jaffre A, Breton J, Baldi I, Vital A, Chapon F, Dutoit S, Lecluse Y, Loiseau H, Lebailly P, Gauduchon P (2005) Screening of TP53 mutations by DHPLC and sequencing in brain tumours from patients with an occupational exposure to pesticides or organic solvents. Mutagenesis 20:365–373

Martin JD, King DM, Slauch JM, Frisque RJ (1985) Differences in regulatory sequences of naturally occurring JC virus variants. J Virol 53:306–311

Moss AR (1985) Occupational exposure and brain tumors. J Toxicol Environ Health 16:703–711

Muller W, Afra D, Schroder R (1977a) Supratentorial recurrences of gliomas. Morphological studies in relation to time intervals with astrocytomas. Acta Neurochir 37:75–91

Muller W, Afra D, Schroder R (1977b) Supratentorial recurrences of gliomas. Morphological studies in relation to time intervals with oligodendrogliomas. Acta Neurochir 39:15–25

Musicco M, Filippini G, Bordo BM, Melotto A, Morello G, Berrino F (1982) Gliomas and occupational exposure to carcinogens: case-control study. Am J Epidemiol 116:782–790

Musicco M, Sant M, Molinari S, Filippini G, Gatta G, Berrino F (1988) A case–control study of brain gliomas and occupational exposure to chemical carcinogens: the risk to farmers. Am J Epidemiol 128:778–785

Neuberger JS, Ward-Smith P, Morantz RA, Tian C, Schmelzle KH, Mayo MS, Chin TD (2003) Brain cancer in a residential area bordering on an oil refinery. Neuroepidemiology 22:46–56

Nomura K, Committee of Brain Tumor Registry of Japan (2003) Report of Brain Tumor Registry of Japan. Neurologia Med Chir 43:1–111

Ohgaki H, Kleihues P (2005) Population-based studies on incidence, survival rates, and genetic alterations in astrocytic and oligodendroglial gliomas. J Neuropathol Exp Neurol 64:479–489

Olin RG, Ahlbom A, Lindberg-Navier I, Norell SE, Spannare B (1987) Occupational factors associated with astrocytomas: a case-control study. Am J Ind Med 11:615–625

Prados MD, Edwards MS, Rabbitt J, Lamborn K, Davis RL, Levin VA (1997) Treatment of pediatric low-grade gliomas with a nitrosourea-based multiagent chemotherapy regimen. J Neuro-oncol 32:235–241

Preston-Martin S (1996) Epidemiology of primary CNS neoplasms. Neurol Clin 14:273–290

Rencic A, Gordon J, Otte J, Curtis M, Kovatich A, Zoltick P, Khalili K, Andrews D (1996) Detection of JC virus DNA sequence and expression of the viral oncoprotein, tumor antigen, in brain of immunocompetent patient with oligoastrocytoma. Proc Natl Acad Sci U S A 93:7352–7357

Rollison DE, Utaipat U, Ryschkewitsch C, Hou J, Goldthwaite P, Daniel R, Helzlsouer KJ, Burger PC, Shah KV, Major EO (2005) Investigation of human brain tumors for the presence of polyomavirus genome sequences by two independent laboratories. Int J Cancer 113:769–774

Saha S, Hoerger TJ, Pignone MP, Teutsch SM, Helfand M, Mandelblatt JS (2001) The art and science of incorporating cost effectiveness into evidence-based recommendations for clinical preventive services. Am J Prev Med 20:36–43

Sakata K, Hareyama M, Komae T, Shirato H, Watanabe O, Watarai J, Takai K, Yamada S, Tsuchida E, Sakai K (2001a) Supratentorial astrocytomas and oligodendrogliomas treated in the MRI era. Jpn J Clin Oncol 31:240–245

Schiffer D, Dutto A, Cavalla P, Bosone I, Chio A, Villani R, Bellotti (1997) Prognostic factors in oligodendroglioma Canadian Journal of Neurological Sciences 24:313–319

Schlehofer B, Blettner M, Preston-Martin S, Niehoff D, Wahrendorf J, Arslan A, Ahlbom A, Choi WN, Giles GG, Howe GR, Little J, Menegoz F, Ryan P (1999) Role of medical history in brain tumour development. Results from the international adult brain tumour study. Int J Cancer 82:155–160

Shaw EG, Scheithauer BW, O'Fallon JR (1993) Management of supratentorial low-grade gliomas. Oncology (Huntingt) 7:97–104

Shaw E, Arusell R, Scheithauer B, O'Fallon J, O'Neill B, Dinapoli R, Nelson D, Earle J, Jones C, Cascino T, Nichols D, Ivnik R, Hellman R, Curran W, Abrams R (2002) Prospective randomized trial of low- versus high-dose radiation therapy in adults with supratentorial low-grade glioma: initial report of a North Central Cancer Treatment Group/Radiation Therapy Oncology Group/Eastern Cooperative Oncology Group study. J Clin Oncol 20:2267–2276

Simpson JR, Horton J, Scott C, Curran WJ, Rubin P, Fischbach J, Isaacson S, Rotman M, Asbell SO, Nelson JS et al (1993) Influence of location and extent of surgical resection on survival of patients with glioblastoma multiforme: results of three consecutive Radiation Therapy Oncology Group (RTOG) clinical trials. Int J Radiat Oncol Biol Phys 26:239–244

Teta MJ, Ott MG, Schnatter AR (1991) An update of mortality due to brain neoplasms and other causes among employees of a petrochemical facility. J Occup Med 33:45–51

Tynes T, Haldorsen T (1997) Electromagnetic fields and cancer in children residing near Norwegian high-voltage power lines. Am J Epidemiol 145:219–226

Winger MJ, Macdonald DR, Cairncross JG (1989) Supratentorial anaplastic gliomas in adults: The prognostic importance of extent of resection and prior low-grade glioma. J Neurosurg 71:487–493

Wrensch M, Lee M, Miike R, Newman B, Barger G, Davis R, Wiencke J, Neuhaus J (1997) Familial and personal medical history of cancer and nervous system conditions among adults with glioma and controls. Am J Epidemiol 145:581–593

Zahm SH, Devesa SS (1995) Childhood cancer: overview of incidence trends and environmental carcinogens. Environ Health Perspect 103 [Suppl 6]:177–184

Part VII   The Future of Cancer (Chemo)Prevention

Angiogenesis and Cancer Prevention: A Vision

Douglas M. Noonan, Roberto Benelli, Adriana Albini

Recent Results in Cancer Research, Vol. 174
© Springer-Verlag Berlin Heidelberg 2007

Abstract

Angiogenesis is necessary for solid tumor growth and dissemination. In addition to angiogenesis, it has become increasingly clear that inflammation is a key component in cancer insurgence that can promote tumor angiogenesis. We noted that angiogenesis is a common and key target of most chemopreventive molecules, where they most likely suppress the angiogenic switch in premalignant tumors, a concept we termed angioprevention. We have shown that various molecules, such as flavonoids, antioxidants, and retinoids, act in the tumor microenvironment, inhibiting the recruitment and/or activation of endothelial cells and phagocytes of the innate immunity. N-acetyl-cysteine, and the green tea flavonoid epigallocatechin-3-gallate (EGCG) and the beer/hops-derived chalcone Xanthohumol all prevent angiogenesis in the Matrigel sponge angiogenic assay in vivo and inhibit the growth of the highly angiogenic Kaposi's sarcoma tumor cells (KS-Imm) in nude mice. The synthetic retinoid 4-hydroxyfenretinide (4HPR) also shows anti-angiogenic effects. We analyzed the regulation of gene expression they exert in primary human umbilical endothelial cells (HUVEC) in culture with functional genomics. Expression profiles obtained through Affymetrix GeneChip arrays identified overlapping sets of genes regulated by anti-oxidants. In contrast, the ROS-producing 4HPR induced members of the TGFβ-ligand superfamily, which, at least in part, explains its anti-angiogenic activity. NAC and the flavonoids all suppressed the IkB/NF-κB signaling pathway even in the presence of NF-κB stimulation by TNFα, and showed reduced expression of many NF-κB target genes. A selective apoptotic effect on transformed cells, but not on endothelial cells, of the anti-oxidants may be related to the reduced expression of the NF-κB-dependent survival factors Bcl2 and Birc5/surviving, which are selectively overexpressed in transformed cells by these factors. The repression of the NF-κB pathway suggests anti-inflammatory effects for the antioxidant compounds that may also represent an indirect role in angiogenesis inhibition. The green tea flavonoid EGCG does target inflammatory cells, mostly neutrophils, and inhibits inflammation-associated angiogenesis. The other angiopreventive molecules are turning out to be effective modulators of phagocyte recruitment and activation, further linking inflammation and vascularization to tumor onset and progression and providing a key target for cancer prevention.

Introduction

It is now well established that growth of a tumor to clinically relevant dimensions requires the ability to induce the formation of new blood vessels (Kerbel and Folkman 2002). Angiogenesis is a rate-limiting step in progression to tumor malignancy (Hanahan and Weinberg 2000), and not only do proliferating cells in nonangiogenic lesions have limited access to the blood and lymphatic systems, but the counterbalancing cell death that ensues because of insufficient oxygen and nutrients reduces the accumulation of cells that may have acquired additional genetic alterations favoring malignancy. Folkman introduced the concept that inhibition of angiogenesis could be a strategy in cancer therapy in 1971 (Folkman 1971). Angiogenesis inhibition is now a clinical reality, the commercially available anti-VEGF antibody Avastin, or bevacizumab, significantly improves survival when combined with standard chemotherapy approaches (Ferrara and Kerbel 2005). Clearly this approach perturbs the VEGF-based tumor-endothelium loops that feed cancer angiogenesis. However, how this contributes to clinical benefit is currently under scrutiny. In addition to the original idea of suffocating tumors by cutting off the lifelines by eliminating new vessel formation, the concept that this therapeutic approach results in vascular normalization (Jain 2005) has been put forth by R. Jain. The vascular normalization hypothesis suggests that blocking the VEGF signal pathway results in less permeable, stabile vessels that paradoxically deliver the associated chemotherapeutics better. Perhaps both may be operational in the clinical setting. While the general goal in development of these drugs was to interrupt the tumor-endothelium crosstalk between tumor-derived VEGF and endothelial VEGF receptors, we may be doing much more than that. In addition to endothelial cells, we are starting to appreciate that other cells also express receptors for, and respond to, VEGF. These include the tumor cells themselves, which in some cases may rely on autocrine loops of VEGF (Carmeliet 2005), hematopoietic cells and leukocytes, and bone marrow-derived progenitors that appear to contribute to the endothelium, although the extent to which they do so is controversial, in newly forming vessels (Rafii et al. 2002).

In spite of the excitement surrounding the clinical success of these agents, the extent of improvement in survival with anti-angiogenics is as yet still only a few months rather than the long-term tumor suppression originally postulated. Furthermore, we must ask why, since we are targeting a normal cell, do tumors soon progress in a therapy-resistant manner? One possibility, among several (Carmeliet 2005), is the numerous roads that may be taken to induce vessel formation: targeting one molecular pathway, or even a few, may not be enough to combat the phenotypic plasticity of an established tumor.

Chemoprevention and Angiogenesis

The acquisition of the capacity to induce angiogenesis, the process necessary for tumor progression, is often a discreet step referred to as the angiogenic switch (Hanahan and Weinberg 2000). Intuitively, it is clear that if we can prevent the angiogenic switch, we should be able to prevent progression of hyperplastic foci, blocking these into a small, benign and clinically indolent state, effectively preventing cancer insurgence (Albini et al. 2005). Furthermore, if we assume that tumor progression depends on the increase in risk for malignant conversion as a function of tumor cell accumulation as suggested above, we could significantly reduce the risk for progression and malignancy.

Given that the principle of cancer chemoprevention is based on the use of agents that interfere with processes associated with malignant progression have limited collateral effects, anti-angiogenesis may be an effective strategy. In fact, while working with diverse chemoprevention agents, we observed that angiogenesis was both a common and key target of most chemopreventive molecules. We termed the concept that effective chemoprevention targets angiogenesis as "angioprevention" (Tosetti et al. 2002). As a corollary to this hypothesis, we would also suggest that many of the antiangiogenesis compounds developed for tumor therapy may be effective as cancer chemoprevention agents. The identification of more effective cancer prevention compounds will be enhanced by inclusion of antiangiogenesis as an endpoint for evaluation. Furthermore, we have begun searching for common pathways targeted by these molecules to identify the key molecular mechanisms and thus highly specific targets.

Molecular Mechanisms in Angioprevention

Our approach to analysis of the effects of angioprevention compounds on endothelial cells has been through employment of microarray analyses (Pfeffer et al. 2005). These studies have demonstrated that the flavonoids and antioxidant compounds all specifically target the NF-κB pathway in endothelial cells (Pfeffer et al. 2005).

This can be expanded to include the vast majority of the numerous potential cancer chemoprevention agents that have been studied by different laboratories; these have been shown interfere with pathways leading to NF-κB activation, and to repress AKT activation (Aggarwal and Shishodia 2004; Dorai and Aggarwal 2004; Pfeffer et al. 2005; Tosetti et al. 2002). The exceptions to this are the compounds devoid of antioxidant activity, such as the retinoid 4HPR (Ferrari et al. 2005) and possibly the steroid analogs. We have shown that repression of the NF-κB and Akt pathways produces downregulation of downstream elements such as p21, p53, and survivin (Dell'Eva et al., unpublished data), that in turn correlate with reduced endothelial cell activation, proliferation, migration, and even survival. Taken together, these data show that the AKT-NF-κB pathway lies at the core of angiogenesis as a common target for the angioprevention molecules. Given the central role of NF-κB in regulating inflammation (Karin 2005; Karin and Greten 2005), these data may also reflect an anti-inflammatory activity of these compounds. This appears to be the case.

Angiogenesis, Inflammation, and Angioprevention

Apart from the traditional and extensively studied tumor-endothelium axis in angiogenesis research, recent data indicate that a tumor–inflammation–endothelium exchange is of critical importance in cancer insurgence and progression (Balkwill and Mantovani 2001; Balkwill et al. 2005; Coussens and Werb 2002; Pollard 2004) and that it represents a potential therapeutic target (Albini et al. 2005; Benelli et al. 2006b; Brigati et al. 2002; Coussens and Werb 2001, 2002). As often observed in the molecular mechanisms mediating tumor cell invasion and metastatic dissemination, the tumor may ask host cells to orchestrate the angiogenic process as well. Recent data suggest that chronic inflammation is a driving force in angiogenesis associated with numerous pathologies, including tumor angiogenesis (Balkwill and Mantovani 2001). Currently, approximately 15% of the world's tumor burden can be ascribed to infectious agents (Coussens

and Werb 2002). If we add clinically recognized chronic inflammation and subclinical chronic inflammation (Balkwill et al. 2005), the percentage of tumors associated with chronic inflammation rises further. These inflammatory components often appear to drive tumor angiogenesis. Inflammatory angiogenesis may be considered part of a normal homeostatic process occurring in conditions of tissue remodeling subsequent to injury. However, since the transformed tumor cells do not cease to proliferate, the injury cannot resolve; this is basically the Dvorak concept of tumors as wounds that never heal (Dvorak 2005). Innate inflammatory cells appear to often play a key role in assisting tumor growth, angiogenesis, and expansion as part of the tissue remodeling process (Benelli et al. 2003, 2006a, b).

The potential growth-promoting role of tumor-infiltrating macrophages has been well established (Pollard 2004), and it is suggested that these assume different phenotypes based on environmental stimuli (Balkwill et al. 2005), one M1 phenotype associated with tissue damage and tumor killing, another M2 phenotype associated with tissue salvage, remodeling and angiogenesis. Substantial data indicate that the M2 phenotype dominates in cancers (Balkwill et al. 2005). Mast cells and neutrophils also provide angiogenic stimuli necessary for tumor progression (Coussens and Werb 2001, 2002). Neutrophils mediate the vessel formation induced by the angiogenic CXC chemokines (Benelli et al. 2002; Scapini et al. 2004) and play a key role in tumor progression related to *ras* oncogene modulation of angiogenic CXC chemokine expression (Karin 2005; Sparmann and Bar-Sagi 2004).

Interestingly, neutrophils have been found to be a target for the angiogenesis inhibitor angiostatin (Benelli et al. 2002). We would extend this to suggest that inhibitors of angiogenesis will inhibit inflammation, and that anti-inflammatory agents will also repress angiogenesis. This has in part been suggested for classic COX inhibitors such as aspirin of specific COX2 inhibitors (Albini and Noonan 2005; Brown and DuBois 2005). These inflammation inhibitors have been shown to be effective in prevention of colon cancer (Brown and DuBois 2005), where the antiangiogenic activity has been postulated to play a role.

Toward Clinical Angioprevention

Development of successful angiogenesis-targeted therapies requires that we know the mechanisms of how tumor cells can induce the formation of new vessels. Knowledge of the diversity of the events occurring and examination of the mechanisms of molecules that interfere with these processes are providing critical insight into future directions for therapy. From the observations discussed here, it becomes clear that compounds that can repress tumor-endothelial cell and inflammation-induced angiogenesis will show promise in chemoprevention settings and perhaps in therapy (Fig. 1). We now need to focus on clinical evaluation of these concepts, potentially initially targeting high-risk groups.

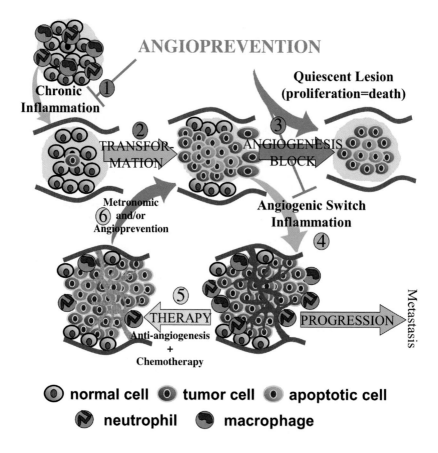

Fig. 1 Points in the carcinogenesis pathway where angioprevention may significantly delay cancer. (*1*) Chronic inflammation clearly predisposes to tumor development; the tight relationship between anti-inflammation and antiangiogenesis suggests that this may a common pathway, potentially reducing step (*2*) transformation. (*3*) Transformed foci of cells devoid of capacity to induce angiogenesis either directly or via inflammation are limited to small hyperplastic foci that are not clinically significant. Acquisition of angiogenic potential and/or inflammation, the angiogenic switch, results in tumor expansion and eventually clinical cancer. Angioprevention represses the angiogenic switch and favors quiescence, thus indirectly limits step (*4*) progression toward malignancy. Antiangiogenic VEGF blockade together with chemotherapy (*5*) reduce tumor burden, further antiangiogenic measures (*6*, metronomic therapy; angioprevention) may further favor maintenance of quiescence

Acknowledgements

These studies were supported by grants from the Compagnia di San Paolo, the Ministero della Salute Progetto Finalizzato, the MIUR Progetto Strategico, Progetto FIRB and PRIN, the Fondi di Ateneo of the University of Insubria, the PNR-Oncologia Citochine & Chemokine.

References

Aggarwal BB, Shishodia S (2004). Suppression of the nuclear factor-kappaB activation pathway by spice-derived phytochemicals: reasoning for seasoning. Ann N Y Acad Sci 1030:434–441

Albini A, Noonan DM (2005) Rescuing COX-2 Inhibitors From the Waste Bin. J Natl Cancer Inst 97:859–860

Albini A, Tosetti F, Benelli R, Noonan DM (2005) Tumor inflammatory angiogenesis and its chemoprevention. Cancer Res 65:10637–10641

Balkwill F, Mantovani A (2001) Inflammation and cancer: back to Virchow? Lancet 357:539–545

Balkwill F, Charles KA, Mantovani A (2005) Smoldering and polarized inflammation in the initiation and promotion of malignant disease. Cancer Cell 7:211–217

Benelli R, Morini M, Carrozzino F, Ferrari N, Minghelli S, Santi L, Cassatella M, Noonan DM, Albini A (2002) Neutrophils as a key cellular target for angiostatin: implications for regulation of angiogenesis and inflammation. FASEB J 16:267–269

Benelli R, Albini A, Noonan D (2003) Neutrophils and angiogenesis: potential initiators of the angiogenic cascade. In: The neutrophil: Cassatella MA (ed) An emerging regulator of inflammatory and immune response. Karger, Basel pp 167–181

Benelli R, Frumento G, Albini A, Noonan DM (2006a) Models of inflammatory processes in cancer. In: Marshall LA, Stevenson CS, Morgan DW (eds) In vivo models of inflammation. Birkhäuser, Basel, pp 83–102

Benelli R, Lorusso G, Albini A, Noonan DM (2006b) Cytokines and Chemokines as regulators of angiogenesis in health and disease. Curr Pharm Des 12:3101–3115

Brigati C, Noonan DM, Albini A, Benelli R (2002) Tumors and inflammatory infiltrates: friends or foes? Clin Exp Metastasis 19:247–258

Brown JR, DuBois RN (2005) COX-2: a molecular target for colorectal cancer prevention. J Clin Oncol 23:2840–2855

Carmeliet P (2005) Angiogenesis in life, disease and medicine. Nature 438:932–936

Coussens LM, Werb Z (2001) Inflammatory cells and cancer: think different! J Exp Med 193:F23–F26

Coussens LM, Werb Z (2002) Inflammation and cancer. Nature 420:860–867

Dell'Eva R, Ambrosini C, Minghelli S, Noonan DM, Albini A, Ferrari N (2006) The Akt inhibitor deguelin, is an angiopreventive agent also acting on the NF-{kappa} B pathway. Carciogenesis, in press

Dorai T, Aggarwal BB (2004) Role of chemopreventive agents in cancer therapy. Cancer Lett 215:129–140

Dvorak HF (2005) Angiogenesis: update 2005. J Thromb Haemost 3:1835–1842

Ferrara N, Kerbel RS (2005) Angiogenesis as a therapeutic target. Nature 438:967–974

Ferrari N, Pfeffer U, Dell'Eva R, Ambrosini C, Noonan DM, Albini A (2005) The transforming growth factor-beta family members bone morphogenetic protein-2 and macrophage inhibitory cytokine-1 as mediators of the antiangiogenic activity of N-(4-hydroxyphenyl) retinamide. Clin Cancer Res 11:4610–4619

Folkman J (1971) Tumor angiogenesis: therapeutic implications. N Engl J Med 285:1182–1186

Hanahan D, Weinberg RA (2000) The hallmarks of cancer. Cell 100:57–70

Jain RK (2005) Normalization of tumor vasculature: an emerging concept in antiangiogenic therapy. Science 307:58–62

Karin M (2005) Inflammation and cancer: the long reach of Ras. Nat Med 11:20–21

Karin M, Greten FR (2005) NF-kappaB: linking inflammation and immunity to cancer development and progression. Nat Rev Immunol 5:749–759

Kerbel R, Folkman J (2002) Clinical translation of angiogenesis inhibitors. Nat Rev Cancer 2:727–739

Pfeffer U, Ferrari N, Dell'eva R, Indraccolo S, Morini M, Noonan DM, Albini A (2005) Molecular mechanisms of action of angiopreventive anti-oxidants on endothelial cells: Microarray gene expression analyses. Mutat Res 591:198–211

Pollard JW (2004) Tumour-educated macrophages promote tumour progression and metastasis. Nat Rev Cancer 4:71–78

Rafii S, Lyden D, Benezra R, Hattori K, Heissig B (2002) Vascular and haematopoietic stem cells: novel targets for anti-angiogenesis therapy? Nat Rev Cancer 2:826–835

Scapini P, Morini M, Tecchio C, Minghelli S, Carlo ED, Tanghetti E, Albini A, Lowell C, Berton G, Noonan DM, Cassatella MA (2004) CXCL1/Macrophage Inflammatory Protein-2-Induced Angiogenesis in Vivo is Mediated by Neutrophil-Derived Vascular Endothelial Growth Factor-A1. J Immunol 172:5032–5040

Sparmann A, Bar-Sagi D (2004) Ras-induced interleukin-8 expression plays a critical role in tumor growth and angiogenesis. Cancer Cell 6:447–458

Tosetti F, Ferrari N, De Flora S, Albini A (2002) Angioprevention: angiogenesis is a common and key target for cancer chemopreventive agents. FASEB J 16:2–14

An Estimate of Cancer Mortality Rate Reductions in Europe and the US with 1,000 IU of Oral Vitamin D Per Day

William B. Grant, Cedric F. Garland, Edward D. Gorham

Recent Results in Cancer Research, Vol. 174
© Springer-Verlag Berlin Heidelberg 2007

Abstract

Solar ultraviolet B (UVB) irradiance and/or vitamin D have been found inversely correlated with incidence, mortality, and/or survival rates for breast, colorectal, ovarian, and prostate cancer and Hodgkin's and non-Hodgkin's lymphoma. Evidence is emerging that more than 17 different types of cancer are likely to be vitamin D-sensitive. A recent meta-analysis concluded that 1,000 IU of oral vitamin D per day is associated with a 50% reduction in colorectal cancer incidence. Using this value, as well as the findings in a multifactorial ecologic study of cancer mortality rates in the US, estimates for reductions in risk of vitamin D-sensitive cancer mortality rates were made for 1,000 IU/day. These estimates, along with annual average serum 25-hydroxyvitamin D levels, were used to estimate the reduction in cancer mortality rates in several Western European and North American countries that would result from intake of 1,000 IU/day of vitamin D. It was estimated that reductions could be 7% for males and 9% for females in the US and 14% for males and 20% for females in Western European countries below 59°. It is proposed that increased fortification of food and increased availability of supplements could help increase vitamin D intake and could augment small increases in production of vitamin D from solar UVB irradiance. Providing 1,000 IU of vitamin D per day for all adult Americans would cost about $1 billion; the expected benefits for cancer would be in the range of $16–25 billion in addition to other health benefits of vitamin D.

Introduction

Numerous epidemiologic studies have found that higher levels of vitamin D are associated with reduced risk of many types of cancer (Grant and Garland, in press; Grant 2006; Holick 2006). The first such study, an ecologic study, suggested that solar ultraviolet-B (UVB) irradiance, through the production of vitamin D, largely explained the factor of nearly two variation in colon cancer mortality rates in the US between the Northeast (high) and the Southwest (low) (Garland and Garland 1980). Later, dietary vitamin D was found inversely associated with colorectal cancer risk (Garland et al. 1985), as was prediagnostic serum 25-hydroxyvitamin D (25(OH)D) (Garland et al. 1989). About that time, risk of breast and ovarian cancer was also linked to lower solar UVB and vitamin D (Gorham et al. 1989, 1990; Garland et al. 1990; Lefkowitz and Garland 1994), and prostate cancer (Hanchette and Schwartz 1992). A more comprehensive ecologic study raised the number of UVB- or vitamin D-sensitive cancers to a total of 14 (Grant 2002). The 14 associations persisted after multivariate analyses that controlled for smoking (based on lung cancer mortality rates), alcohol consumption, urban compared to rural residence, Hispanic heritage, and fraction of the population living below the poverty level. Further analyses revealed that there are 17 different vitamin D-sensitive cancers (Grant and Garland, in press). While diet also plays a very important role in cancer risk (Doll and Peto 1981; Donaldson 2004), there are no data on dietary variations by state (Nutrition Monitoring Division 1978).

There are many mechanisms whereby vitamin D and its metabolites reduce the risk of cancer. These have been extensively investigated and include increasing cell differentiation, suppression of growth stimulatory signals, amplification of growth inhibitory signals, induction of apoptosis, suppression of cellular proliferation, suppression of angiogenesis around tumors, increased intercellular adherence, and reduced tumor metastasis (Palmer et al. 2001; van den Bemd and Chang 2002; Krishnan et al. 2003; Lamprecht and Lipkin 2003).

It is also known that many tissues can convert circulating 25(OH)D to 1,25-dihydroxyvitamin D (1,25(OH)$_2$D), potentially suppressing carcinogenesis (Cross et al. 1997; Zehnder et al. 2001). The action of 1,25(OH)$_2$D is mediated by vitamin D receptors (VDR) and different allelic forms of polymorphims of the VDRare associated with substantially different risks of cancer (John et al. 2005; Slattery et al. 2006).

More recently, there have been several papers reporting that cancer survival is dependent on solar UVB irradiance and vitamin D. A series of studies in Norway found that 18-month survival with breast, colon, and prostate cancer and Hodgkin's lymphoma was 30% higher for cases discovered in the fall compared to those discovered in winter or spring, and that factors other than solar UVB and vitamin D were unlikely to explain the findings (Robsahm et al. 2004; Moan et al. 2005; Porojnicu et al. 2005). In addition, a study in Boston found that patients with non-small-cell lung cancer who were operated on in summer and had a high vitamin D index considering all sources, had a 72% 5-year survival rate, while those who were operated on in winter and had a low vitamin D index had only a 29% 5-year survival rate (Zhou et al. 2005). These findings indicate that vitamin D plays an important role in inhibiting growth and metastasis of cancer after it has reached the stage where it can be detected.

There is rapidly mounting evidence that vitamin D reduces the risk of both cancer incidence and mortality for a large variety of cancers. The goal of this paper is to provide the framework for estimating the reduction in cancer mortality rates if the vitamin D levels are raised at the population level for adults, especially the elderly, by adding 1,000 IU per day to present oral intake and that produced through casual solar UVB irradiance in North America and several Western European countries.

Data and Methods

Determination of Cancer Risk Reduction from Vitamin D

The dose–response relationship between vitamin D and cancer has been determined through nested case–control studies in large cohorts. There have been a sufficient number of such studies of oral vitamin D intake and serum 25(OH)D with respect to colorectal cancer incidence that the relationship between vitamin D and risk reduction can be determined. A recent meta-analysis found that 1,000 IU (25 µg) per day may reduce the incidence of colorectal cancer by 50%, based on logarithmic extrapolation of measurements to 500 IU per day (Gorham et al. 2005). The p value for the trend was <0.0001. The determination was made based on 8,816 cases and 342,211 controls in 14 studies. The same study also found that a serum 25(OH)D level of 38 ng/ml was associated with a 50% reduction in colorectal cancer risk. The p value for trend was 0.01. There were 387 cases and 768 controls. This finding did not require extrapolation.

It was estimated that similar vitamin D intake and serum 25(OH)D levels would reduce breast and ovarian cancer by 33% (Garland et al. 2006). There is also evidence that intake of 1,000 IU/day would reduce incidence non-Hodgkin's lymphoma (NHL) (Hughes et al. 2004; Smedby et al. 2005). There were fewer studies of the association of these cancers with UVB or vitamin D, so there is greater uncertainty in the determinations.

These findings can be extended to other cancers using multifactorial ecological studies of cancer mortality rates for US whites for the periods 1950–1969 and 1970–1994 (Grant and Garland, in press). The cancer mortality maps in Devesa et al. (1999) indicate that many cancers had geographic variations that were similar to breast, colon, and ovarian cancers, i.e., high in the Northeast, low in the Southwest There is substantially lower UVB irradiance in the Northeast

Table 1 Estimates of cancer mortality rate reductions for oral intake of 1,000 IU of vitamin D per day based on beta (β) times the adjusted R^2 in Grant and Garland (2006)

Cancer	β*Adjusted R^2 Males, 1970–1994	β*Adjusted R^2 Females, 1970–1994	β*Adjusted R^2 Males, 1950–1969	β*Adjusted R^2 Females, 1950–1969	Reductions estimated for 1,000 IU/day	Uncertainty
Bladder	0.22	0.29	0.27	0.20	0.20	0.05
Breast		0.60		0.53	0.35	0.07
Cervical		0.20		0	0.10	0.05
Colon	0.53	0.44	0.54	0.55	0.50	0.05
Esophageal	0.42	0.26	0.50	0.14	0.20	0.07
Gastric	0.18	0.14	0.42	0.40	0.20	0.07
Hodgkin's	0.47	0.45	0.11	0.32	0.25	0.10
Laryngeal	0.64	0.23	0.29	0.18	0.20	0.07
Lung					0.10	0.07
Melanoma					0.20	0.07
NHL	0.29	0.22	0.33	0.28	0.20	0.07
Ovarian		0.50		0.56	0.30	0.07
Pancreatic	0.18	0.09	0.15	0.37	0.10	0.05
Prostate					0.10	0.07
Rectal	0.59	0.48	0.53	0.50	0.50	0.05
Renal	0.26	0.25	0.43	0.43	0.25	0.05
Uterine, corpus		0.53		0.31	0.20	0.07

than the Southwest based on known patterns of solar UVB irradiance (Leffell and Brash 1996; Grant 2002).

There are two tables of normalized coefficients (beta) for all of the factors, as well as the adjusted coefficient of determination (R^2) of the regression model in Grant and Garland (2006). Beta gives the relative contribution of a particular factor to the regression model and the adjusted R^2 gives the fraction of the data explained by the model (Riffenburgh 1999). The product of the beta for solar UVB times the adjusted R^2 was determined for each cancer, sex, and time period (Table 1). For colon cancer, the product varied from 0.44 to 0.55, while for rectal cancer, the range was 0.48–0.53. These values are very similar to the value of 0.5 for the reduction factor for 1,000 IU of vitamin D per day in Gorham et al. (2005). The values for breast and ovarian cancer were in the range of 0.50–0.63, which are higher

than the 33% reduction estimated by Garland et al. (2006). While the results from the calculation may be correct, the more conservative estimate of Garland et al. (2006) will be used in this study. In general, the estimate for cancer risk reduction due to vitamin D is taken for the low range of the 2 or 4 determinations of the product.

No product estimate is given for melanoma or lung and prostate cancer. However, there is evidence that higher vitamin D status is associated with lower risk of melanoma (Millen et al. 2004) and that solar UVA (315–400 nm) is the important risk factor for melanoma, rather than solar UVB (Moan et al. 1999). There is also evidence that vitamin D reduces the risk of lung cancer (Nakagawa et al. 2005; Zhou et al. 2005). For prostate cancer, there is evidence that higher vitamin D status is associated with lower incidence and mortality rates (Krishnan et al. 2003; Schwartz 2005).

Table 2 Values of annual average serum 25(OH)D levels consulted for this study

Country	Latitude (degrees)	Sex, mean age or range (years)	Serum 25(OH)D, standard deviation (ng/ml)	Reference
Belgium	51	M, 72	19, 7	Boonen et al. 1997
Canada	51	M, F, 27–89	26, 9	Rucker et al. 2002
Italy	42	F, 59	18, 8	Bettica et al. 1999
Netherlands	52.5	M, F, 74	13, 6	Lips et al. 1987
UK	52	M, F, >65	22, 11	Bates et al. 1999
US	26–46	White M, F, >18	38.5, 10	Grant and Holick 2005

In addition, data from the Surveillance, Epidemiology and End Results (SEER) Program indicate that 5-year survival rates for melanoma, lung and prostate cancers were slightly higher in the states with higher UVB levels in the 1970s, diminishing somewhat in later decades as screening and treatment programs increased survival rates for most people. In the 1970s, 5-year survival rates in Hawaii for males were 10%, 100%, and 15%–30% higher than in Connecticut and Iowa for melanoma, lung and prostate cancer, respectively (Grant and Garland 2006).

The estimates in Table 1 are considered to have from 10%–70% uncertainty as indicated for each cancer.

Vitamin D Levels by Country

Oral vitamin D intake is generally much lower in most European countries than in North America and Nordic countries (Punnonen et al. 1988; McKenna 1992). Serum 25(OH)D data were obtained from several papers. The review by Ovensen et al. (2003) provided serum 25(OH)D levels for European countries. Annual average values for several countries primarily from the papers reviewed in Ovensen et al. (2003) are given in Table 2.

From published values for serum 25(OH)D, it was determined that Southern European countries would benefit from 1,000 IU/day by a 50% reduction in colorectal cancer mortality rates, while the US would benefit by about a 35% reduction, due to higher baseline serum 25(OH)D levels in the US population.

Cancer Mortality Rate Data

Recent cancer mortality rate data were obtained from GLOBOCAN 2002 (Ferlay et al. 2004).

Results

Estimates of cancer risk reductions for 1,000 IU of vitamin D per day are shown in detail for Belgium, as an example of a European country, and the US (Table 3). The largest savings in lives from additional vitamin D are estimated to result from reductions in incidence of from breast, colorectal, and lung cancer, with substantial reductions also predicted for esophageal, gastric, ovarian, and renal cancer and non-Hodgkin's lymphoma. The estimates of total premature deaths prevented in all countries studied are presented in Table 4. For Europe, the mean cancer mortality rate reduction is 14% for males and 20% for females.

The uncertainties of the estimates were determined as follows. First, the uncertainties in Table 1 were used to calculate the uncertainties of each cancer for each sex and country. Second, the uncertainty of the effect of 1,000 IU of vitamin D per day was estimated at 20% of the number of premature deaths. The total uncertainty was then estimated as the square root of the sum of the squares of the two uncertainties.

Discussion

These results provide additional estimates of the effects of vitamin D in reducing the burden of

Table 3 Estimates for cancer risk reduction in Belgium and the US for 1,000 IU of oral vitamin D per day

Cancer	Reduction for 1,000 IU/day	Belgium Males Deaths in 2000	Belgium Females Deaths in 2000	US Males Deaths in 2000	US Females Deaths in 2000
Bladder	0.20	153	60	846	389
Breast	0.35		949	7510	7510
Cervical	0.10		33	261	
Colorectal	0.50	866	882	7429	7407
Esophageal	0.20	93	32	972	297
Gastric	0.20	147	108	776	541
Hodgkin's	0.25	10	7	96	78
Laryngeal	0.20	66	7	319	85
Lung	0.10	624	105	4732	3290
Melanoma	0.20	21	24	481	284
NHL	0.20	78	66	1242	1126
Ovarian	0.30		240		2169
Pancreatic	0.10	69	68	748	763
Prostate	0.10	203		1622	
Renal	0.25	104	76	975	598
Uterine, corpus	0.20		55		585
Total, vitamin D-sensitive		2,434	2,712	20,239	25,382
Total cancer deaths		17,718	12,669	295,630	270,105
Premature deaths, %		14	21	7	9

cancer. The results for the US are about twice that estimated in Grant (2002), but very similar to the 45,000 premature deaths estimated in Grant (2004). The fraction of cancer deaths that 1,000 IU of vitamin D might reduce in the US is about half that in Western European countries (other than Nordic countries), where solar UVB irradiance and oral intake levels are lower. While the uncertainties associated with these estimates are about 30%–40%, they do indicate that significant public health gains in cancer risk reduction could accrue from raising the serum 25(OH)D.

One way to increase serum 25(OH)D levels is through increased casual solar UVB irradiance. During times of the year when vitamin D can be produced from solar UVB irradiance (Webb et al. 1988), 10–15 min of casual exposure of 25%

of the body can produce about 1,000 IU for those with pale skin (Holick 2004a). The time near solar noon is optimal for such exposure for two reasons: one, the time required is reduced and two, the ratio of solar UVB to UVA is highest. UVA is considered most responsible for both melanoma (Moan et al. 1999; Garland et al. 2003) and basal cell carcinoma (Agar et al. 2004; Halliday et al. 2005) through generation of free radicals deep in the epidermis (Garland et al. 2003; Agar et al. 2004; Halliday et al. 2005). Since sunscreen can totally block vitamin D production (Matsuoka et al. 1988), it is recommended that those going into the sun for extended periods not apply sunscreen until after 10–15 min in the sun without sunscreen. In addition, if the UVA blocking is weak, total time in the sun with sunscreen should be limited as well.

Table 4 Fractions of cancer deaths that might be reduced if the population average oral vitamin D intake was 1,000 IU/day

Country	Fraction	Vitamin D preventable deaths, males	Vitamin D preventable deaths, females	Vitamin D preventable deaths, males (%)	Vitamin D preventable deaths, females (%)
Austria	1.0	1540	1,970	15±6	21±6
Canada	0.8	3,920	4,610	11±5	15±5
Belgium	1.0	2,430	2,710	14±6	21±6
France	1.0	11,850	12,100	13±6	21±6
Germany	1.0	17,130	22,120	15±5	21±6
Greece	1.0	1,770	1,640	12±5	18±5
Italy	1.0	12,550	12,420	13±5	19±6
Netherlands	1.0	3,170	3,740	18±6	17±6
Spain	1.0	8,470	7,010	15±6	20±5
Switzerland	1.0	1,300	1,440	14±5	20±6
UK	1.0	11,760	14,440	14±6	19±6
US	0.5	20,240	25,380	7±3	9±3
Simple mean, Europe				14±6	20±6

However, the easiest way to increase vitamin D levels in Europe and the US is through oral intake, both of fortified food and supplements. There are a number of recent reviews on dietary intake of vitamin D and the role that fortification could play (Calvo et al. 2004, 2005; Whiting and Calvo 2005a, b). Dairy products are the largest food source of vitamin D in the US, and orange juice is also fortified in the US (Tangpricha et al. 2003). Milk is now fortified in Finland with demonstrated benefits (Laaksi et al. 2006). However, milk should be fortified with more than 400 IU of vitamin D per quart (Daly et al. 2006) in order to be useful in reducing the risk of cancer since the benefits are only observed at daily consumption of more than 400 IU per day (Grant and Garland 2004; Gorham et al. 2005).

Another food group that should be viewed favorably in this regard is cereal and grain products. They comprise a large fraction of all national dietary supplies. Bread fortified with vitamin D has been demonstrated to increase serum 25(OH)D levels as well as supplements (Natri et al. 2006). While there is generally reluctance to fortify food in European countries, hopefully the OPTIFORD research will determine if fortification of food with vitamin D is a feasible strategy to remedy the insufficient vitamin D status of large population groups in Europe, and to determine at what level fortification should be pitched (Andersen et al. 2001).

Supplements could also supply 1,000 IU of vitamin D per day in a safe and reliable manner. Vitamin D dietary supplement use may contribute 6%–47% of the average vitamin D intake in some countries (Calvo et al. 2005). Vitamin D supplements of at least 2,000 IU per day are considered safe (Institute of Medicine 1997), and the toxic level is probably 40,000 IU/day (Vieth 1999). However, large-dose supplements such as 50,000 IU could be safely consumed at least once a month for the same benefit (Goldzieher et al. 1999) and might be more convenient for some people. It is estimated that an annual supply of 1,000 IU of vitamin D for each American would cost approximately $1 billion. This cost is far lower than the estimated $16–25 billion a year in premature cancer deaths and $24–31 billion in other avoidable health costs from this level of additional oral vitamin D intake in the US (Grant et al. 2005).

Unfortunately, despite the 26-year history of the UVB/vitamin D/cancer hypothesis (Garland and Garland 1980, 2006), the health agencies and organizations that would be expected to embrace vitamin D as an inexpensive, safe, and effective way to reduce cancer incidence and mortality rates are still reluctant to do so, in spite of the growing body of evidence supporting the hypothesis. The primary reason given is that the hypothesis is unproven using the prospective, placebo double-blind method usually employed to confirm the efficacy of any health intervention as well as look for adverse side effects. However, in the authors' opinion, such a study is unnecessary for at least two reasons. First, vitamin D is a natural substance that man has coexisted with since the origin of the species, so that there are plenty of data available on the health benefits. Ecologic studies offer a convenient way to organize and interpret these data (e.g., Garland and Garland 1980, in press; Freedman et al. 2002; Grant 2002; Grant and Garland, in press). Second, there are few, if any, adverse side effects for vitamin D supplementation at levels below 2,000–4,000 IU/day, and the toxic level may be as high as 40,000 IU/day over an extended period (Vieth 1999).

In addition, there is concern that endorsing vitamin D as a cancer-fighting substance would lead to more solar UVB irradiance and, hence, increased incidence of melanoma and non-melanoma skin cancer. An example of the concerns expressed by dermatologists is found in reading a recent review of the health benefits of vitamin D and risks of solar UV irradiance by two dermatologists (Wolpowitz and Gilchrest 2006). They selectively reviewed the literature in a manner that permitted them to state that the benefits of vitamin D for many diseases were less well-established but purported. However, the bias with which they selected and interpreted the literature greatly diminished the value of this review. Their concern is overblown in that the strongest risk factor for melanoma and basal cell carcinoma is intermittent solar UV irradiance and sunburning, not normal UV irradiance short of sunburning (Kennedy et al. 2003), and sunburning is not required for vitamin D production. However, we concede that while many of the studies regarding the health benefits of vitamin D are based on data in which solar UVB provided much of the vitamin D, oral intake of fortified food and supplements can be effective in providing the vitamin D and does not entail the risks of skin cancer or immunosuppression (Halliday 2005; Schwarz 2005; Ullrich 2005).

It should also be noted that vitamin D has benefits for many conditions and diseases, as discussed in a number of recent reviews (Heaney 2003; Plotnikoff and Quigley 2003; Holick 2004a, b, 2006; Grant and Holick 2005; Mosekilde 2005; Peterlik and Cross 2005; Zittermann et al. 2005; Grant 2006).

Summary and Conclusion

Sufficient epidemiologic data with supporting laboratory data on mechanisms are now available so that quantitative estimates can be made of the beneficial role of vitamin D in reducing the burden of cancer. The estimates presented in this paper indicate that the reductions could be in the range of 10%–20% in Western Europe and North America. The cost of a program to provide 1,000 IU of oral vitamin D to all adults in such countries would be a small fraction of the expected benefits for cancer, and there would be significant benefits for many other conditions and diseases as well. It is hoped that public health policies will move in the direction of recommending increased vitamin D levels sooner rather than later.

References

Agar NS, Halliday GM, Barnetson RS et al (2004) The basal layer in human squamous tumors harbors more UVA than UVB fingerprint mutations: a role for UVA in human skin carcinogenesis. Proc Natl Acad Sci U S A 101:4954–4959

Andersen R, Brot C, Ovesen L et al (2001) Towards a strategy for optimal vitamin D fortification (OPTI-FORD). Nutr Metab Cardiovasc Dis 11:74–77

Bates CJ, Prentice A, Cole TJ et al (1999) Micronutrients: highlights and research challenges from the 1994–5 National Diet and Nutrition Survey of people aged 65 years and over. Br J Nutr 82:7–15

Bettica P, Bevilacqua M, Vago T et al (1999) High prevalence of hypovitaminosis D among free-living postmenopausal women referred to an osteoporosis outpatient clinic in northern Italy for initial screening. Osteoporos Int 9:226–229

Boonen S, Vanderschueren D, Cheng XG et al (1997) Age-related (type II) femoral neck osteoporosis in men: biochemical evidence for both hypovitaminosis D-and androgen deficiency-induced bone resorption J Bone Miner Res 12:2119–2126

Calvo MS, Whiting SJ, Barton CN et al (2004) Vitamin D fortification in the United States and Canada: current status and data needs. Am J Clin Nutr 80:1710S–1716S

Calvo MS, Whiting SJ, Barton CN et al (2005) Vitamin D intake: a global perspective of current status. J Nutr 135:310–316

Cross HS, Peterlik M, Reddy GS, Schuster I (1997) Vitamin D metabolism in human colon adenocarcinoma-derived Caco-2 cells: expression of 25-hydroxyvitamin D3-1alpha-hydroxylase activity and regulation of side-chain metabolism. J Steroid Biochem Mol Biol 62:21–28

Daly RM, Brown M, Bass S et al (2006) Calcium- and vitamin D(3)-fortified milk reduces bone loss at clinically relevant skeletal sites in older men: a 2-year randomized controlled trial. J Bone Miner Res 21:397–405

Devesa SS, Grauman DJ, Blot WJ, Pennello G, Hoover RN, Fraumeni JF Jr (1999) Atlas of Cancer Mortality in the United States, 1950–1994. NIH Publication No. 99–4564. US Govt Print Office, Washington, DC: http://cancer.gov/atlasplus/new.html. Cited 24 August 2006

Doll R, Peto R (1981)The causes of cancer: quantitative estimates of avoidable risks of cancer in the United States today. J Natl Cancer Inst 66:1191–308

Donaldson MS (2004) Nutrition and cancer: a review of the evidence for an anti-cancer diet. Nutr J 3:19

Ferlay J, Bray F, Pisani P et al (2002) GLOBOCAN: Cancer incidence, mortality and prevalence worldwide IARC CancerBase No. 5. version 2.0, IARC-Press, Lyon, http://www-dep.iarc.fr. Cited 24 August 2006

Freedman DM, Dosemeci M, McGlynn K et al (2002) Sunlight and mortality from breast, ovarian, colon, prostate, and non-melanoma skin cancer: a composite death certificate based case-control study. Occup Environ Med 51:257–262

Garland CF, Garland FC (1980) Do sunlight and vitamin D reduce the likelihood of colon cancer? Int J Epidemiol 9:227–231

Garland CF, Garland FC (2006) Do sunlight and vitamin D reduce the likelihood of colon cancer? Int J Epidemiol 35:217–220

Garland C, Shekelle RB, Barrett-Connor E et al (1985) Dietary vitamin D and calcium and risk of colorectal cancer: a 19-year prospective study in men. Lancet 1:307–309

Garland CF, Comstock GW, Garland FC et al (1989) Serum 25-hydroxyvitamin D and colon cancer: eight-year prospective study. Lancet 2:1176–1178

Garland FC, Garland CF, Gorham ED et al (1990) Geographic variation in breast cancer mortality in the United States: a hypothesis involving exposure to solar radiation. Prev Med 19:614–622

Garland CF, Garland FC, Gorham ED et al (2003) Epidemiologic evidence for different roles of ultraviolet A and B radiation in melanoma mortality rates. Ann Epidemiol 13:395–404

Garland CF, Garland FC, Gorham ED et al (2006) The role of vitamin D in cancer prevention. Am J Public Health 96:252–261

Goldzieher JW, Zerwekh JE, Castracane VD et al (1999) Single-monthly-dose vitamin D supplementation in elderly patients. Endocr Pract 5:229–232

Gorham ED, Garland FC, Garland CF et al (1990) Sunlight and breast cancer incidence in the USSR. Int J Epidemiol 19:820–824

Gorham ED, Garland CF, Garland FC et al (2005) Vitamin D and prevention of colorectal cancer. J Steroid Biochem Mol Biol 97:179–194

Grant WB (2002) An estimate of premature cancer mortality in the United States due to inadequate doses of solar ultraviolet-B radiation. Cancer 94:1867–1875

Grant WB (2004) Insufficient sunlight may kill 45,000 Americans each year from internal cancer. J Cos Dermatol 3:176–178

Grant WB (2006) Epidemiology of disease risks in relation to vitamin D insufficiency. Progress Biophys Molec Biol 92:65–79

Grant WB, Garland CF (2004) A critical review of studies on vitamin D in relation to colorectal cancer. Nutr Cancer 48:115–123

Grant WB, Garland CF (2006) The association of solar ultraviolet B (UVB) with reducing risk of cancer: multifactorial ecologic analysis of geographic variation in age-adjusted cancer mortality rates. Anticancer Res 26:2687–2699

Grant WB, Holick MF (2005) Benefits and requirements of vitamin D for optimal health: a review. Altern Med Rev 10:94–111

Grant WB, Garland CF, Holick, MF et al (2005) Comparisons of estimated economic burdens due to insufficient solar ultraviolet irradiance and vitamin D and excess solar UV irradiance for the United States. Photochem Photobiol 81:1276–1286

Halliday GM (2005) Inflammation, gene mutation and photoimmunosuppression in response to UVR-induced oxidative damage contributes to photocarcinogenesis. Mutat Res 571:107–120

Halliday GM, Agar NS, Barnetson RS et al (2005) UV-A fingerprint mutations in human skin cancer. Photochem Photobiol 81:3–8

Hanchette CL, Schwartz GG (1992) Geographic patterns of prostate cancer mortality. Evidence for a protective effect of ultraviolet radiation. Cancer 70:2861–2869

Heaney RP (2003) Long-latency deficiency disease: insights from calcium and vitamin D. Am J Clin Nutr 78:912–919

Hill AB (1965) The environment and disease: Association or causation? Proc R Soc Med 58:295–300

Holick MF (2004a) Sunlight and vitamin D for bone health and prevention of autoimmune diseases, cancers, and cardiovascular disease. Am J Clin Nutr 80:1678S–1688S

Holick MF (2004b) Vitamin D: importance in the prevention of cancers, type 1 diabetes, heart disease, and osteoporosis. Am J Clin Nutr 79:362–371

Holick MF (2006) High prevalence of vitamin D inadequacy and implications for health. Mayo Clin Proc 81:353–373

Hughes AM, Armstrong BK, Vajdic CM et al (2004) Sun exposure may protect against non-Hodgkin lymphoma: a case-control study. Int J Cancer 112:865–871

Institute of Medicine, National Academy of Sciences (1997) Dietary reference intakes for calcium, phosphorous, magnesium, vitamin D, and fluoride. National Academy Press, Washington, DC

John EM, Schwartz GG, Koo J et al (2005) Sun exposure, vitamin D receptor gene polymorphisms, and risk of advanced prostate cancer. Cancer Res 65:5470–5479

Kennedy C, Bajdik CD, Willemze R et al (2003) The influence of painful sunburns and lifetime sun exposure on the risk of actinic keratoses, seborrheic warts, melanocytic nevi, atypical nevi, and skin cancer. J Invest Dermatol 120:1087–1093

Krishnan AV, Peehl DM, Feldman D et al (2003) The role of vitamin D in prostate cancer. Recent Results Cancer Res 164:205–221

Laaksi IT, Ruohola JP, Ylikomi TJ et al (2006) Vitamin D fortification as public health policy: significant improvement in vitamin D status in young Finnish men. Eur J Clin Nutr 60:1035–1038

Lamprecht SA, Lipkin M (2003) Chemoprevention of colon cancer by calcium, vitamin D and folate: molecular mechanisms. Nat Rev Cancer 3:601–614

Leffell DJ, Brash DE (1996) Sunlight and skin cancer. Sci Am 275:52–53, 56–59

Lefkowitz ES, Garland CF (1994) Sunlight, vitamin D, and ovarian cancer mortality rates in US women. Int J Epidemiol 23:1133–1136

Lips P (1987) Determinants of vitamin D status in patients with hip fracture and in elderly control subjects. Am J Clin Nutr 46:1005–1010

Matsuoka LY, Wortsman J, Hanifan N et al (1988) Chronic sunscreen use decreases circulating concentrations of 25-hydroxyvitamin D. A preliminary study. Arch Dermatol 124:1802–1804

McKenna MJ (1992) Differences in vitamin D status between countries in young adults and the elderly. Am J Med 93:69–77

Millen AE, Tucker MA, Hartge P et al (2004) Diet and melanoma in a case-control study. Cancer Epidemiol Biomarkers Prev 13:1042–1051

Moan J, Porojnicu AC, Robsahm, Dahlback A et al. (2005) Solar radiation, vitamin D and survival rate of colon cancer in Norway. J Photochem Photobiol B 78:189–193

Mosekilde L (2005) Vitamin D and the elderly. Clin Endocrinol (Oxf) 62:265–281

Nakagawa K, Kawaura A, Kato S et al (2005) 1 alpha,25-Dihydroxyvitamin D(3) is a preventive factor in the metastasis of lung cancer. Carcinogenesis 26:429–440

National Cancer Institute (2006) Surveillance Research Program, SEER*Stat software (seer.cancer.gov/seerstat) version 6.1.4

Natri AM, Salo P, Vikstedt T et al (2006) Bread fortified with cholecalciferol increases the serum 25-hydroxyvitamin D concentration in women as effectively as a cholecalciferol supplement. J Nutr 136:123–127

Nutrition Monitoring Div., Human Nutrition Information Service, U.S. Dept. of Agriculture (1985) Food and nutrient intakes: individuals in four regions, year 1977-78. Report No. I-3. U.S. Dept. of Agriculture, Hyattsville, MD

Ovesen L, Andersen R, Jakobsen J et al (2003) Geographical differences in vitamin D status, with particular reference to European countries. Proc Nutr Soc 62:813–821

Palmer HG, Gonzalez-Sancho JM et al (2001) Vitamin D3 promotes the differentiation of colon carcinoma cells by the induction of E-cadherin and the inhibition of beta-catenin signaling. J Cell Biol 154:369–387

Peterlik M, Cross HS (2005) Vitamin D and calcium insufficiencies predispose for multiple chronic diseases. Eur J Clin Invest 35:290–304

Plotnikoff GA, Quigley JM (2003) Prevalence of severe hypovitaminosis D in patients with persistent, nonspecific musculoskeletal pain. Mayo Clin Proc 78:1463–1470

Porojnicu AC, Robsahm TE, Ree AH et al (2005) Season of diagnosis is a prognostic factor in Hodgkin's lymphoma: a possible role of sun-induced vitamin D. Br J Cancer 93:571–574

Punnonen R, Gillepsy M, Hahl M et al (1988) Serum 25-OHD, vitamin A and vitamin E concentrations in healthy Finnish and Floridian women. Int J Vitam Nutr Res 58:37–39

Riffenburgh RH (1999) Statistics in medicine. Academic Press, San Diego

Rucker D, Allan JA, Fick GH, Hanley DA (2002) Vitamin D insufficiency in a population of healthy western Canadians. CMAJ 166:1517–1524

Robsahm TE, Tretli S, Dahlback A, Moan J (2004) Vitamin D3 from sunlight may improve the prognosis of breast-, colon- and prostate cancer (Norway). Cancer Causes Control 15:149–158

Schwartz GG (2005) Vitamin D and the epidemiology of prostate cancer. Semin Dial 18:276–289

Schwarz T (2005) Mechanisms of UV-induced immunosuppression. Keio J Med 54:165–171

Slattery ML, Sweeney C, Murtaugh M et al (2006) Associations between vitamin D, vitamin D receptor gene and the androgen receptor gene with colon and rectal cancer. Int J Cancer 118:3140–3146

Smedby KE, Hjalgrim H, Melbye M et al (2005) Ultraviolet radiation exposure and risk of malignant lymphomas. J Natl Cancer Inst 97:199–209

Tangpricha V, Koutkia P, Rieke SM et al (2003) Fortification of orange juice with vitamin D: a novel approach for enhancing vitamin D nutritional health. Am J Clin Nutr 77:1478–1483

Ullrich SE (2005) Mechanisms underlying UV-induced immune suppression. Mutat Res 571:185–205

Van den Bemd GJ, Chang GT (2002) Vitamin D and vitamin D analogs in cancer treatment. Curr Drug Targets 3:85–94

Vieth R (1999) Vitamin D supplementation, 25-hydroxyvitamin D concentrations, and safety. Am J Clin Nutr 69:842–856

Webb AR, Kline L, Holick MF (1988) Influence of season and latitude on the cutaneous synthesis of vitamin D3: exposure to winter sunlight in Boston and Edmonton will not promote vitamin D3 synthesis in human skin. J Clin Endocrinol Metab 67:373–378

Whiting SJ, Calvo MS (2005a) Dietary recommendations for vitamin D: a critical need for functional end points to establish an estimated average requirement. J Nutr 135:304–309

Whiting SJ, Calvo MS (2005b) Dietary recommendations to meet both endocrine and autocrine needs of Vitamin D. J Steroid Biochem Mol Biol 97:7–12

Wolpowitz D, Gilchrest BA (2006) The vitamin D questions: how much do you need and how should you get it? J Am Acad Dermatol 54:301–317

Zehnder D, Bland R, Williams MC, McNinch RW, Howie AJ, Stewart PM, Hewison M (2001) Extrarenal expression of 25-hydroxyvitamin d(3)-1 alpha-hydroxylase. J Clin Endocrinol Metab 86:888–894

Zhou W, Suk R, Liu G, Park S, Neuberg DS, Wain JC, Lynch TJ, Giovannucci E, Christiani DC (2005) Vitamin D is associated with improved survival in early-stage non-small cell lung cancer patients. Cancer Epidemiol Biomarkers Prev 14:2303–2309

Zittermann A, Schleithoff SS, Koerfer R et al (2005) Putting cardiovascular disease and vitamin D insufficiency into perspective. Br J Nutr 94:483–492

21

Uncovering Novel Targets for Cancer Chemoprevention

Konstantin H. Dragnev, Qing Feng, Yan Ma, Sumit J. Shah,
Candice Black, Vincent Memoli, William Nugent, James R. Rigas,
Sutisak Kitareewan, Sarah Freemantle, Ethan Dmitrovsky

Recent Results in Cancer Research, Vol. 174
© Springer-Verlag Berlin Heidelberg 2007

Abstract

Tobacco carcinogen treatment of immortalized human bronchial epithelial (HBE) cells has uncovered novel targets for cancer chemoprevention. Experiments were conducted with HBE cells and independent treatments with tobacco carcinogens along with the chemopreventive agent all-*trans*-retinoic acid (RA). That work highlighted D-type and E-type cyclins as novel molecular pharmacologic targets of several chemopreventive agents. G1 cyclins are often aberrantly expressed in bronchial preneoplasia and lung cancers. This implicated these species as targets for clinical cancer chemoprevention. Retinoid regulation mechanisms of D-type cyclins in lung cancer chemoprevention have been comprehensively explored. Retinoid chemoprevention has been mechanistically linked to proteasomal degradation of cyclin D1 and cyclin D3. Threonine 286 mutation stabilized cyclin D1, implicating phosphorylation in this retinoid chemoprevention. Studies with a phospho-specific anti-cyclin D1 antibody confirmed this hypothesis. Glycogen synthase kinase (GSK) inhibitors established a role for this kinase in the retinoid regulation of cyclin D1, but not cyclin D3. Involvement of D-type cyclins in this chemoprevention was shown using small interfering RNAs (siRNAs). Gene profiling experiments highlighted the E1-like ubiquitin-activating enzyme (UBE1L) in the retinoid regulation of cyclin D1. Proof of principle trials have translated these studies into the clinic and established that chemopreventive agents can target D-type cyclins. These findings have been built upon with a targeted combination regimen that cooperatively affects D-type cyclins. Taken together, these preclinical and clinical findings strongly implicate these cyclins as novel molecular pharmacological targets for cancer chemoprevention.

Introduction

Carcinogenesis is a chronic process involving multiple genetic, cellular, and tissue alterations, resulting from changes in critical growth regulating genes and their products. This ultimately leads to development of invasive or metastatic cancer, as reviewed (Weston and Harris 1997). Several steps contribute to carcinogenesis and these include promotion, progression, and invasion steps. Each of these represents potential pharmacological targets for cancer chemoprevention, as previously reviewed (Weston and Harris 1997). The cancer chemoprevention concept emphasizes interventions at early stages of carcinogenesis, even before malignancy becomes clinically evident (Sporn et al. 1976). An improved understanding of the basic biology of carcinogenesis remains essential for the development of effective cancer chemoprevention measures. Lifestyle interventions are known to play critical roles in cancer prevention. Yet the focus of this chapter is to review how preclinical models and proof-of-principle clinical trials can be used to uncover novel chemopreventive targets.

Carcinogenesis steps can be targeted by antiproliferative, differentiation-inducing, pro-apoptotic, or anti-angiogenic agents, as previously reviewed (Dmitrovsky and Sporn 2002). Indeed, an empirical approach to cancer chemoprevention has been replaced by targeted therapeutic strategies. These emphasize a mechanistic approach to validate chemopreventive agents in preclinical models and in clinical trials. This builds on the basic scientific understanding of biomarkers of carcinogenesis. As will be shown here, some of these are not only biomarkers of the carcinogenesis process, but are also molecular pharmacological targets for cancer chemoprevention. Examples include the D-type cyclins, which are novel targets for cancer chemoprevention, as will be discussed.

Several features make a target attractive for chemoprevention (Dragnev et al. 2003a). For instance, a validated target is often viewed as one required for the maintenance of a preneoplastic lesion or for its progression to a malignancy. In vitro studies as well as carcinogen-induced or genetically engineered animal models have all proven useful for validating a molecular pharmacological target in chemoprevention. Differential expression of a candidate target in preneoplastic or malignant cells and tissues as compared to histopathologically normal cells and tissues should provide simultaneous evidence for a role of the highlighted species not only in carcinogenesis

but also as a candidate target for cancer therapy or chemoprevention. Likewise, for a therapeutic agent to be attractive to consider for use in clinical cancer chemoprevention, it is helpful to have available pharmacological data from preclinical testing in in vitro as well as animal models. This review focuses on how preclinical models have proven useful for uncovering novel chemopreventive targets. Proof of principle clinical trials are being used to validate these targets. Attention will be placed on discussing how D-type cyclins were found as novel targets for cancer chemoprevention. Notably, specific chemopreventive agents have been shown to target G1 cyclin proteins for destruction. This is proposed as a potential chemopreventive mechanism.

Targets Uncovered Using Preclinical Models

One approach to uncover potential chemoprevention targets is to evaluate their functional roles in relevant preclinical models. These include cellular models (Langenfeld et al. 1996), carcinogen-induced animal models (Moon et al. 1994), as well as genetically engineered mouse models (Johnson et al. 2001). Cell culture models are useful to pursue mechanistic studies in can-

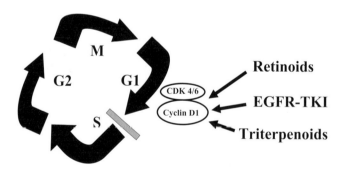

Fig. 1 The cell cycle is a target for some chemopreventive agents. This figure summarizes that specific chemopreventive agents (classical and certain nonclassical retinoids), epidermal growth factor receptor-tyrosine kinase inhibitors (EGFR-TKIs), and the triterpenoids are each able to repress cyclin D1 expression. Transcriptional as well as post-transcriptional mechanisms are engaged in this repression, as discussed in the text. Although not displayed in this figure, repression of cyclin E expression also follows treatment with certain retinoids and triterpenoids. The G1 cell cycle arrest that follows this repression (depicted as a *gray bar* in this figure) is hypothesized to result in chemoprevention, as this delay permits repair of carcinogenic damage to genomic DNA

cer chemoprevention. To establish a model relevant for studies of lung carcinogenesis, BEAS-2B immortalized human bronchial epithelial (HBE) cells were transformed after independent exposure to the tobacco-derived carcinogens N-nitrosamine-4-(methylnitrosamino)-1-(3-pyridyl)-1-butanone (NNK) or cigarette smoke condensate (CSC). All-*trans*-retinoic acid (RA) treatment was found to prevent NNK or CSC-mediated carcinogenic transformation of these cells (Langenfeld et al. 1996). This chemopreventive activity in HBE cells was linked to triggering of G1 cell cycle arrest, concomitant growth suppression, and a decline in expression of G1 cyclin proteins (Langenfeld et al. 1996, 1997; Boyle et al. 1999). This signaling of G1 arrest was proposed as a chemoprevention mechanism, as this would permit repair of carcinogenic damage to genomic DNA. Posttranslational mechanisms were shown to trigger cyclin degradation. Inhibitors of the proteasome-dependent degradation pathway blocked retinoid repression of G1 cyclin expression (Langenfeld et al. 1997; Boyle et al. 1999). In this way, G1 cyclins were highlighted as candidate chemopreventive targets in the lung and induced cyclin proteolysis was hypothesized as a chemopreventive mechanism (Langenfeld et al. 1996, 1997; Boyle et al. 1999), as summarized in Fig. 1.

Studies of the D-type cyclins revealed that retinoid-treatment activated both transcriptional and post-transcriptional mechanisms that regulated their individual expression profiles (Ma et al. 2005). RA modestly increased cyclin D2 and substantially decreased cyclin D3 mRNA expression, without an observed effect on cyclin D1 mRNA expression (Ma et al. 2005). However, RA-treatment substantially repressed both cyclin D1 and cyclin D3 protein expression. Co-treatment with proteasomal inhibitors was found to prevent degradation of both cyclin D1 and cyclin D3 proteins (Langenfeld et al. 1997; Boyle et al. 1999; Ma et al. 2005). To better understand the precise mechanisms involved in triggering this degradation, mutation of cyclin D1 was engineered to substitute threonine 286 with an alanine residue. This stabilized cyclin D1 expression, despite RA treatment, and this in turn implicated phosphorylation of this cyclin D1 resi-

due as playing a key role in the post-translational retinoid regulation of this species. Use of a phospho-specific anti-cyclin D1 antibody that recognized threonine 286 cyclin D1 phosphorylation confirmed this hypothesis. Notably, homologous mutation of threonine 283 within cyclin D3 did not affect the stability of cyclin D3, establishing that a different kinase was likely involved in the phosphorylation of cyclin D3 at this site (Ma et al. 2005).

Pharmacological inhibitors were used to uncover a candidate kinase involved in the phosphorylation of cyclin D1 at threonine 286. Independent glycogen synthase kinase 3 (GSK3) inhibitors were found to antagonize the retinoid repression of cyclin D1, but not of cyclin D3 proteins. Notably, phospho-T286 cyclin D1 expression was also inhibited by lithium chloride (a GSK3 inhibitor), directly implicating GSK3 in this phosphorylation of cyclin D1 (Ma et al. 2005). Functional screens of D-type cyclins were performed using small interfering RNAs (siRNAs) to repress expression of each D-type cyclin and this confirmed an important growth regulatory role for each of these species (Ma et al. 2005). The simultaneous targeting of all the D-type cyclins was also accomplished in HBE cells and showed cooperative repression of bronchial epithelial cell growth (Ma et al. 2005). Together, these findings helped established these cyclins as novel targets for cancer chemoprevention.

Proteasomal Degradation as a Chemopreventive Target

Regulation of proteolysis is critical for homeostasis of diverse cellular processes. The ubiquitin-proteasome pathway plays an important role in this process. Ubiquitin and its related proteins are responsible for post-translational modification of targeted proteins. Several enzymes are involved in ubiquitination, including the E1, E2, and E3 enzymes, as reviewed (Pickart 2001a). Ubiquitin is a polypeptide highly conserved in eukaryotes. It is activated in an ATP-dependent manner by a thiol ester linked to the ubiquitin-activating enzyme, E1. Activated ubiquitin is then bound to the conjugating enzyme, E2.

Ubiquitin is transferred to specific proteins by E2, requiring an E3 ligase for final modification. Attachment of ubiquitin monomers to substrates results in mono-ubiquitination that confers distinct functions. Multi-ubiquitinated species also occur and this signals proteasomal degradation. Several ubiquitin-related proteins exist such as Sumo, Nedd8, and ISG15 (Pickart 2001b). Conjugation of these species to target proteins can trigger protein degradation as well as other effects, as reviewed (Pickart 2001b).

Components of the ubiquitin-proteasome pathway are pharmacological targets of chemopreventive agents. For example, the E1-like ubiquitin-activating enzyme (UBE1L) is a nonclassical E1 that is induced by retinoid treatments (Tamayo et al. 1999; Kitareewan et al. 2002; Pitha-Rowe et al. 2004b). This component of the ubiquitin-proteasome pathway was uncovered by microarray analyses of several cell contexts (Tamayo et al. 1999; Pitha-Rowe et al. 2004b). Notably, microarray analyses of immortalized, tobacco-carcinogen-transformed and retinoid-chemoprevented HBE cells revealed increase expression of several RA-target genes as well as interferon-stimulated genes, including UBE1L during chemoprevention (Pitha-Rowe et al. 2004b). Biochemical studies recently uncovered involvement of UBE1L in the ISG15 conjugation pathway induced by RA treatment (Pitha-Rowe et al. 2004a). ISG15 also becomes conjugated to intracellular substrates after interferon treatment (Loeb and Haas 1992; Narasimhan et al. 1996).

UBE1L expression is reported as repressed in lung cancer cell lines and some lung cancers, directly implicating UBE1L in lung carcinogenesis (Pitha-Rowe et al. 2004b; Kok et al. 1993). Immunoblot expression of UBE1L has been shown to be reduced in some examined malignant as compared to adjacent normal lung tissues (Pitha-Rowe et al. 2004b). In the histologically normal human bronchial epithelium, immunohistochemical analyses revealed abundant UBE1L but low levels of cyclin D1, implicating an inverse relationship between these species (Pitha-Rowe et al. 2004b). A direct relationship between these species was confirmed by co-transfection experiments conducted in HBE cells, where UBE1L was shown to repress cyclin D1 expression in a UBE1L dose-dependent manner (Pitha-Rowe et al. 2004b). This finding mechanistically linked UBE1L to retinoid chemoprevention by conferring repression of cyclin D1 protein expression (Pitha-Rowe et al. 2004b). This has also directly implicated UBE1L as a retinoid pharmacologic target for lung cancer chemoprevention.

G1 Cyclins and Premalignancy

One hypothesis from these in vitro chemopreventive studies that highlighted G1 cyclins was that the same species would be aberrantly expressed in premalignancy as well as malignancy. Cyclin D1 and cyclin E are often overexpressed in lung cancers (Lonardo et al. 1999; Schauer et al. 1994; Mate et al. 1996; Betticher et al. 1996, 1997; Hayashi et al. 2001; Vonlanthen et al. 2000; Ratschiller et al. 2003). Bronchial preneoplastic lesions have been examined for G1 cyclin expression. It was proposed that expression of these species would be deregulated early during lung carcinogenesis. Immunohistochemical analyses revealed that both cyclin D1 and cyclin E deregulation was frequently detected in bronchial preneoplasia (Lonardo et al. 1999). Aberrant expression of these species was even more frequently detected than either for p53 or the retinoblastoma gene product (Rb) (Lonardo et al. 1999). These findings implicated altered expression of these cyclins as playing critical roles in the maintenance or progression of a preneoplastic bronchial lesion. These observations also implicated these species as potential targets for cancer chemoprevention. This possibility has been confirmed by analysis of bronchial epithelial cellular models (Dragnev et al. 2004), carcinogen-induced lung tumors in animal models (Witschi et al. 2002), as well as examination of cyclin expression in tissues harvested during a retinoid proof of principle clinical trial (Papadimitrakopoulou et al. 2001). These findings directly indicate that cyclin D1 and perhaps other G1 cyclins are chemopreventive targets. Treatments with effective chemopreventive agents should repress aberrant G1 cyclin expression found in tissues at high risk for malignant progression of preneoplastic lesions. Future clinical trials will address this possibility.

EGFR as a Chemoprevention Target

The described bronchial epithelial chemopreventive model has proven useful to highlight the epidermal growth factor receptor (EGFR) as another chemoprevention target (Lonardo et al. 2002). Carcinogen-transformed bronchial epithelial cells, as compared to RA-chemoprevented cells, overexpressed EGFR (Lonardo et al. 2002). EGFR activation promotes cellular growth and transformation and signals other biological effects (Salomon et al. 1995). EGFR overexpression is frequently observed in malignancies, including non-small-cell lung cancer (NSCLC) as well as in premalignant lung lesions (Rusch et al. 1995, 1996). Overexpression of EGFR and its ligand(s) often enhances EGFR-associated tyrosine kinase activity and triggers EGFR-dependent effects that regulate tumorigenesis (Salomon et al. 1995). RA is known to repress EGFR expression through a transcriptional mechanism (Lonardo et al. 2002). In bronchial epithelial cells treated with the epidermal growth factor (EGF), RA also prevented induction of mitogenesis and cyclin D1 protein expression (Lonardo et al. 2002). Thus, retinoids inhibit EGFR expression through a transcriptional mechanism and also reduce cyclin D1 expression through a post-transcriptional mechanism.

EGF augments cyclin D1 expression through several pathways (Mendelsohn 2001). Targeting EGFR with the small molecule tyrosine kinase inhibitor (TKI) erlotinib (tarceva) confers G1 arrest and inhibits EGF-mediated induction of cyclin D1 expression in erlotinib-sensitive cancer cells (Petty et al. 2004). It is notable that cyclin D1 expression was repressed by erlotinib treatment in erlotinib-sensitive, but not -resistant NSCLC cell lines (Petty et al. 2004). There is also a favorable clinical toxicity profile observed in the advanced disease setting with EGFR inhibitors. This highlights that targeting EGFR should be considered for specific cancer chemoprevention trials.

Proof-of-Principle Clinical Trials

There is a clinical need to establish whether those pathways activated in vitro are also activated in vivo. If candidate chemoprevention agents are unable to activate expected pharmacodynamic pathways in relevant clinical tissues or tumors, inactivity of a candidate chemopreventive agent is an expected clinical outcome. If pathways are affected in clinical tissues, this supports use of these agents in chemopreventive (or therapeutic) trials either as single agents or as part of combination therapy. Proof of principle trials are needed to establish the precise relationship in pretreatment and post-treatment biopsies between pharmacodynamic and pharmacokinetic effects in target cells or tissues, as summarized in Fig. 2. The proof-of-principle approach would validate therapeutic or chemopreventive effects on a desired molecular pharmacological target. These trials might also yield early objective tumor responses that would offer another strong rationale for use of a pharmacological agent in cancer therapeutic or chemopreventive trials. A validated biomarker of response would prove useful to monitor clinical responses. A biomarker could also represent a target for cancer therapy or chemoprevention. The D-type cyclins are examples of this based on prior published work (Petty et al. 2004; Rigas et al. 2005).

We recently completed two mechanistic proof-of-principle trials. In a proof-of-principle study of the EGFR-TKI erlotinib (tarceva), patients with aerodigestive tract tumors each had a pretreatment tumor biopsy and then received

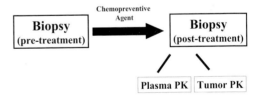

Fig. 2 The proof-of-principle trial platform is used to evaluate chemopreventive agents in the clinic. This trial approach is typically conducted in the perioperative period, which permits pretreatment as well as post-treatment biopsies where expression of a molecular pharmacological target (such as cyclin D1) is assessed. At the time of surgical resection, a second biopsy is obtained. Since the length of treatment is sufficient to achieve steady-state drug levels, it is possible to relate plasma to tumoral pharmacokinetic (PK) levels. In this way, it becomes possible to learn whether the chemopreventive agent affects the expected intratumoral pharmacodynamic target

short-term erlotinib (tarceva) therapy before undergoing a repeat post-treatment biopsy (Petty et
al. 2004). Cyclin D1 was identified as a biomarker
of clinical response as there was a decrease in
expression of cyclin D1 in cases whose tumors
underwent necrosis in a post-treatment biopsy
and also had substantial accumulation of intratumoral erlotinib (tarvceva). In contrast, this effect
was not observed in those cases whose tumors
had low levels of this agent and in turn did not
exhibit necrosis in the resected tumors (Petty et
al. 2004). Since activating EGFR mutations were
infrequently detected in the responding cases
(Petty et al. 2004), these pharmacodynamic and
pharmacokinetic effects have added clinical impact.

In another phase II trial, the rexinoid bexarotene was administered before resection of stage
I and II NSCLC cases (Rigas et al. 2005). The effects of this agent in resected lung tumors after
short-term therapy were evaluated along with
the relationship of changes in D-type cyclin expression to plasma and tumor tissue bexarotene
levels. Cyclin D1 expression was only decreased
in those cases exhibiting the highest detected intratumoral bexarotene concentrations (Rigas et
al. 2005).

Taken together, these two clinical trials un-
derscore the value of the proof-of-principle trial
platform as well as the importance of measuring
plasma and tissue drug levels and relating these
pharmacokinetic effects to the expected changes
in pharmacodynamic targets of the studied
agent. These findings also set the stage for targeted combination regimens in cancer therapy or
chemoprevention.

Combination Therapy

Effective clinical chemoprevention may require
combination therapy rather than single-agent
regimens (Dragnev et al. 2003c). One way to
limit clinical toxicities of cancer chemopreventive agents would be through combining agents
targeting different chemopreventive pathways,
each administered at dosages lower than when
these are typically used as single agents. For each
chemopreventive agent used in a combination

regimen, a validated target can be selected based
on preclinical and clinical activities. An active
combination regimen should be associated with
a tolerable toxicity profile as well as a safe and
convenient schedule of chronic administration.
Ideally, synergistic or additive effects would first
be observed in in vitro and animal models. Animal model testing could establish that a combination regimen is potentially safe for clinical use.
If available, clinical evidence for drug synergy in
treatment of advanced stage cancer might provide a basis for use of a regimen in cancer chemoprevention.

The findings already summarized directly
implicated cyclin D1 as a key downstream signaling species in the EGFR pathway (Lonardo
et al. 2002; Petty et al. 2004). This indicated that
targeting cyclin D1 with a combination regimen
that independently affected this cyclin would
augment clinical activity of an EGFR-TKI. It was
hypothesized that combining an EGFR inhibitor with a rexinoid would coordinately repress
cyclin D1 expression and thereby confer cooperative clinical anti-tumor effects (Dragnev et al.
2003b, 2004; Petty et al. 2004; Fan et al. 2004). To
explore this mechanistically, in vitro studies revealed that combining the rexinoid, bexarotene,
with the EGFR-TKI, erlotinib (tarceva), yielded
at least additive growth inhibitory effects and
cooperative repression of cyclin D1 immunoblot expression in examined bronchial epithelial
and lung cancer cells (Dragnev et al. 2005). This
regimen has the added therapeutic advantage
of using a nonclassical retinoid, a rexinoid that
activates the retinoid X receptor (RXR) pathway
and thereby overcomes the block to classical retinoids that occurs in cells that aberrantly express
the retinoic acid receptor-β (RARβ), as has been
reported to occur in lung carcinogenesis (Petty et
al. 2005). The clinical rationale for this regimen
is summarized in Fig. 3.

A recent clinical trial investigated bexarotene
(targretin) and erlotinib (tarceva) in patients
with advanced aerodigestive tract cancers and
demonstrated clinical efficacy of this hypoth-
esis-driven combination regimen (Dragnev et al.
2005). Clinical findings indicated that combining
these agents broadened activity of single agent
erlotinib (tarceva). Results from this trial pro-

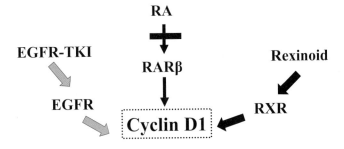

Fig. 3 Use of combination regimens for cancer therapy or chemoprevention. A combination chemopreventive regimen has been developed that involves use of a nonclassical retinoid (a rexinoid, retinoid X receptor, RXR, agonist) depicted by the *black arrows* and an epidermal growth factor receptor-tyrosine kinase inhibitor (EGFR-TKI), depicted by the *gray arrows*. This regimen has been shown preclinically to exert at least additive growth inhibitory activity against lung cancer cell lines. This occurs at least partly by targeting cyclin D1 expression (Dragnev et al. 2005). The same combination regimen has been shown in the clinic to cause objective responses in advanced-stage lung cancer cases, including cases that were resistant to combination chemotherapy (Dragnev et al. 2005). Notably, cyclin D1 expression in surrogate cells was targeted by these agents (Dragnev et al. 2005). As depicted by the *black bar* in this figure, an RXR agonist can by-pass the block to classical retinoids such as to all-*trans*-retinoic acid (RA). RA treatment requires activation of the retinoic acid receptor-β (RARβ) in the case of lung carcinogenesis (Petty et al. 2005). Whether the same combination regimen is active in cancer chemoprevention is the subject of ongoing studies

vided evidence that clinical cooperation between these agents might overcome a requirement for activating EGFR mutations to achieve clinical responses to EGFR-TKIs in NSCLC (Dragnev et al. 2005). Whether this targeted combination regimen is active in cancer chemoprevention is the subject of future work.

Conclusions

Identification of validated molecular pharmacological targets enhances a molecular understanding of mechanisms of response or resistance to cancer chemoprevention agents. Preclinical models are useful to explore these mechanisms. Candidate target genes should uncover known or previously unrecognized therapeutic or chemopreventive pathways. These could become surrogate markers of clinical response or even novel pharmacological targets. The preclinical and clinical findings presented here strongly implicate cyclin D1 and other species as novel molecular targets for cancer chemoprevention. Future work will determine whether targeting these species inhibits clinical carcinogenesis.

Acknowledgements

This work was supported by the National Institutes of Health grants RO1-CA087546 (E.D.), R01-CA111422, and RO1-CA62275 (E.D.), the Community Clinical Oncology Program Grant CA37447–21 (K.H.D.), a Samuel Waxman Foundation Cancer Research Award (E.D.), and the Oracle Giving Fund (E.D.).

References

Betticher DC, Heighway J, Hasleton PS, Altermatt HJ, Ryder WD, Cerny T, Thatcher N (1996) Prognostic significance of CCND1 (cyclin D1) overexpression in primary resected non-small-cell lung cancer. Br J Cancer 73:294–300

Betticher DC, White GR, Vonlanthen S, Liu X, Kappeler A, Altermatt HJ, Thatcher N, Heighway J (1997) G1 control gene status is frequently altered in resectable non-small cell lung cancer. Int J Cancer 74:556–562

Boyle JO, Langenfeld J, Lonardo F, Sekula D, Reczek P, Rusch V, Dawson MI, Dmitrovsky E (1999) Cyclin D1 proteolysis: a retinoid chemoprevention signal in normal, immortalized, and transformed human bronchial epithelial cells. J Natl Cancer Inst 91:373–379

Dmitrovsky E, Sporn MB (2002) Pharmacology of cancer chemoprevention. In: Bertino JB (ed) Encyclopedia of cancer. Academic, San Diego, pp 449–456

Dragnev KH, Petty WJ, Dmitrovsky E (2003a) Retinoid targets for cancer therapy and prevention. Cancer Biol Ther 2:S150–S156

Dragnev KH, Petty WJ, Dmitrovsky E (2003b) Targeted combination lung cancer therapy with a non-classical retinoid and an EGFR inhibitor. Proc AACR, 44:617

Dragnev KH, Stover D, Dmitrovsky E (2003c) Lung cancer prevention: the guidelines. Chest 123:60S–71S

Dragnev KH, Pitha-Rowe I, Ma Y, Petty WJ, Sekula D, Murphy B, Rendi M, Suh N, Desai NB, Sporn MB, Freemantle SJ, Dmitrovsky E (2004) Specific chemopreventive agents trigger proteasomal degradation of G1 cyclins: implications for combination therapy. Clin Cancer Res 10:2570–2577

Dragnev KH, Petty WJ, Shah S, Biddle A, Desai NB, Memoli V, Rigas JR, Dmitrovsky E (2005) Bexarotene and erlotinib for aerodigestive tract cancer. J Clin Oncol 23:8757–8764

Fan B, Negro-Vilar A, Lamph WW, Bissonnette RP (2004) A retinoid X receptor (RXR)-selective agonist bexarotene produces synergistic growth inhibitory activity with gefitinib in non-small cell lung cancer (NSCLC) cell lines. Proc ASCO 23:652

Hayashi H, Ogawa N, Ishiwa N, Yazawa T, Inayama Y, Ito T, Kitamura H (2001) High cyclin E and low p27/Kip1 expressions are potentially poor prognostic factors in lung adenocarcinoma patients. Lung Cancer 34:59–65

Johnson L, Mercer K, Greenbaum D, Bronson RT, Crowley D, Tuveson DA, Jacks T (2001) Somatic activation of the K-ras oncogene causes early onset lung cancer in mice. Nature 410:1111–1116

Kitareewan S, Pitha-Rowe I, Sekula D, Lowrey CH, Nemeth MJ, Golub TR, Freemantle SJ, Dmitrovsky E (2002) UBE1L is a retinoid target that triggers PML/RARα degradation and apoptosis in acute promyelocytic leukemia. Proc Natl Acad Sci U S A 99:3806–3811

Kok K, Hofstra R, Pilz A, van den Berg A, Terpstra P, Buys CH, Carritt B (1993) A gene in the chromosomal region 3p21 with greatly reduced expression in lung cancer is similar to the gene for ubiquitin-activating enzyme. Proc Natl Acad Sci U S A 90:6071–6075

Langenfeld J, Lonardo F, Kiyokawa H, Passalaris T, Ahn MJ, Rusch V, Dmitrovsky E (1996) Inhibited transformation of immortalized human bronchial epithelial cells by retinoic acid is linked to cyclin E down-regulation. Oncogene 13:1983–1990

Langenfeld J, Kiyokawa H, Sekula D, Boyle J, Dmitrovsky E (1997) Posttranslational regulation of cyclin D1 by retinoic acid: a chemoprevention mechanism. Proc Natl Acad Sci U S A 94:12070–12074

Loeb KR, Haas AL (1992) The interferon-inducible 15-kDa ubiquitin homolog conjugates to intracellular proteins. J Biol Chem 267:7806–7813

Lonardo F, Rusch V, Langenfeld J, Dmitrovsky E, Klimstra DS (1999) Overexpression of cyclins D1 and E is frequent in bronchial preneoplasia and precedes squamous cell carcinoma development. Cancer Res 59:2470–2476

Lonardo F, Dragnev KH, Freemantle SJ, Ma Y, Memoli N, Sekula D, Knauth EA, Beebe JS, Dmitrovsky E (2002) Evidence for the epidermal growth factor receptor as a target for lung cancer prevention. Clin Cancer Res 8:54–60

Ma Y, Feng Q, Sekula D, Diehl JA, Freemantle SJ, Dmitrovsky E (2005) Retinoid targeting of different D-type cyclins through distinct chemopreventive mechanisms. Cancer Res 65:6476–6483

Mate JL, Ariza A, Aracil C, Lopez D, Isamat M, Perez-Piteira J, Navas-Palacios JJ (1996) Cyclin D1 overexpression in non-small cell lung carcinoma: correlation with Ki67 labeling index and poor cytoplasmic differentiation. J Pathol 180:395–399

Mendelsohn J (2001) The epidermal growth factor receptor as a target for cancer therapy. Endocr Relat Cancer 8:3–9

Moon RC, Mehta RG, Rao KVN (1994) Retinoids and cancer in experimental animals. In: Sporn MB, Roberts AB, Goodman DS (eds) The retinoids: biology, chemistry, and medicine, 2nd edn. Raven Press, New York, pp 573–595

Narasimhan J, Potter JL, Haas AL (1996) Conjugation of the 15-kDa interferon-induced ubiquitin homolog is distinct from that of ubiquitin. J Biol Chem 271:324–330

Papadimitrakopoulou VA, Izzo J, Mao L, Keck J, Hamilton D, Shin DM, El-Naggar A, den Hollander P, Liu D, Hittelman WN, Hong WK (2001) Cyclin D1 and p16 alterations in advanced premalignant lesions of the upper aerodigestive tract: role in response to chemoprevention and cancer development. Clin Cancer Res 7:3127–3134

Petty WJ, Dragnev KH, Memoli VA, Ma Y, Desai NB, Biddle A, Davis TH, Nugent WC, Memoli N, Hamilton M, Iwata KK, Rigas JR, Dmitrovsky E (2004) Epidermal growth factor receptor tyrosine kinase inhibition represses cyclin D1 in aerodigestive tract cancers. Clin Cancer Res 10:7547–7554

Petty WJ, Li N, Biddle A, Bounds R, Nitkin C, Ma Y, Dragnev KH, Freemantle SJ, Dmitrovsky E (2005) A novel retinoic acid receptor β isoform and retinoid resistance in lung carcinogenesis. J Natl Cancer Inst 97:1645–1651

Pickart CM (2001a) Mechanisms underlying ubiquitination. Ann Rev Biochem 70:503–533

Pickart CM (2001b) Ubiquitin enters the new millennium. Mol Cell 8:499–504

Pitha-Rowe I, Hassel BA, Dmitrovsky E (2004a) Involvement of UBE1L in ISG15 conjugation during retinoid-induced differentiation of acute promyelocytic leukemia. J Biol Chem 279:18178–18187

Pitha-Rowe I, Petty WJ, Feng Q, Koza-Taylor PH, Dimattia DA, Pinder L, Dragnev KH, Memoli N, Memoli V, Turi T, Beebe J, Kitareewan S, Dmitrovsky E (2004b) Microarray analyses uncover UBE1L as a candidate target gene for lung cancer chemoprevention. Cancer Res 64:8109–8115

Ratschiller D, Heighway J, Gugger M, Kappeler A, Pirnia F, Schmid RA, Borner MM, Betticher DC (2003) Cyclin D1 overexpression in bronchial epithelia of patients with lung cancer is associated with smoking and predicts survival. J Clin Oncol 21:2085–2093

Rigas JR, Dragnev KH, Petty WJ, Nugent WC, Memoli VA, Black CC, Lewis LD, Loewen G, Negro-Vilar A, Dmitrovsky E (2005) A proof-of-principle trial of bexarotene in patients (pts) with resectable non-small cell lung cancer (NSCLC). Proc Am Soc Clin Onc 23:654s

Rusch V, Klimstra D, Linkov I, Dmitrovsky E (1995) Aberrant expression of p53 or the epidermal growth factor receptor is frequent in early bronchial neoplasia and coexpression precedes squamous cell carcinoma development. Cancer Res 55:1365–1372

Rusch V, Mendelsohn J, Dmitrovsky E (1996) The epidermal growth factor receptor and its ligands as therapeutic targets in human tumors. Cytokine Growth Factor Rev 7:133–141

Salomon DS, Brandt R, Ciardiello F, Normanno N (1995) Epidermal growth factor-related peptides and their receptors in human malignancies. Crit Rev Oncol Hematol 19:183–232

Schauer IE, Siriwardana S, Langan TA, Sclafani RA (1994) Cyclin D1 overexpression vs. retinoblastoma inactivation: implications for growth control evasion in non-small cell and small cell lung cancer. Proc Natl Acad Sci U S A 91:7827–7831

Sporn MB, Dunlop NM, Newton DL, Smith JM (1976) Prevention of chemical carcinogenesis by vitamin A and its synthetic analogs (retinoids). Fed Proc 35:1332–1338

Tamayo P, Slonim D, Mesirov J, Zhu Q, Kitareewan S, Dmitrovsky E, Lander ES, Golub TR (1999) Interpreting patterns of gene expression with self-organizing maps: methods and application to hematopoietic differentiation. Proc Natl Acad Sci U S A 96:2907–2912

Vonlanthen S, Heighway J, Kappeler A, Altermatt HJ, Borner MM, Betticher DC (2000) p21 is associated with cyclin D1, p16INK4a and pRb expression in resectable non-small cell lung cancer. Int J Oncol 16:951–957

Weston A, Harris CC (1997) Chemical carcinogenesis. In: Holland JF, Frei E, Bast RC, Kufe DW, Morton DL, Weichselbaum RR (eds) Cancer medicine, 4th edn., Vol. 1, Williams and Wilkins, Baltimore, pp 261–276

Witschi H, Espiritu I, Suffia M, Pinkerton KE (2002) Expression of cyclin D1/2 in the lungs of strain A/J mice fed chemopreventive agents. Carcinogenesis 23:289–294

Part VIII Conclusions and Summary

Conference Summary

Ursula Kapp, Hans-Jörg Senn

Recent Results in Cancer Research, Vol. 174
© Springer-Verlag Berlin Heidelberg 2007

A total of 188 international experts from 32 countries met at the University of St. Gallen, Switzerland for a 3-day conference to discuss the recent developments in the field of cancer prevention. The meeting was organized and co-sponsored by St. Gallen Oncology Conferences, the European School of Oncology (Milan, Italy), the International Society of Cancer Prevention (New York, NY, USA), the European Cancer Prevention Organisation (Brussels, Belgium), and this year for the first time by the European Society of Medical Oncology (Lugano, Switzerland). The local organizers were Prof. Hans-Jörg Senn, MD, and Prof. Ursula Kapp, MD, both from the Center for Tumor Detection, Treatment and Prevention (ZeTuP) in St. Gallen, Switzerland.

In a rather provocative opening lecture, cancer survivor Clifton Leaf, editor of Fortune Magazine, New York, USA tried to answer the question "Why we are in danger of losing the war on cancer?", which was meant to encourage scientists, clinicians, and the general public to spend more work and money on cancer prevention. He made it very clear that because of demographic development, global cancer rates could increase by 50% to 15 million a year by 2020. The age-adjusted cancer death rate per 100,000 population has remained constant since 1950, with about 200 cases per year. In contrast, the age-adjusted death rate from heart disease decreased significantly due to efficient means of prevention. Clifton Leaf tried to give a wake-up call encouraging greater effort on cancer prevention because of the terrifying loss of human potential, especially in view of the rapidly increasing economic cost of cancer treatment, which in the future might possibly paralyze any public health system.

Peter Greenwald (NCI, Bethesda, MD, USA) responded with a more optimistic lecture on the "Progress in Cancer Prevention" and discussed how public guidance (smoke-free environment, diet), chemopreventive drugs (e.g., statins, finasteride), bioactive food, and screening programs could be successfully applied in the prevention of lung, breast, colon, and prostate cancer. Other epidemiologists and scientists working in basic research gave insights in strategies, how biological knowledge can elucidate potential new targets for cancer prevention or for the definition of certain risk groups.

Tak W. Mak (Toronto, Canada) emphasized the emerging concept in cancer research that cancer therapeutics should be targeting cell survival genes that prevent cancer cells from dying and discussed research projects that have dissected these signaling pathways, activating cell survival via NFkappaB or PI3K activation, or via activation of anti-apoptotic genes. Helmut Bartsch (Heidelberg, Germany) investigated polymorphisms in metabolic and repair genes in a lung cancer case–control study and concluded that specific metabolic and DNA repair gene variants can affect cancer risk and therapy outcome. But large population-based studies have to follow. Michael Pollak (Montreal, Canada) gave an update on insulin-like growth factor and insulin-related signaling, which initiates signal transduction via PI3K or MAPK, key components in the control of cell survival and proliferation. He described how IGF-serum levels correlate with the risk of epithelial cancer, particularly advanced prostate and postmenopausal breast cancer, especially if the serum level is elevated at an early age. He also discussed the question of whether

IGF-I inhibiting drugs such as metformin could be candidates for cancer prevention.

Chemoprevention is an important issue in cancer prevention. In hormone-responsive tumors such as prostate and breast cancer, blockade of the hormonal stimulus is used as a target for preventive intervention. Peter Greenwald (Bethesda, MD, USA) and Hans-Peter Schmid (St. Gallen, Switzerland) discussed data from the prostate cancer prevention trial (PCPT), which investigates the effect of the testosterone inhibitor finasteride on prevention of prostate cancer. Treatment with finasteride in this study reduces the incidence of prostate cancer by 25%, but the cancers occurring in the treatment group more commonly present with a higher Gleason score of 7–10 and might be more aggressive. Therefore finasteride is not yet ready for clinical use as a chemopreventive agent against prostate cancer outside of clinical trials.

The role of estrogen in the development of breast cancer was extensively discussed by Anthony Howell (Manchester, UK), Irma and José Russo (Philadelphia, PA, USA), Per Hall (Stockholm, Sweden), and Trevor Powles (London, UK). As Anthony Howell pointed out, estrogen withdrawal for prevention of breast cancer, inducing early menopause, results in a significant reduction of breast cancer incidence. Trevor Powles gave a nice overview of current trials investigating the use of selective estrogen receptor modulators (SERMS) for breast cancer prevention. It is well known that tamoxifen reduces the early incidence of breast cancer by about 40%. It also reduces bone loss and serum cholesterol, but on the other hand increases the risk of endometrial cancer and thromboembolism. The benefit of tamoxifen intake is limited to high-risk premenopausal and younger postmenopausal women after hysterectomy. A new generation of SERMs – e.g., raloxifene, arzoxifene and lasofoxifene – has been developed, which have been shown to be more potent than tamoxifen and might have fewer side effects. It is possible to substantially reduce the incidence of breast cancer in healthy women using SERMS. Numerous trials are under way.

Promising data were shown by Vikas Khurana, Shreveport, LA, USA, who gave a talk on a retrospective case–control study, showing a correlation between the incidence of pancreatic cancer and intake of statins. Statins are known to suppress cell growth and cause inhibition of carcinogen-induced tumors in animal models. In presenting this study, he noted that the use of statins was associated with a 63% risk reduction for pancreatic cancer after controlling for age, gender, smoking, alcohol use, and diabetes. A correlation with the duration of statin use could also be shown. However, prospective studies are still missing.

The use of celecoxib for prevention of colon cancer was discussed by Monica Bertagnolli (Boston, MA, USA). It is well known that treatment of familial adenomatous polyposis (FAP) by the COX-2 inhibitor celecoxib leads to a significant reduction in polyp number and polyp burden. Thus chemoprevention trials with COX-2 inhibitors were initiated in 1999 for prevention of colorectal adenomas, Barrett's esophagus, and bladder cancer. Since unfortunately an elevated cardiovascular toxicity was detected with the use of COX-2 inhibitors in these chemoprevention trials, the human trial on celecoxib was suspended. This is a major drawback for the investigation of useful preventive drugs such as COX-2 inhibitors. Work on these agents should be continued, since many questions remain unanswered. We must identify subsets of patients for whom the risk-benefit-balance could be favorable. In addition, the question remains of whether successful chemoprevention requires long, continuous drug administration.

In contrast, prevention of cervical cancer has made better progress. Brad Monk (Orange, CA, USA) presented promising results of vaccination strategies against human papilloma virus (HPV). In a phase III trial, a HPV 16/18 vaccine could prevent more than 70% of cervical cancers. This vaccine will be available for routine clinical use in late 2006.

Another important topic of the conference was the role of lifestyle and food components for cancer prevention. Cheryl Rock (San Diego, CA, USA) discussed primary dietary prevention of colon cancer. Four intervention studies have tested the effect of fiber supplementation. Unfortunately no effect was shown on adenoma recurrence. A specific link between fiber intake and colon cancer risk could not be established. But there might be indirect benefits of dietary fiber relevant to colon cancer, because dietary fiber is a key feature of a diet low in energy density. For prostate cancer, the impact of lycopenes, which can be found in tomatoes, as well as phytoestrogens, selenium, and vitamin E was discussed by Peter Greenwald (Bethesda, MD, USA) and Hans-Peter Schmid (St. Gallen, Switzerland). Vitamin E and selenium are presently being investigated in the SELECT trial; especially selenium might be a promising food supplement for prevention of prostate cancer in the near future.

Clarissa Gerhäuser (DKFZ, Heidelberg, Germany) and collaborators presented their work on food components with cancer preventive potential. One of those components is xanthohumol, which is a flavonoid derived from hop and was identified as an interesting chemopreventive agent with antiestrogenic activity and as an antiangiogenic agent. Also, cloudy apple juice contains polyphenols that could be shown to prevent intestinal adenoma formation in the APC Min/+ mouse model for colon cancer prevention. William Grant (San Francisco, CA, USA) talked about the role of vitamin D in cancer prevention. He promoted vitamin D as a food supplement that has been shown to increase cell differentiation, suppress genes responsible for enhancing cellular proliferation, and possibly of reducing metastasis.

As a future perspective, Anna Barker (Bethesda, MD, USA) gave a keynote lecture on the potential use of nanotechnology in cancer prevention. In nanotechnology molecules smaller than 50 nanometers, which can easily enter cells and react with molecules inside the cell, could potentially be used for repair of DNA, killing of cancer cells and many other applications. Nanotechnology is a future technology. We do not yet know how long it takes until this would constitute a safe technology for everyday clinical use, and it remains unclear which potentially dangerous side effects might be involved in this technology. However, it may very well revolutionize medical practice, also in cancer prevention.

Finally Peter Boyle (IARC, Lyon, France) in his closing lecture, presented a summarizing overview of the current issues in cancer prevention. He pointed out the crucial problems with the increasing worldwide cancer burden and cost because of the demographic development. He concluded that there is an important role for chemoprevention in the future and a great need to develop nontoxic compounds. In addition, better biological (surrogate) markers and statistical methodologies are required. "We no longer wait for cardiovascular disease to develop before intervening." It should be the same for malignant disease. Thus effort and money must be spent on the development of equivalent safe and effective drugs, and informative biomarkers for the progress of cancer prevention. This would be a constructive investment in the future.

The organizers and the international scientific committee of this bi-annual meeting on cancer prevention are carefully monitoring the progress in this field over the next 2 years and plan to invite dedicated scientists, epidemiologists, and clinicians currently interested in primary and secondary cancer prevention to the next conference to be held in St. Gallen in early 2008.

Printing: Krips bv, Meppel
Binding: Stürtz, Würzburg